Colorectal Polyps

Editor

AASMA SHAUKAT

GASTROINTESTINAL ENDOSCOPY
CLINICS OF NORTH AMERICA

www.giendo.theclinics.com

Consulting Editor
CHARLES J. LIGHTDALE

April 2022 • Volume 32 • Number 2

ELSEVIER

1600 John F. Kennedy Boulevard • Suite 1800 • Philadelphia, Pennsylvania, 19103-2899

http://www.theclinics.com

GASTROINTESTINAL ENDOSCOPY CLINICS OF NORTH AMERICA Volume 32, Number 2
April 2022 ISSN 1052-5157, ISBN-13: 978-0-323-98673-1

Editor: Kerry Holland
Developmental Editor: Jessica Cañaberal

Gastrointestinal Endoscopy Clinics of North America (ISSN 1052-5157) is published quarterly by Elsevier Inc., 360 Park Avenue South, New York, NY 10010-1710. Months of issue are January, April, July, and October. Business and Editorial Offices: 1600 John F. Kennedy Blvd., Suite 1800, Philadelphia, PA, 19103-2899. Periodicals postage paid at New York, NY and additional mailing offices. Subscription prices are $370.00 per year for US individuals, $837.00 per year for US institutions, $100.00 per year for US and Canadian students/residents, $407.00 per year for Canadian individuals, $862.00 per year for Canadian institutions, $486.00 per year for international individuals, $862.00 per year for international institutions, and $245.00 per year for international students/residents. To receive student/resident rate, orders must be accompanied by name of affiliated institution, date of term, and the *signature* of program/residency coordinator on institution letterhead. Orders will be billed at individual rate until proof of status is received. Foreign air speed delivery is included in all *Clinics* subscription prices. All prices are subject to change without notice. **POSTMASTER:** Send address change to *Gastrointestinal Endoscopy Clinics of North America*, Elsevier Health Sciences Division, Subscription Customer Service, 3251 Riverport Lane, Maryland Heights, MO 63043. **Customer Service: 1-800-654-2452 (US). From outside the United States, call 1-314-447-8871. Fax: 1-314-447-8029. E-mail: JournalsCustomerService-usa@elsevier.com (for print support) or JournalsOnlineSupport-usa@elsevier.com (for online support).**

Reprints. For copies of 100 or more, of articles in this publication, please contact the Commercial Reprints Department, Elsevier Inc., 360 Park Avenue South, New York, NY 10010-1710. Tel. 212-633-3874; Fax: 212-633-3820; E-mail: reprints@elsevier.com.

Gastrointestinal Endoscopy Clinics of North America is covered in *Excerpta Medica, MEDLINE/PubMed (Index Medicus), and MEDLINE/MEDLARS.*

Contributors

CONSULTING EDITOR

CHARLES J. LIGHTDALE, MD
Professor of Medicine, Division of Digestive and Liver Diseases, Columbia University Medical Center, New York, New York, USA

EDITOR

AASMA SHAUKAT, MD, MPH
Robert M. and Mary H. Glickman Professor of Medicine and Gastroenterology, Professor of Population Health, Director of Outcomes Research, Division of Gastroenterology and Hepatology, Department of Medicine, NYU Grossman School of Medicine, New York, New York, USA

AUTHORS

NEENA S. ABRAHAM, MD, MSc (Epi), FACG, FASGE, AGAF
Professor of Medicine, Division of Gastroenterology and Hepatology, Department of Medicine, Mayo Clinic, Scottsdale, Arizona, USA

NABEEL AZEEM, MD
Division of Gastroenterology, Hepatology and Nutrition, University of Minnesota, Minneapolis, Minnesota, USA

MOHAMMAD BILAL, MD
Division of Gastroenterology, Hepatology and Nutrition, Assistant Professor of Medicine, University of Minnesota, Advanced Endoscopy, Division of Gastroenterology and Hepatology, Minneapolis Veterans Affairs Medical Center, Minneapolis, Minnesota, USA

SETH D. CROCKETT, MD, MPH
Associate Professor, Division of Gastroenterology and Hepatology, University of North Carolina School of Medicine, Chapel Hill, North Carolina, USA

JOHN A. DAMIANOS, MD
Department of Internal Medicine, Yale New Haven Health System, Yale School of Medicine, New Haven, Connecticut, USA

ROUPEN DJINBACHIAN, MD
Department of Internal Medicine, University of Montreal Hospital Center (CHUM), Department of Gastroenterology, University of Montreal Hospital Research Center (CRCHUM), Montreal, Canada

ANNA M. DULOY, MD
Division of Gastroenterology and Hepatology, University of Colorado Anschutz Medical Center, Aurora, Colorado, USA

HASHROOP GURM, MD
Veterans Affairs Medical Center, Gastroenterology Fellow, Division of Digestive Diseases and Nutrition, University of Oklahoma Health Sciences Center, Oklahoma City, Oklahoma, USA

MAHAM HAYAT, MD
Section of Digestive Diseases and Nutrition, University of Oklahoma Health Sciences Center, Oklahoma City, Oklahoma, USA

RAJESH N. KESWANI, MD, MS
Division of Gastroenterology and Hepatology, Northwestern University Feinberg School of Medicine, Chicago, Illinois, USA

KARL KWOK, MD, FASGE
Assistant Clinical Professor of Medicine, David Geffen School of Medicine at UCLA, Interventional Endoscopy, Division of Gastroenterology, Kaiser Permanente, Los Angeles Medical Center, Los Angeles, California, USA

ANGELA Y. LAM, MD
Department of Gastroenterology, Kaiser Permanente, San Francisco Medical Center, San Francisco, California, USA

BRITON LEE, MD
Department of Medicine, NYU Langone Health, New York, New York, USA

DANIEL LEW, MD
Division of Gastroenterology, Cedars Sinai Medical Center, Los Angeles, California, USA

PETER S. LIANG, MD, MPH
Department of Medicine, NYU Langone Health, Department of Medicine, VA New York Harbor Health Care, New York, New York, USA

KEVIN LIN, MD
Department of Medicine, NYU Langone Health, New York, New York, USA

GABRIEL V. LUPU, MD
Department of Medicine, Internal Medicine, University of North Carolina School of Medicine, The University of North Carolina at Chapel Hill, Chapel Hill, North Carolina, USA

MOHAMMAD F. MADHOUN, MD, MS
Veterans Affairs Medical Center, Chief, Gastroenterology and Hepatology, Associate Professor of Medicine, Division of Digestive Diseases and Nutrition, University of Oklahoma Health Sciences Center, Oklahoma City, Oklahoma, USA

SULTAN MAHMOOD, MD
Division of Gastroenterology, Hepatology and Nutrition, University at Buffalo, Buffalo General Medical Center, Buffalo, New York, USA

KARL MARETH, MD
Veterans Affairs Medical Center, Gastroenterology Fellow, Division of Digestive Diseases and Nutrition, University of Oklahoma Health Sciences Center, Oklahoma City, Oklahoma, USA

HECTOR MESA, MD
Associate Professor, Department of Pathology and Laboratory Medicine, Indiana University School of Medicine, Indianapolis, Indiana, USA

QUINN MILLER, MD
Department of Pathology and Laboratory Medicine, Indiana University School of Medicine, Indianapolis, Indiana, USA

CHARLES MULLER, MD
Instructor of Medicine, Division of Gastroenterology and Hepatology, Northwestern University, Chicago, Illinois, USA

MICHAEL NOUJAIM, MD
Division of Gastroenterology, Department of Medicine, Duke University School of Medicine, Division of Gastroenterology, Durham Veterans Affairs Medical Center, Durham, North Carolina, USA

VIJAYA L. RAO, MD
Assistant Professor of Medicine, Section of Gastroenterology, Hepatology and Nutrition, University of Chicago Medicine, Chicago, Illinois, USA

JATIN ROPER, MD
Division of Gastroenterology, Department of Medicine, Duke University School of Medicine, Division of Gastroenterology, Durham Veterans Affairs Medical Center, Durham, North Carolina, USA

OMER SAEED, MD
Assistant Professor, Department of Pathology and Laboratory Medicine, Indiana University School of Medicine, Indianapolis, Indiana, USA

BRANDON M. SHORE, MD
Department of Medicine, Internal Medicine, University of North Carolina School of Medicine, The University of North Carolina at Chapel Hill, Chapel Hill, North Carolina, USA

JARED A. SNINSKY, MD
Division of Gastroenterology and Hepatology, University of North Carolina School of Medicine, The University of North Carolina at Chapel Hill, Chapel Hill, North Carolina, USA

BRIAN A. SULLIVAN, MD, MHS
Division of Gastroenterology, Department of Medicine, Duke University School of Medicine, Division of Gastroenterology, Durham Veterans Affairs Medical Center, Durham, North Carolina, USA

JENNIFER J. TELFORD, MD, MPH, FRCPC, FCAG, FACG
Clinical Professor of Medicine, Division of Gastroenterology, Department of Medicine, University of British Columbia, Vancouver, British Columbia, Canada

SANJEEVANI K. TOMAR, MD
Department of Internal Medicine, University at Buffalo, Erie County Medical Center, David K. Miller Building, Buffalo, New York, USA

TRI TRAN, MD
Department of Medicine, Kaiser Permanente, Los Angeles Medical Center, Los Angeles, California, USA

DANIEL VON RENTELN, MD
Department of Gastroenterology, University of Montreal Hospital Research Center (CRCHUM), Division of Gastroenterology, Montreal University Hospital Center (CHUM), Montreal, Canada

MELISSA ZARANDI-NOWROOZI, MD
Department of Internal Medicine, University of Montreal Hospital Center (CHUM),
Department of Gastroenterology, University of Montreal Hospital Research Center
(CRCHUM), Montreal, Canada

Contents

Colorectal cancer is the second leading cause of cancer-associated mortality, with a lifetime risk of approximately 4% to 5%. Colorectal cancer develops from the sequential acquisition of defined genetic mutations in the colonic epithelium. Tumorigenesis from normal tissue to cancer occurs largely through 3 pathways: the chromosomal instability pathway, the microsatellite instability pathway, and the sessile serrated pathway. Colorectal cancer incidence and mortality have decreased by approximately 35% since the beginning of screening programs in the 1990s, although other factors such as use of aspirin for coronary disease prevention and decreased smoking rates may also be important. In this review, we discuss the etiology, epidemiology, and histology of colorectal polyps and cancer.

Colorectal cancer (CRC) is a common malignancy in the U.S. and worldwide. Most CRC cases arise from precancerous adenomatous and serrated polyps. Established risk factors for conventional adenomas and CRC include age, male sex, family history, obesity and physical inactivity, and red meat intake. White race and tobacco and alcohol use are important risk factors for serrated polyps, which have a distinct risk factor profile compared to conventional adenomas. A history of abdominopelvic radiation, acromegaly, hereditary hemochromatosis, or prior ureterosigmoidostomy also increases CRC risk. Understanding these risk factors allows for targeted screening of high-risk groups to reduce CRC incidence.

Colorectal cancer screening incorporates various testing modalities. Factors including effectiveness, harms, cost, screening interval, patient preferences, and test availability should be considered when determining which test to use. Fecal occult blood testing and endoscopic screening have the most robust evidence, while newer blood- and imaging-based techniques require further evaluation. In this review, we compare the effectiveness, harms, and costs of the various screening strategies.

Colonoscopy allows the performing endoscopist to thoroughly evaluate superficial colon lesions based on morphologic features such as size, location, shape, and surface pattern and also perform endoscopic resection where appropriate. Different elements of polyp characterization have been incorporated into systems that standardize this evaluation process and elucidate the likelihood of submucosal invasion or malignancy. Lesions which have invaded the submucosa are more likely to metastasize and are often not appropriate for endoscopic resection. It is, therefore, essential for the proceduralist to understand the multiple elements of lesion characterization and how they fit into the existing classification schemes.

Diminutive and small colorectal polyps are common findings during colonoscopies, and rarely contain dysplastic elements and progress to colorectal cancer. With improving technology and the advent of artificial intelligence, detection rates of small or diminutive polyps and adenomas are rising, resulting in increasing costs associated with colonoscopy. Incomplete resection rates are an outcome of interest because it correlates with interval colorectal cancer. More effort is warranted to standardize training programs and sensitize endoscopists to the importance of personal performance as a quality metric of colonoscopy. This article reviews indications, methods, and recent developments in polypectomy for small and diminutive polyps.

Beginning in 1955, when the saline injection was first described to prevent transmural injury during polyp fulguration, endoscopic mucosal resection (EMR) has grown exponentially, both in scope and in practice. Because EMR is an organ-preserving technique even for large polyps, this allows for comparable outcomes to surgery, but substantially improved cost savings and significantly reduced morbidity and mortality. To achieve this, however, one must master the 4 fundamental components that are critical to the success of EMR— time, team, tools, and technique. This article aims to provide a compendium of state of the art updates within the field of endoluminal resection.

Endoscopic resection has become the gold standard for the management of most of the large colorectal polyps. Various endoscopic resection techniques include endoscopic mucosal resection (EMR), endoscopic submucosal dissection (ESD), and endoscopic full-thickness resection (EFTR). ESD is a minimally invasive method for the resection of advanced lesions in the gastrointestinal (GI) tract to achieve en-bloc resection. While, EFTR is more commonly used in lesions with suspected deeper submucosal invasion, lesions originating from muscularis propria, or those with advanced fibrosis. This article reviews the indications, technique, and adverse events for use of ESD and EFTR in the colon.

Antithrombotic medications, including antiplatelet drugs and anticoagulants, are widely prescribed to treat and prevent thromboembolic disease. There is limited evidence informing gastroenterologists of the management of patients on antithrombotic medications undergoing colonoscopy and polypectomy. A patient's risk of thromboembolism versus postpolypectomy bleeding should be carefully considered, incorporating patient preferences concerning benefits and harms of temporary antithrombotic interruption. We will review the available consensus guidelines, current literature, and strategies to mitigate the risk of bleeding following polypectomy. These will be interpreted in the framework of shared decision-making with the patient to arrive at the safest solution best aligned with the patient's preferences.

Most colorectal cancer arises from epithelial polyps. Polyps can be the result of acquired, germline, or inflammation-associated mutations in colonic stem cells (CSC). Their incidence and risk of progression are determined by factors that modify the baseline rate of spontaneous mutations occurring in CSC. In sporadic polyps, factors are primarily environmental; in individuals with germline mutations, it is the specific mutation, and in inflammation-associated polyps, it correlates with the extent, duration, and severity of the process. The different clinicopathologic and molecular genetic abnormalities underlying the different types of polyps are discussed.

Modifiable risk factors for postcolonoscopy colorectal cancer include suboptimal lesion detection (missed neoplasms) and inadequate lesion removal (incomplete polypectomy) during colonoscopy. Competent detection and removal of colorectal polyps are thus fundamental to ensuring adequate colonoscopy quality. Several well-researched quality metrics for polyp detection have been implemented into clinical practice, chief among these the adenoma detection rate. Less data are available on quality indicators for polyp removal, which currently include complete resection rates and skills assessment tools. This review summarizes the available literature on quality indicators for the detection and removal of colorectal polyps, as well as interventions to improve them.

Video content accompanies this article at http://www.giendo.
theclinics.com

The 2 most significant complications of colonoscopy with polypectomy are bleeding and perforation. Although the incidence rates are generally low (<1%), these can be avoided by recognizing pertinent risk factors, which can be patient, polyp, and technique/device related. Endoscopists should be equipped to manage bleeding and perforation. Currently available devices and techniques to achieve hemostasis and manage colon perforations are reviewed.

The incidence and mortality of colorectal cancer (CRC) have declined over the past several decades, largely due to improvement and uptake in screening, particularly with colonoscopy. The US Multi-Society Task Force on CRC published guidelines for surveillance after polypectomy in 2012, which were updated in 2020 with some important changes, and this review will provide an updated overview of evidence and outcomes of surveillance after polypectomy. Notable modifications to surveillance guidelines include increasing interval time between colonoscopies from 5 to 7 to 10 years for 1 to 2 low-risk adenomas (<10 mm) and from 3 years to 3 to 5 years when 3 to 4 low-risk adenomas are identified.

GASTROINTESTINAL ENDOSCOPY CLINICS OF NORTH AMERICA

RELATED CLINICS SERIES

Gastroenterology Clinics
(www.gastro.theclinics.com)
Clinics in Liver Disease
(www.liver.theclinics.com)

THE CLINICS ARE AVAILABLE ONLINE!
Access your subscription at:
www.theclinics.com

GASTROINTESTINAL ENDOSCOPY CLINICS OF NORTH AMERICA

FORTHCOMING ISSUES

July 2022
Advances in Biliary Endoscopy
Mouen Kashab, Editor

October 2022
Interventional Inflammatory Bowel
Disease: Endoscopic Treatment of
Complications
Bo Shen, Editor

January 2023
Submucosal Endoscopy
Amrita Sethi, Editor

RECENT ISSUES

January 2021
Inherited GI Cancers: Identification,
Management and the Role of Genetic
Evaluation and Testing
Fay Kastrinos, Editor

October 2021
Optimizing Endoscopic Operations
Sunguk N. Jang and John J. Vargo, Editors

July 2021
Gastric Cancer
Chin Hur, Editor

RELATED CLINICS SERIES

Gastroenterology Clinics
(www.gastro.theclinics.com)
Clinics in Liver Disease
(www.liver.theclinics.com)

THE CLINICS ARE AVAILABLE ONLINE!
Access your subscription at:
www.theclinics.com

Foreword

Colorectal Polyps: Coin of the Realm for Colonoscopists

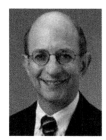

Charles J. Lightdale, MD
Consulting Editor

Pathology observations of the colon adenoma-carcinoma sequence by Morson, innovations in colonoscopy and polypectomy by Shinya and Wolff and by Waye, colonoscopic classification of polyps by Kudo, definitive findings that adenoma removal by colonoscopic polypectomy significantly decreased the incidence of colon cancer by Winawer and Zauber, insistence on colonoscopy and polypectomy quality by Rex, and contributions of many others have led us to the point where we are today: colonoscopy screening is the gold standard for colon cancer prevention, and colon adenoma detection and removal is the coin of the realm.

The torch of colon cancer prevention has been passed to a new generation. I am so gratified that Aasma Shaukat, a key new leader in this field with a focus on population health and patient outcomes, is the Guest Editor for this issue of the *Gastrointestinal Endoscopy Clinics of North America* devoted to a "Comprehensive Guide on Management of Colorectal Polyps." She has compiled a terrific and truly comprehensive list of topics for this issue and has gathered an amazing group of authors who have produced an outstanding state-of-the-art review with a look at the future. You would not go on a journey without a guide, and every colonoscopist should consider having this issue, digital or hard copy, so jam packed with important information. Don't miss it.

Charles J. Lightdale, MD
Department of Medicine
Columbia University Irving Medical Center
161 Fort Washington Avenue
New York, NY 10032, USA

E-mail address:
cjl18@cumc.columbia.edu

Gastrointest Endoscopy Clin N Am 32 (2022) xiii
https://doi.org/10.1016/j.giec.2022.01.001
1052-5157/22/© 2022 Published by Elsevier Inc.

giendo.theclinics.com

Preface

Comprehensive Guide on Management of Colorectal Polyps

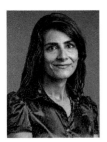

Aasma Shaukat, MD, MPH
Editor

Colorectal polyps are common and known precursors for majority of colorectal cancers. Our understanding of the pathogenesis, natural history, detection, and resection has rapidly increased over the last 2 decades. The purpose of this issue of *Gastrointestinal Endoscopy Clinics of North America* was to comprehensively review the current and upcoming knowledge on colorectal polyps and their management, making it an essential guide for gastroenterologists, colorectal surgeons, and providers that take care of patients with polyps. In particular, we review the latest polypectomy techniques that are effective and safe and discuss management of anticoagulation and quality indicators for colonoscopy. The overarching goal is to render a deeper understanding of the field and provide tools for high-quality colonoscopy and effective colorectal cancer prevention.

Aasma Shaukat, MD, MPH
Division of Gastroenterology
Department of Medicine
NYU Grossman School of Medicine
240 East 38th Street, Floor 23
New York, NY 10016, USA

E-mail address:
Aasma.shaukat@nyulangone.org

Gastrointest Endoscopy Clin N Am 32 (2022) xv
https://doi.org/10.1016/j.giec.2021.12.013
1052-5157/22/© 2021 Published by Elsevier Inc.

giendo.theclinics.com

Cause, Epidemiology, and Histology of Polyps and Pathways to Colorectal Cancer

Brian A. Sullivan, MD, MHS[a,b], Michael Noujaim, MD[a,b,1],
Jatin Roper, MD[a,b],*

KEYWORDS

- Colorectal cancer • Colon polyp • Adenoma • Colon cancer screening

KEY POINTS

- Colorectal cancer (CRC) is a genetic disease that develops from precursor colon lesions/polyps that progress through various tumorigenesis pathways.
- Clinical and genetic epidemiologic studies of colon polyps inform CRC screening programs, which aim to detect and remove precancerous colon polyps to prevent CRC.
- The incidence of CRC has increased markedly in younger individuals, but the epidemiology of young onset neoplasia remains unclear.

INTRODUCTION

Gilbertson first suggested in the 1960s that colorectal cancer (CRC) may arise from intermediary lesions in the colon.[1] Subsequent studies demonstrated foci of adenocarcinoma in adenomatous polyps, termed "adenomas," which suggested these polyps might develop into cancers.[2] In the late 1980s, Fearon and Vogelstein described CRC as a genetic disease, with the polyp-to-carcinoma progression as a sequence of specific genetic mutations.[3] Some of these mutations may be preexisting in the blood (ie, the germline), whereas others accumulate over time in the colonic epithelium due to environmental or other factors (i.e., somatic mutations) and drive the tumorigenesis pathways from a precursor lesion to CRC. Given the length of time it takes to progress through the polyp-to-carcinoma sequence, it was suggested that CRC could be prevented by detecting and removing these precancerous colon polyps.[3]

[a] Division of Gastroenterology, Department of Medicine, Duke University School of Medicine, 200 Trent Drive, Suite 03,107 Basement Orange Zone, Durham, NC 27710, USA; [b] Division of Gastroenterology, Durham Veterans Affairs Medical Center, 508 Fulton Street, Durham, NC 27705, USA
[1] Present address: 200 Trent Drive, Suite 03,107 Basement Orange Zone, Durham NC 27710.
* Corresponding author. 905 South LaSalle Street, GSRB-1 Room 1033B, Durham, NC 27710.
E-mail address: jatin.roper@duke.edu

Gastrointest Endoscopy Clin N Am 32 (2022) 177–194
https://doi.org/10.1016/j.giec.2021.12.001
1052-5157/22/Published by Elsevier Inc.

Since then, several studies have demonstrated that CRC screening and removal of precancerous colon adenomas leads to a reduction in CRC incidence and mortality by approximately 50%.[4–12] Ongoing research into the cause and epidemiology of these precancerous colon lesions continues to inform CRC prevention by helping to refine optimal screening strategies, create new screening modalities, and identify new therapeutic targets.

CAUSE

In the mid-1970s, pathology studies of polyps and CRCs suggested that colorectal adenocarcinoma may progress from adenomatous polyps. Areas of adenomatous tissue are sometimes found in cancers, whereas conversely, foci of cancer are often observed in larger adenomas (i.e., greater than 1 cm).[2] A natural history study of unresected colonic polyps greater than 1 cm in size in patients who declined surgical resection reported a 24% risk of invasive adenocarcinoma at the site of the index polyp and a 35% risk of carcinoma at any colonic site after 20 years.[13] In addition, familial adenomatous polyposis (FAP), an inherited disease, is caused by germline mutations in the adenomatous polyposis coli (APC) tumor suppressor gene and is associated with numerous colonic adenomas. Patients with FAP almost universally develop CRC by age 40 years if they are not managed with total proctocolectomy.[14] Inactivating mutations in the APC tumor suppressor gene are also commonly found in sporadic nonhereditary lesions, such as small adenomas and larger carcinomas, whereas oncogenic KRAS and loss-of-function TP53 mutations are mostly limited to adenomas greater than 1 cm in size and carcinomas.[3] Based on these studies and others, in 1990 Fearon and Vogelstein proposed a multistep genetic model of colorectal carcinogenesis in which inactivation of the APC tumor suppressor gene occurs first in normal colonic mucosa, followed by activating mutations in the KRAS oncogene and subsequent additional mutations. Recent efforts to classify CRCs by gene expression profiles have resulted in 4 consensus molecular subtypes (CMS1–4), each associated with distinct molecular features and clinical outcomes (**Fig. 1**).[15]

Chromosomal Instability Pathway

Somatic mutations accumulate with aging in the normal intestine and colon at a rate of approximately 40 novel mutations per year.[16] Colonic stem cell division is correlated with cancer risk in epidemiologic analyses, which suggests that mutagenesis in normal colonic stem cells underlies cancer initiation.[17] However, the rate of spontaneous mutagenesis is believed to be too low to account for the multiple mutations required for CRC development (proposed to be 3 mutations).[18] Rather, up to 70% of CRCs exhibit chromosomal changes such as somatic copy number alterations caused by aneuploidy, deletions, insertions, amplifications, or loss of heterozygosity. These changes are caused by defective chromosomal segregation that results in karyotypic variability between cells.

Karyotypic instability typically results in mutations in the tumor suppressor genes APC and TP53 and in the oncogene KRAS. Mutations in APC result in activation of the Wnt signaling pathway and are typically the earliest event in the initiation of colon adenomas in the chromosomal instability pathway. CMS2 CRC are characterized by activation of the Wnt signaling pathway.[15] Studies in animal models and patient-derived colon cultures or "organoids" have demonstrated that loss of APC transforms intestinal or colonic stem cells (located at the base of crypts) into adenomas by activating the Wnt signaling pathway and that additional mutations in oncogenic KRAS and TP53 then accelerate progression to cancer.[19–22] Indeed, mutations in KRAS

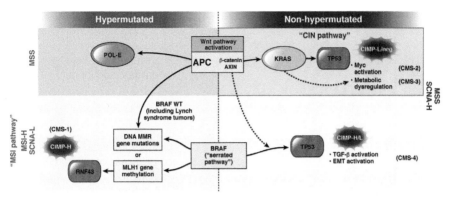

Fig. 1. Pathways of colorectal carcinogenesis. Activation of the Wnt pathway (primarily via *APC* mutation) or a mutation in *BRAF* can initiate colorectal tumorigenesis. *BRAF* mutations promote tumorigenesis via the serrated neoplasia pathway, leading to microsatellite instability (MSI) with hypermutation or microsatellite stable (MSS) without hypermutation (indicated in the figure). Colorectal tumor classifications include chromosomal instability (CIN), MSI, and the serrated pathway (see CMS). EMT, epithelial to mesenchymal transition; H, high; L, low; neg, negative. (*From* Nguyen LH, Goel A, Chung DC. Pathways of Colorectal Carcinogenesis. Gastroenterology. 2020 Jan;158(2):291-302.)

often arise after inactivating *APC* mutations and are found in approximately 40% of tumors.[3] Oncogenic *KRAS* mutations result in constitutive activation of the ectodermal growth factor receptor (EGFR) signaling pathway. Inhibitors of EGFR are used to treat metastatic CRC but are ineffective in *KRAS*-mutant cancer.[23] CMS3 cancers exhibit metabolic dysregulation such as sugar, amino acid, and fatty acid metabolism.[15] Other commonly mutated genes in the chromosomal instability pathway that occur late in the adenoma-carcinoma sequence include *PIK3CA* (found in 10%–20% of colorectal tumors) and *TP53* (found in greater than 60% of colorectal cancers).[24,25] Mutations in genes that encode proteins in the transforming growth factor pathway such as *SMAD2* and *SMAD4* explain only a small portion of the 70% of advanced cancers with loss of heterozygosity in chromosome arm 18q.[25,26] Recent deep sequencing studies of mutations in CRC have confirmed previously identified cancer-associated genes and have revealed many uncharacterized somatic mutations that could be either "driver" mutations with an essential role in disease pathogenesis or "passenger" mutations that are incidental (**Fig. 2**).[25,27,28]

Microsatellite Instability Pathway

The microsatellite instability (MSI) pathway is observed in approximately 15% of CRCs. Our current understanding of the MSI pathway of CRC is based on the discovery, first made in yeast by Paul Modrich, that DNA microsatellite sequence fidelity after DNA replication is maintained by a DNA mismatch repair (MMR) system.[29] The MMR genes are *MSH2, MLH1, MSH6, MSH3, PMS2,* and *EPCAM*; the MSH2 protein forms heterodimers with MSH6 as well as MSH3, MLH1 pairs with PMS2, and *EPCAM* encodes a protein that regulates MSH2. MSI (i.e., MSI-high) refers to the presence of frameshifted microsatellite sequences from genomic DNA due to defective MMR of DNA replication mistakes at microsatellites.[30] Defective MMR due to a germline mutation in an MMR gene causes accelerated colorectal tumorigenesis in an autosomal dominant inherited condition known as Lynch syndrome. Lynch syndrome is the most common hereditary CRC syndrome and accounts for approximately 3% of CRC. These patients

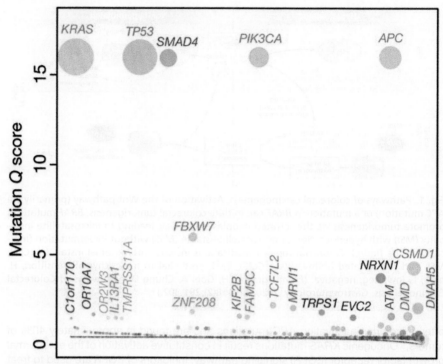

Fig. 2. Mutational landscape in microsatellite stable (MSS) colorectal cancer. Seshagiri and colleagues performed somatic exome sequencing of 57 MSS colorectal cancers. Genes were evaluated for significance using Q score criteria. Each circle represents a gene, and the size of the circle is proportional to the mutation count for that gene. The genes are represented in order of increasing number of expected mutations from left to right on the x axis. Genes with a statistically significant Q score are labeled. *(From* Seshagiri S, Stawiski EW, Durinck S, Modrusan Z, Storm EE, Conboy CB, Chaudhuri S, Guan Y, Janakiraman V, Jaiswal BS, Guillory J, Ha C, Dijkgraaf GJ, Stinson J, Gnad F, Huntley MA, Degenhardt JD, Haverty PM, Bourgon R, Wang W, Koeppen H, Gentleman R, Starr TK, Zhang Z, Largaespada DA, Wu TD, de Sauvage FJ. Recurrent R-spondin fusions in colon cancer. Nature. 2012 Aug 30;488(7413):660-4.)

often present 10 to 30 years younger than patients with sporadic CRC.[31] These tumors are classified as CMS1 (i.e., hypermethylation of DNA, MSI-high, and immune cell infiltration).[29] Colorectal tumors in patients with Lynch syndrome that arise from germline defects in MMR genes have MSI but typically do not have *BRAF* mutations. In contrast, the most common cause of the sporadic MSI phenotype is epigenetic silencing of *MLH1* because of promoter methylation. These MSI pathway cancers often manifest with *BRAF* mutations and a lower frequency of *APC* and *TP53* mutations.[32] In addition, the MSI pathway is characterized by a high level of methylation at regulator regions in the genome, known as the cytosine/guanine (CpG) island methylator phenotype (CIMP).

Serrated Pathway

Recent advances in endoscopic technology have led to the detection of flat or sessile polyps that pathologically have a serrated or saw-toothed appearance. Serrated neoplasia may account for 15% of CRCs. Hyperplastic polyps comprise approximately two-thirds of serrated lesions but rarely progress to cancer.[33] Hyperplastic polyps feature narrow crypt bases with serration confined to the upper region. On the other hand, sessile serrated lesions (SSLs) are distinguished from hyperplastic polyps by abnormal proliferation, branching or dilated T-/L-shaped crypts, and are often challenging to diagnose by pathologists. Traditional serrated adenomas are serrated lesions with villiform projections and are less common than sessile serrated lesions.[34]

A distinguishing feature of the sessile serrated pathway is an activating mutation in the *BRAF* oncogene, which is rare in convention adenomas from the chromosomal instability pathway; *BRAF* and *KRAS* mutations are mutually exclusive.[35] *BRAF*-mutant serrated lesions can progress into cancer either through the MSI pathway, via mutations in an MMR gene or *MLH1* methylation causing an MSI-high phenotype, or with additional mutations in *TP53* and other cancer-associated genes that result in a traditional serrated adenoma and then an microsatellite stable (MSS) cancer.[36] Serrated lesions that progress on the MSI-high pathway are often classified as CMS1. Serrated lesions that progress along the MSS pathway typically develop into CMS4 cancers, with an immunosuppressive microenvironment that facilitates tumor invasion, immune evasion, and poor survival.[15] The Wnt signaling pathway is often activated in SSLs, via inactivating mutations in *RNF43* (a gene encoding an E3 ubiquitin ligase that negatively regulates Wnt signaling) rather than missense mutations in *APC*.[37] Serrated pathway cancers (both MSI-high and MSS) also feature high levels of cytosine/guanine (CpG) island methylation or CIMP; hypermethylation of these promoter-rich regions leads to inactivation of nearby tumor suppressor genes and subsequent tumorigenesis.[38] *BRAF*-mutant cancers that arise from the sessile serrated pathway may respond to treatment with dual BRAF/MEK inhibition.[39,40]

EPIDEMIOLOGY
Prevalence Rates in the United States and Internationally

Although CRC is a preventable disease, it remains the second leading cause of cancer death in the United States and globally, with a lifetime risk of approximately 4% to 5%.[41–43] Current models that inform the United States Preventative Services Task Force (USPSTF) guidelines on CRC screening estimate that, in the absence of screening, between 7.7% and 8.5% of 40-year-olds would develop CRC in their lifetimes, and 3.2% to 3.4% would die from this disease.[44] Incidence rates are highest in developed countries, but increasing westernization of diet and lifestyle in developing countries is expected to significantly increase the global burden of disease by 2030.[42,45] Fortunately, CRC incidence and mortality is decreasing in the United States (**Fig. 3**), most European countries, and much of the Asia-Pacific.[45–48] CRC incidence has decreased in the United States by greater than 35% since the widespread use of screening in the 1990s.[49] Indeed, detecting precancerous lesions is now an important goal of CRC screening,[44,50,51] as removal of polyps during colonoscopy or sigmoidoscopy has been shown to effectively prevent CRC in observational and randomized studies.[5,9,10,12,52–56] Other factors also explain this decline in CRC incidence, such as decreased tobacco use, improved diet, more widespread use of aspirin for cardioprotection, more effective surgical techniques, and advances in chemotherapy.[57] Therefore, understanding the epidemiology of precancerous lesions in the colon is critical to developing effective CRC prevention programs.

Models that inform adenoma prevalence data are based on global autopsy studies before the dissemination of screening programs. These models estimate the prevalence of adenomas from approximately 20% at age 45 years to greater than 50% to

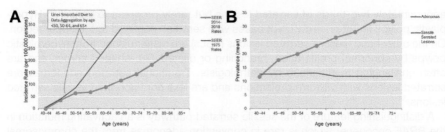

Fig. 3. Incidence rates of colorectal cancer and prevalence rates of adenomas/SSLs by age. (*A*) CRC incidence rates by age and compared across time periods (screening era of 2014–2018 vs an unscreened era in 1975). (*B*) Prevalence rates of adenomas on screening colonoscopy compared with SSLs on index colonoscopy by age. Figure was produced from data found in References [49,70,76,142]

60% by age 85 years.[58–68] Contemporary estimates of adenoma prevalence are based on studies of colonoscopy, which generally report adenomas in 20% to 53% of individuals 50 years or older, including up to 9.7% with advanced adenomas (defined as an adenoma sized ≥10 mm or with villous features or with high-grade dysplasia).[4,11,12,54,55,57,69–75] Meta-analyses of colonoscopy studies (age ≥50 years) suggest an overall adenoma prevalence rate of approximately 24% and advanced adenoma prevalence rate of about 4.5%.[76,77] However, rates of adenomas are also estimated to be higher in men and increase with age (see **Fig. 3**).[70,77] Recent evidence has also suggested a trend toward a greater proportion of adenomas in the proximal colon with increasing age, although it is unclear if this is a true increase or related to recent improvements in methods of detection for proximal polyps.[70,77–79]

Between a quarter to one-third of all CRCs develop from the sessile serrated pathway.[80–82] Serrated lesions include both SSLs and hyperplastic polyps.[57,81,82] Although it remains inconclusive whether hyperplastic polyps and SSLs arise independently,[83] and whether hyperplastic polyps have malignant potential (particularly if >5 mm and/or proximally located),[81,82,84,85] current evidence indicates that SSLs may develop into cancer. .[81,82] Rates of SSL detection vary between 1% and 18%; the true prevalence remains uncertain.[33,86–93] The high variability in prevalence estimates is likely due to differences in detection, resection, and classification practices across studies. For example, sessile and flat lesions are approximately 5 times more likely to be missed than pedunculated polyps, and when detected, there is variability among pathologists in distinguishing hyperplastic from SSLs.[94–96] Importantly, almost half of patients with SSLs are found to have adenomas on the same examination.[89–93] Yet, in contrast to adenomas, prevalence rates of SSLs generally do not substantially vary by age (see **Fig. 3**) or sex (despite conflicting evidence suggesting either sex may have higher risk[88,97]). On the other hand, hyperplastic polyps have prevalence rates on colonoscopy studies generally between 10% and 15% but can be up to 30% in certain populations.[11,33,90,97–102] Hyperplastic polyps are typically less than or equal to 5 mm and occur in the distal colon, whereas SSLs are larger and have a predilection for the proximal colon.[81] Finally, traditional serrated adenomas are villous polyps, often erythematous and (semi-)pedunculated, and located in the distal colon (with an average size of about 15 mm). These polyps have prevalence rates of less than 1% at screening colonoscopy.[86,89,91,101–104]

Table 1 summarizes the epidemiology of different colon polyps. Most importantly, detection of colon polyps is critical to preventing CRC. In landmark studies by Corley and colleagues and Kaminski and colleagues, increased adenoma detection rates

Table 1
Summary of colon polyp epidemiology

Features	Adenomas	Sessile Serrated Lesions	Hyperplastic Polyps
Prevalence	Up to 60%	1%–18%[a]	Up to 30%
Age≥50 y	20%–60%	No data	No data
Age<50 y	20%	No data	No data
Cause	Chromosomal instability or microsatellite instability pathways	Sessile serrated pathway	Sessile serrated pathway
Location	Evenly distributed[b] (34% rectum, 32% distal colon, and 34% proximal colon)	Up to 90% proximal colon	Up to 80% distal colon
Natural history	If size <10 mm, typically with low risk of progression to CRC. Higher risk of progression if size ≥10 mm or with villous or high-grade dysplasia, with ~1%–5% annual progression to CRC.	Possibly slower growth rate compared with adenomas, with annual progression to CRC of <1%. SSLs ≥10 mm with similar risk of CRC compared with large adenomas.	Unlikely neoplastic, although size >5–10 mm and/or proximally location may increase risk.

[a] True prevalence unknown.
[b] In individuals younger than 50 years, location is shifted to rectum (42%), distal colon (31%), and proximal colon (27%).

(ADR) in the highest quintile on screening colonoscopy were associated with a linear decrease in incidence of interval CRC by 48% to 82%.[71,74] These findings led to the development of ADR as an important quality metric of screening colonoscopy, with recommendations for ADR of greater than or equal to 25% for the general screening population. Similar efforts are ongoing to establish benchmark detection rates for SSLs.[80,89,90] Given an increasing focus on quality metrics emphasizing adenoma detection, together with advances in colonoscopy technology and technique, prevalence rates of adenoma and SSL are expected to increase.[71,74,105] However, it remains unclear whether increased detection of diminutive and nonadvanced polyps will translate to further decreases in CRC incidence and mortality or whether the benefits will be outweighed by the cost and risks of increased utilization of follow-up colonoscopy.[106–109] Therefore, significant efforts are also ongoing to improve CRC screening uptake among the unscreened population and address important disparities and barriers that remain to optimal primary prevention, especially given that most CRC diagnoses are in unscreened populations.[110–113]

Natural History

Cancer prevention by detecting and removing a precancerous lesion is a feature unique to CRC and only a few other malignancies (e.g., cervical cancer). IThe mean overall time from adenoma incidence to cancer development ranges from 10.6 to 25.8 years across all age groups, and the time from preclinical cancer development to (symptomatic) cancer detection is estimated at approximately 1.6 to 4.0 years.[44,58,114,115] However, understanding the natural history of colon polyps, or the "window" of the precancerous lesion's existence, has important implications for CRC screening and surveillance programs. For example, slower progression rates would lead to increased effectiveness of screening and decreased utility of surveillance, whereas increased progression rates would have the opposite impact.

Growth rates are believed to be highest in adenomas with size greater than or equal to 10 mm or with villous or high-grade dysplasia. These "advanced adenomas" are felt to be nearing CRC in progression, as studies estimate approximately 1% to 5% annual progression rates of advanced adenomas to CRC, with rates in the lower range for women overall, and rates typically on the higher end in older age groups.[116] A longitudinal barium enema study of polyps greater than or equal to 10 mm in size estimated the cumulative risk of invasive CRC at 1, 5, and 10 years of 1%, 2.5%, and 8%, respectively.[13] i Longitudinal barium enema studies also found that most of polyps less than 10 mm in size grew so slow that "they could not have achieved a significant size during the longest human life span."[117,118] However, although some argue that polyps greater than or equal to 5 mm may be of little or no clinical import, given that less than 1% contain advanced features, studies suggest that up to 10% of small (6–9 mm) polyps actually harbor advanced histology, including 1% with CRC[106,108,119–122]; this would argue the importance of colonoscopy with polypectomy in patients with small polyps, though this is an area of ongoing investigation.

Finally, despite increasing recognition of the contribution of the sessile serrated pathway to a relevant proportion of CRCs, flat SSLs were largely unobservable or unrecognized in the past and are not included in the current models that inform national guidelines. Yet, a recent study that incorporated the SSL pathway into modeling estimates found that predictions of screening effectiveness were similar to models that assume all CRCs arise only from adenomas. This finding is likely related to the fact that many patients with SSLs also have adenomas (and thus undergo complete resection of both lesions) and improved recognition of these lesions in practice is now effectively mitigating risk from both lesions.[123] This study also estimated that annual rates of progression from SSLs to CRC were less than 1% across age groups and sex (much less than rates for advanced adenomas).[116] A recent CT colography study confirmed the suggestion of slower growth rates for SSLs: when comparing SSLs (mean size 9.3 mm) with adenomas (mean size 6.3 mm), only 22% of SSLs achieved a 20% growth increase over mean 5.3 years compared with 41% of adenomas.[124] Stratifying the malignant potential of various SSLs is currently uncertain and an area of ongoing research.

YOUNG-ONSET NEOPLASIA

Incidence and mortality of young-onset (YO) CRC, defined as CRC occurring in individuals younger than 50 years, has been increasing worldwide over the past 3 decades.[125–127] In 1992 the incidence of CRC among young adults was 8.6 per 100,000, which has increased by 45% to 12.5 per 100,000 in 2015.[128] Furthermore, the CRC mortality rate among young adults has increased by 1.3% annually from 2008 through 2017, compared with a decrease of 3% annually in adults aged 65 years and older.[129] Patients with YO CRC have a higher prevalence (53%–72%) of advanced-stage (III–IV) disease at the time of diagnosis compared with average-onset (AO) CRC patients (41%–63%).[130–132] This disparity has been suggested to be related to either delays in diagnosis[125,130] versus more aggressive tumor biology.[132–136] However, a large retrospective analysis that excluded patients with syndromic or genetic predispositions for CRC found no difference in the tumor histopathology or mutational burden of sporadic YO CRC compared with sporadic AO CRC.[135] Furthermore, although CRC in individuals older than 50 years is generally equally distributed throughout the colon, YO CRC occurs most frequently in the rectum, then distal colon, and least commonly in the proximal colon (42%, 31%, and 27%, respectively).[125,137,138] In fact, patients with YO CRC commonly present with rectal bleeding or other symptoms associated with left-sided disease.[135] However, colonoscopy is still recommended in adults younger than 50 years with other "alarm" symptoms, such as unexplained hematochezia and/or iron deficiency anemia, given the significant association with YO CRC (5-year cumulative incidence for YO CRC of 0.45% if these signs or symptoms are present).[139]

In 2018, the American Cancer Society issued a qualified recommendation to start CRC screening at the age of 45 years for average-risk persons.[140] Although this statement was based on modeling data, emerging observational data support the suggestion that individuals aged 40 to 49 years may benefit from screening to detect and remove precancerous adenomas. A recent meta-analysis by Kolb and colleagues of average-risk patients undergoing colonoscopy younger than 50 years found that the rates of any colorectal neoplasm and advanced neoplasm were 14% and 2%, respectively.[76] Furthermore, this study showed that the rate of advanced neoplasia was statistically similar in the 45 to 49 years age group compared with the 50 to 59 years population (3.6% vs 4.2%, respectively). Another systemic review studying the yield of screening colonoscopy in both average risk and symptomatic individuals younger than 50 years (18–49 years) found that the prevalence of YO adenoma was 9%, with increasing age being the most consistent risk factor.[141] And although there is a paucity of data related to SSL prevalence in those younger than 50 years, Anderson and colleagues found a similar prevalence rate of SSL in those aged between 40 and 49 years and older than 50 years.[142] Taken together, these studies have informed recent CRC screening guidelines, which suggest that expanding screening to individuals aged 45 years may yield a similar impact on the reduction of CRC incidence as has been observed in those aged 50 years and older.[44,143] Nevertheless, the true impact of screening and surveillance on YO CRC is still unknown and more studies are required to address this question.

SUMMARY

Studies of the cause and epidemiology of precancerous colon polyps have significantly affected clinical practice and public policy in the last few decades. This research has informed public health initiatives for education and risk mitigation, screening recommendations across various populations, new (and often less-invasive) screening modalities, and potential chemotherapeutic options. However, despite the increasing detection of precancerous colon polyps, the lifetime risk for CRC remains approximately 4% to 5%.[49] In the future, personalized risk assessment tools based on clinical and genetic epidemiologic insights could help better target screening and surveillance resources to truly high-risk individuals, while reducing exposure to the costs and risks inherent to large-scale screening (particularly with invasive procedures) among those at low risk of CRC.

CLINICS CARE POINTS

- Understanding the epidemiology of colon polyps will help providers have informed discussions with patients regarding personalized colorectal cancer risk assessments.

- Insights in the natural history of colon polyps, including the long latency period of tumorigenesis pathways, will allow providers to make recommendations for appropriate colorectal cancer risk reduction strategies, including follow-up intervals for screening.

- Knowledge about the increasing burden of young-onset colorectal cancer will help providers advise patients on the timing of CRC screening and follow-up studies. Furthermore, providers must have a low threshold to investigate any 'alarm" symptoms in patients, particularly those younger than 50 years.

DISCLOSURE

B.A. Sullivan reports support from Exact Sciences, which is outside the scope of the this work. J. Roper reports support from Fractyl, Karl Storz, Gilead, and Zentalis, which are outside the scope of this article.

REFERENCES

1. Gilbertsen VA, Knatterud GL, Lober PH, et al. Invasive carcinoma of the large intestine: A preventable disease? Surgery 1965;57:363–5.
2. Morson B. The polyp-cancer sequence in the large bowel. Proc R Soc Med 1974;67:451–7.
3. Vogelstein B, Fearon ER, Hamilton SR, et al. Genetic alterations during colorectal-tumor development. N Engl J Med 1988;319(9):525–32.
4. Zauber AG, Winawer SJ, O'Brien MJ, et al. Colonoscopic polypectomy and long-term prevention of colorectal-cancer deaths. N Engl J Med 2012;366(8): 687–96.
5. Holme Ø, Løberg M, Kalager M, et al. Effect of flexible sigmoidoscopy screening on colorectal cancer incidence and mortality: A randomized clinical trial. JAMA 2014;312(6):606–15.
6. Shaukat A, Mongin SJ, Geisser MS, et al. Long-term mortality after screening for colorectal cancer. N Engl J Med 2013;369(12):1106–14.

7. Kronborg O, Jørgensen OD, Fenger C, et al. Randomized study of biennial screening with a faecal occult blood test: Results after nine screening rounds. Scand J Gastroenterol 2004;39(9):846–51.

8. Scholefield JH, Moss SM, Mangham CM, et al. Nottingham trial of faecal occult blood testing for colorectal cancer: A 20-year follow-up. Gut 2012;61(7): 1036–40.

9. Atkin W, Wooldrage K, Parkin DM, et al. Long term effects of once-only flexible sigmoidoscopy screening after 17 years of follow-up: The UK Flexible Sigmoidoscopy Screening randomised controlled trial. Lancet 2017;389(10076): 1299–311.

10. Schoen RE, Pinsky PF, Weissfeld JL, et al. Colorectal-cancer incidence and mortality with screening flexible sigmoidoscopy. N Engl J Med 2012;366(25): 2345–57.

11. Lieberman DA, Weiss DG, Bond JH, et al. Use of colonoscopy to screen asymptomatic adults for colorectal cancer. N Engl J Med 2000;343(3):162–8.

12. Nishihara R, Wu K, Lochhead P, et al. Long-term colorectal-cancer incidence and mortality after lower endoscopy. N Engl J Med 2013;369(12):1095–105.

13. Stryker SJ, Wolff BG, Culp CE, et al. Natural history of untreated colonic polyps. Gastroenterology 1987;93(5):1009–13.

14. Peltomaki P, Olkinuora A, Nieminen TT. Updates in the field of hereditary nonpolyposis colorectal cancer. Expert Rev Gastroenterol Hepatol 2020;14(8):707–20.

15. Guinney J, Dienstmann R, Wang X, et al. The consensus molecular subtypes of colorectal cancer. Nat Med 2015;21(11):1350–6.

16. Blokzijl F, de Ligt J, Jager M, et al. Tissue-specific mutation accumulation in human adult stem cells during life. Nature 2016;538(7624):260–4.

17. Tomasetti C, Li L, Vogelstein B. Stem cell divisions, somatic mutations, cancer etiology, and cancer prevention. Science 2017;355(6331):1330–4.

18. Tomasetti C, Marchionni L, Nowak MA, et al. Only three driver gene mutations are required for the development of lung and colorectal cancers. Proc Natl Acad Sci U S A 2015;112(1):118–23.

19. Drost J, van Jaarsveld RH, Ponsioen B, et al. Sequential cancer mutations in cultured human intestinal stem cells. Nature 2015;521(7550):43–7.

20. Matano M, Date S, Shimokawa M, et al. Modeling colorectal cancer using CRISPR-Cas9-mediated engineering of human intestinal organoids. Nat Med 2015;21(3):256–62.

21. Barker N, Ridgway RA, van Es JH, et al. Crypt stem cells as the cells-of-origin of intestinal cancer. Nature 2009;457(7229):608–11.

22. Roper J, Tammela T, Cetinbas NM, et al. In vivo genome editing and organoid transplantation models of colorectal cancer and metastasis. Nat Biotechnol 2017;35(6):569–76.

23. Van Cutsem E, Kohne CH, Hitre E, et al. Cetuximab and chemotherapy as initial treatment for metastatic colorectal cancer. N Engl J Med 2009;360(14):1408–17.

24. Samuels Y, Wang Z, Bardelli A, et al. High frequency of mutations of the PIK3CA gene in human cancers. Science 2004;304(5670):554.

25. Cancer Genome Atlas N. Comprehensive molecular characterization of human colon and rectal cancer. Nature 2012;487(7407):330–7.

26. Lengauer C, Kinzler KW, Vogelstein B. Genetic instabilities in human cancers. Nature 1998;396(6712):643–9.

27. Seshagiri S, Stawiski EW, Durinck S, et al. Recurrent R-spondin fusions in colon cancer. Nature 2012;488(7413):660–4.

28. Wood LD, Parsons DW, Jones S, et al. The genomic landscapes of human breast and colorectal cancers. Science 2007;318(5853):1108–13.
29. Parsons R, Li GM, Longley MJ, et al. Hypermutability and mismatch repair deficiency in RER+ tumor cells. Cell 1993;75(6):1227–36.
30. Boland CR, Thibodeau SN, Hamilton SR, et al. A National Cancer Institute workshop on Microsatellite Instability for cancer detection and familial predisposition: Development of international criteria for the determination of microsatellite instability in colorectal cancer. Cancer Res 1998;58(22):5248–57.
31. Stoffel EM, Boland CR. Genetics and genetic testing in hereditary colorectal cancer. Gastroenterology 2015;149(5):1191–203.
32. Davies H, Bignell GR, Cox C, et al. Mutations of the BRAF gene in human cancer. Nature 2002;417(6892):949–54.
33. Hazewinkel Y, de Wijkerslooth TR, Stoop EM, et al. Prevalence of serrated polyps and association with synchronous advanced neoplasia in screening colonoscopy. Endoscopy 2014;46(3):219–24.
34. Farris AB, Misdraji J, Srivastava A, et al. Sessile serrated adenoma: Challenging discrimination from other serrated colonic polyps. Am J Surg Pathol 2008; 32(1):30–5.
35. Rajagopalan H, Bardelli A, Lengauer C, et al. Tumorigenesis: RAF/RAS oncogenes and mismatch-repair status. Nature 2002;418(6901):934.
36. Spring KJ, Zhao ZZ, Karamatic R, et al. High prevalence of sessile serrated adenomas with BRAF mutations: A prospective study of patients undergoing colonoscopy. Gastroenterology 2006;131(5):1400–7.
37. Yan HHN, Lai JCW, Ho SL, et al. RNF43 germline and somatic mutation in serrated neoplasia pathway and its association with BRAF mutation. Gut 2017;66(9):1645–56.
38. Fang M, Ou J, Hutchinson L, et al. The BRAF oncoprotein functions through the transcriptional repressor MAFG to mediate the CpG Island Methylator phenotype. Mol Cell 2014;55(6):904–15.
39. Prahallad A, Sun C, Huang S, et al. Unresponsiveness of colon cancer to BRAF(V600E) inhibition through feedback activation of EGFR. Nature 2012; 483(7387):100–3.
40. Corcoran RB, Andre T, Atreya CE, et al. Combined BRAF, EGFR, and MEK inhibition in patients with BRAF(V600E)-mutant colorectal cancer. Cancer Discov 2018;8(4):428–43.
41. Centers for Disease Control and Prevention. An update on cancer deaths in the United States. Atlanta, (GA): US Department of Health and Human Services, Centers for Disease Control and Prevention, Division of Cancer Prevention and Control; 2021.
42. Sung H, Ferlay J, Siegel RL, et al. Global cancer statistics 2020: GLOBOCAN estimates of incidence and mortality worldwide for 36 cancers in 185 countries. CA Cancer J Clin 2021;71(3):209–49.
43. American Cancer Society. Cancer facts & Figures 2018. Atlanta: American Cancer Society; 2018.
44. Davidson KW, Barry MJ, Mangione CM, et al. Screening for colorectal cancer: US Preventive Services Task Force recommendation statement. JAMA 2021; 325(19):1965–77.
45. Rabeneck L, Chiu HM, Senore C. International perspective on the burden of colorectal cancer and public health effects. Gastroenterology 2020;158(2): 447–52.

46. Welch HG, Robertson DJ. Colorectal cancer on the decline - Why screening can't explain it all. N Engl J Med 2016;374(17):1605–7.
47. Malvezzi M, Carioli G, Bertuccio P, et al. European cancer mortality predictions for the year 2018 with focus on colorectal cancer. Ann Oncol 2018;29(4): 1016–22.
48. Murphy CC, Sandler RS, Sanoff HK, et al. Decrease in incidence of colorectal cancer among individuals 50 years or older after recommendations for population-based screening. Clin Gastroenterol Hepatol 2017;15(6):903–9.
49. Surveillance, Epidemiology, and End Results (SEER) Program (www.seer. cancer.gov) SEER*Stat Database: Incidence - SEER Research Data, 9 Registries, Nov 2020 Sub (1975-2018) - Linked To County Attributes - Time Dependent (1990-2018) Income/Rurality, 1969-2019 Counties, National Cancer Institute, DCCPS, Surveillance Research Program, released April 2021, based on the November 2020 submission.
50. Gupta S, Lieberman D, Anderson JC, et al. Recommendations for follow-up after colonoscopy and polypectomy: A consensus update by the US Multi-Society Task Force on colorectal cancer. Gastrointest Endosc 2020;91(3):463–85.
51. Rex DK, Boland CR, Dominitz JA, et al. Colorectal cancer screening: Recommendations for physicians and patients from the U.S. Multi-Society Task Force on colorectal cancer. Gastroenterology 2017;153(1):307–23.
52. He X, Hang D, Wu K, et al. Long-term risk of colorectal cancer after removal of conventional adenomas and serrated polyps. Gastroenterology 2020;158(4): 852–61.
53. Lee JK, Jensen CD, Levin TR, et al. Long-term risk of colorectal cancer and related death after adenoma removal in a large, community-based population. Gastroenterology 2020;158(4):884–94.
54. Loberg M, Kalager M, Holme O, et al. Long-term colorectal-cancer mortality after adenoma removal. N Engl J Med 2014;371(9):799–807.
55. Martinez ME, Baron JA, Lieberman DA, et al. A pooled analysis of advanced colorectal neoplasia diagnoses after colonoscopic polypectomy. Gastroenterology 2009;136(3):832–41.
56. Wieszczy P, Kaminski MF, Franczyk R, et al. Colorectal cancer incidence and mortality after removal of adenomas during screening colonoscopies. Gastroenterology 2020;158(4):875–883 e875.
57. Strum WB. Colorectal adenomas. N Engl J Med 2016;375(4):389–90.
58. Kuntz KM, Lansdorp-Vogelaar I, Rutter CM, et al. A systematic comparison of microsimulation models of colorectal cancer: the role of assumptions about adenoma progression. Med Decis Making 2011;31(4):530–9.
59. Arminski TC, McLean DW. Incidence and distribution of adenomatous polyps of the colon and rectum based on 1,000 autopsy examinations. Dis Colon Rectum 1964;7:249–61.
60. Blatt LJ. Polyps of the colon and rectum. Dis Colon Rectum 1961;4(4):277–82.
61. Bombi JA. Polyps of the colon in Barcelona, Spain. An autopsy study. Cancer 1988;61(7):1472–6.
62. Chapman I. Adenomatous polypi of large intestine: incidence and distribution. Ann Surg 1963;157(2):223–6.
63. Clark JC, Collan Y, Eide TJ, et al. Prevalence of polyps in an autopsy series from areas with varying incidence of large-bowel cancer. Int J Cancer 1985;36(2): 179–86.

64. Jass JR, Young PJ, Robinson EM. Predictors of presence, multiplicity, size and dysplasia of colorectal adenomas. A necropsy study in New Zealand. Gut 1992; 33(11):1508–14.
65. Johannsen LG, Momsen O, Jacobsen NO. Polyps of the large intestine in Aarhus, Denmark. An autopsy study. Scand J Gastroenterol 1989;24(7):799–806.
66. Rickert RR, Auerbach O, Garfinkel L, et al. Adenomatous lesions of the large bowel: An autopsy survey. Cancer 1979;43(5):1847–57.
67. Vatn MH, Stalsberg H. The prevalence of polyps of the large intestine in Oslo: An autopsy study. Cancer 1982;49(4):819–25.
68. Williams AR, Balasooriya BA, Day DW. Polyps and cancer of the large bowel: A necropsy study in Liverpool. Gut 1982;23(10):835–42.
69. Bretthauer M, Kaminski MF, Løberg M, et al. Population-based colonoscopy screening for colorectal cancer: A randomized clinical trial. JAMA Intern Med 2016;176(7):894–902.
70. Corley DA, Jensen CD, Marks AR, et al. Variation of adenoma prevalence by age, sex, race, and colon location in a large population: implications for screening and quality programs. Clin Gastroenterol Hepatol 2013;11(2):172–80.
71. Corley DA, Levin TR, Doubeni CA. Adenoma detection rate and risk of colorectal cancer and death. N Engl J Med 2014;370(26):2541.
72. Heitman SJ, Ronksley PE, Hilsden RJ, et al. Prevalence of adenomas and colorectal cancer in average risk individuals: A systematic review and meta-analysis. Clin Gastroenterol Hepatol 2009;7(12):1272–8.
73. Imperiale TF, Ransohoff DF, Itzkowitz SH, et al. Multitarget stool DNA testing for colorectal-cancer screening. N Engl J Med 2014;370(14):1287–97.
74. Kaminski MF, Wieszczy P, Rupinski M, et al. Increased rate of adenoma detection associates with reduced risk of colorectal cancer and death. Gastroenterology 2017;153(1):98–105.
75. Quintero E, Castells A, Bujanda L, et al. Colonoscopy versus Fecal Immunochemical Testing in colorectal-cancer screening. N Engl J Med 2012;366(8): 697–706.
76. Kolb JM, Hu J, DeSanto K, et al. Early-age onset colorectal neoplasia in average-risk individuals undergoing screening colonoscopy: A systematic review and meta-analysis. Gastroenterology 2021;161(4):1145–55.
77. Wong MCS, Huang J, Huang JLW, et al. Global prevalence of colorectal neoplasia: A systematic review and meta-analysis. Clin Gastroenterol Hepatol 2020;18(3):553–61.e510.
78. Fenoglio L, Castagna E, Comino A, et al. A shift from distal to proximal neoplasia in the colon: a decade of polyps and CRC in Italy. BMC Gastroenterol 2010; 10:139.
79. Patel K, Hoffman NE. The anatomical distribution of colorectal polyps at colonoscopy. J Clin Gastroenterol 2001;33(3):222–5.
80. Anderson JC, Butterly LF, Robinson CM, et al. Risk of metachronous high-risk adenomas and large serrated polyps in individuals with serrated polyps on index colonoscopy: Data from the New Hampshire Colonoscopy Registry. Gastroenterology 2018;154(1):117–27.
81. Crockett SD, Nagtegaal ID. Terminology, molecular features, epidemiology, and management of serrated colorectal neoplasia. Gastroenterology 2019;157(4): 949–66.e944.
82. Rex DK, Ahnen DJ, Baron JA, et al. Serrated lesions of the colorectum:/review and recommendations from an expert panel. Am J Gastroenterol 2012;107(9): 1315–29.

83. Bettington M, Walker N, Clouston A, et al. The serrated pathway to colorectal carcinoma: Current concepts and challenges. Histopathology 2013;62(3): 367–86.
84. Bensen SP, Cole BF, Mott LA, et al. Colorectal hyperplastic polyps and risk of recurrence of adenomas and hyperplastic polyps. Polyps Prevention Study. Lancet 1999;354(9193):1873–4.
85. Laiyemo AO, Murphy G, Sansbury LB, et al. Hyperplastic polyps and the risk of adenoma recurrence in the polyp prevention trial. Clin Gastroenterol Hepatol 2009;7(2):192–7.
86. Hetzel JT, Huang CS, Coukos JA, et al. Variation in the detection of serrated polyps in an average risk colorectal cancer screening cohort. Am J Gastroenterol 2010;105(12):2656–64.
87. Kahi CJ, Hewett DG, Norton DL, et al. Prevalence and variable detection of proximal colon serrated polyps during screening colonoscopy. Clin Gastroenterol Hepatol 2011;9(1):42–6.
88. Sanaka MR, Gohel T, Podugu A, et al. Adenoma and sessile serrated polyp detection rates: Variation by patient sex and colonic segment but not specialty of the endoscopist. Dis Colon Rectum 2014;57(9):1113–9.
89. Abdeljawad K, Vemulapalli KC, Kahi CJ, et al. Sessile serrated polyp prevalence determined by a colonoscopist with a high lesion detection rate and an experienced pathologist. Gastrointest Endosc 2015;81(3):517–24.
90. Anderson JC, Butterly LF, Weiss JE, et al. Providing data for serrated polyp detection rate benchmarks: an analysis of the New Hampshire Colonoscopy Registry. Gastrointest Endosc 2017;85(6):1188–94.
91. JE IJ, de Wit K, van der Vlugt M, et al. Prevalence, distribution and risk of sessile serrated adenomas/polyps at a center with a high adenoma detection rate and experienced pathologists. Endoscopy 2016;48(8):740–6.
92. Ohki D, Tsuji Y, Shinozaki T, et al. Sessile serrated adenoma detection rate is correlated with adenoma detection rate. World J Gastrointest Oncol 2018; 10(3):82–90.
93. Payne SR, Church TR, Wandell M, et al. Endoscopic detection of proximal serrated lesions and pathologic identification of sessile serrated adenomas/ polyps vary on the basis of center. Clin Gastroenterol Hepatol 2014;12(7): 1119–26.
94. Vennelaganti S, Cuatrecasas M, Vennalaganti P, et al. Interobserver agreement among pathologists in the differentiation of sessile serrated From hyperplastic polyps. Gastroenterology 2021;160(1):452–4.
95. Vennelaganti S, Hassan C, Patil DT, et al. Inter-observer agreement among pathologists in the diagnosis of sessile serrated polyps: a multi-center international study. Gastroenterology 2017;152(5):S538.
96. van Rijn JC, Reitsma JB, Stoker J, et al. Polyp miss rate determined by tandem colonoscopy: a systematic review. Am J Gastroenterol 2006;101(2):343–50.
97. Carr NJ, Mahajan H, Tan KL, et al. Serrated and non-serrated polyps of the colorectum: Their prevalence in an unselected case series and correlation of BRAF mutation analysis with the diagnosis of sessile serrated adenoma. J Clin Pathol 2009;62(6):516–8.
98. DiSario JA, Foutch PG, Mai HD, et al. Prevalence and malignant potential of colorectal polyps in asymptomatic, average-risk men. Am J Gastroenterol 1991;86(8):941–5.
99. Hassan C, Pickhardt PJ, Marmo R, et al. Impact of lifestyle factors on colorectal polyp detection in the screening setting. Dis Colon Rectum 2010;53(9):1328–33.

100. Provenzale D, Garrett JW, Condon SE, et al. Risk for colon adenomas in patients with rectosigmoid hyperplastic polyps. Ann Intern Med 1990;113(10):760–3.
101. Bettington M, Walker N, Rahman T, et al. High prevalence of sessile serrated adenomas in contemporary outpatient colonoscopy practice. Intern Med J 2017; 47(3):318–23.
102. Schramm C, Janhsen K, Hofer JH, et al. Detection of clinically relevant serrated polyps during screening colonoscopy: results from seven cooperating centers within the German colorectal screening program. Endoscopy 2018;50(10): 993–1000.
103. Bettington ML, Walker NI, Rosty C, et al. A clinicopathological and molecular analysis of 200 traditional serrated adenomas. Mod Pathol 2015;28(3):414–27.
104. Hasegawa S, Mitsuyama K, Kawano H, et al. Endoscopic discrimination of sessile serrated adenomas from other serrated lesions. Oncol Lett 2011;2(5): 785–9.
105. Rex DK, Schoenfeld PS, Cohen J, et al. Quality indicators for colonoscopy. Am J Gastroenterol 2015;110(1):72–90.
106. Vleugels JLA, Hassan C, Senore C, et al. Diminutive polyps with advanced histologic features do not increase risk for metachronous advanced colon neoplasia. Gastroenterology 2019;156(3):623–34.
107. Sekiguchi M, Otake Y, Kakugawa Y, et al. Incidence of advanced colorectal neoplasia in individuals with untreated diminutive colorectal adenomas diagnosed by magnifying image-enhanced endoscopy. Am J Gastroenterol 2019; 114(6):964–73.
108. Vleugels JLA, Hazewinkel Y, Fockens P, et al. Natural history of diminutive and small colorectal polyps: A systematic literature review. Gastrointest Endosc 2017;85(6):1169–76.
109. Lieberman D, Gupta S. Does colon polyp surveillance improve patient outcomes? Gastroenterology 2020;158(2):436–40.
110. Dougherty MK, Brenner AT, Crockett SD, et al. Evaluation of interventions intended to increase colorectal cancer screening rates in the United States: A systematic review and meta-analysis. JAMA Intern Med 2018;178(12):1645–58.
111. Melson JE, Imperiale TF, Itzkowitz SH, et al. AGA White Paper: Roadmap for the future of colorectal cancer screening in the United States. Clin Gastroenterol Hepatol 2020;18(12):2667–78.
112. May FP, Yang L, Corona E, et al. Disparities in colorectal cancer Sscreening in the United States before and after implementation of the affordable care act. Clin Gastroenterol Hepatol 2020;18(8):1796–804.
113. Doubeni CA, Fedewa SA, Levin TR, et al. Modifiable failures in the colorectal cancer screening process and their association with risk of death. Gastroenterology 2019;156(1):63–74.
114. Knudsen AB, Zauber AG, Rutter CM, et al. Estimation of benefits, burden, and harms of colorectal cancer screening strategies: Modeling study for the US Preventive Services Task Force. JAMA 2016;315(23):2595–609.
115. Morson BC. The evolution of colorectal carcinoma. Clin Radiol 1984;35(6): 425–31.
116. Greuter MJ, Xu XM, Lew JB, et al. Modeling the Adenoma and Serrated pathway to Colorectal CAncer (ASCCA). Risk Anal 2014;34(5):889–910.
117. Welin S, Youker J, Spratt JS. The rates and patterns of growth of 375 tumors of the large intestine and rectum observed serially by double contrast enema study (Malmoe technique). Am J Roentgenol 1963;90:673–87.

118. Pickhardt PJ. The natural history of colorectal polyps and masses: Rediscovered truths from the barium enema era. Am J Roentgenol 2007;188(3):619–21.

119. Butterly LF, Chase MP, Pohl H, et al. Prevalence of clinically important histology in small adenomas. Clin Gastroenterol Hepatol 2006;4(3):343–8.

120. O'Brien MJ, Winawer SJ, Zauber AG, et al. The National Polyp Study. Patient and polyp characteristics associated with high-grade dysplasia in colorectal adenomas. Gastroenterology 1990;98(2):371–9.

121. Schoenfeld P. Small and diminutive polyps: implications for colorectal cancer screening with computed tomography colonography. Clin Gastroenterol Hepatol 2006;4(3):293–5.

122. Lieberman D, Moravec M, Holub J, et al. Polyp size and advanced histology in patients undergoing colonoscopy screening: Implications for CT colonography. Gastroenterology 2008;135(4):1100–5.

123. Greuter MJ, Demirel E, Lew JB, et al. Long-term impact of the dutch colorectal cancer screening program on cancer incidence and mortality-model-based exploration of the serrated pathway. Cancer Epidemiol Biomarkers Prev 2016; 25(1):135–44.

124. Pickhardt PJ, Pooler BD, Matkowskyj KA, et al. Volumetric growth rates of sessile serrated adenomas/polyps observed in situ at longitudinal CT colonography. Eur Radiol 2019;29(9):5093–100.

125. Akimoto N, Ugai T, Zhong R, et al. Rising incidence of early-onset colorectal cancer - a call to action. Nat Rev Clin Oncol 2021;18(4):230–43.

126. Burnett-Hartman AN, Lee JK, Demb J, et al. An update on the epidemiology, molecular characterization, diagnosis, and screening strategies for early-onset colorectal cancer. Gastroenterology 2021;160(4):1041–9.

127. Stoffel EM, Murphy CC. Epidemiology and mechanisms of the increasing incidence of colon and rectal cancers in young adults. Gastroenterology 2020; 158(2):341–53.

128. Murphy CC, Wallace K, Sandler RS, et al. Racial disparities in incidence of young-onset colorectal cancer and patient survival. Gastroenterology 2019; 156(4):958–65.

129. Siegel RL, Miller KD, Goding Sauer A, et al. Colorectal cancer statistics, 2020. CA Cancer J Clin 2020;70(3):145–64.

130. Chen FW, Sundaram V, Chew TA, et al. Advanced-stage colorectal cancer in persons younger than 50 years not associated with longer duration of symptoms or time to diagnosis. Clin Gastroenterol Hepatol 2017;15(5):728–37.

131. Myers EA, Feingold DL, Forde KA, et al. Colorectal cancer in patients under 50 years of age: A retrospective analysis of two institutions' experience. World J Gastroenterol 2013;19(34):5651–7.

132. Kneuertz PJ, Chang GJ, Hu CY, et al. Overtreatment of young adults with colon cancer: More intense treatments with unmatched survival gains. JAMA Surg 2015;150(5):402–9.

133. Chang DT, Pai RK, Rybicki LA, et al. Clinicopathologic and molecular features of sporadic early-onset colorectal adenocarcinoma: An adenocarcinoma with frequent signet ring cell differentiation, rectal and sigmoid involvement, and adverse morphologic features. Mod Pathol 2012;25(8):1128–39.

134. Fu J, Yang J, Tan Y, et al. Young patients (</= 35 years old) with colorectal cancer have worse outcomes due to more advanced disease: A 30-year retrospective review. Medicine 2014;93(23):e135.

135. Cercek A, Chatila WK, Yaeger R, et al. A comprehensive comparison of early-onset and average-onset colorectal cancers. J Natl Cancer Inst 2021;113(12): 1683–92.

136. Manjelievskaia J, Brown D, McGlynn KA, et al. Chemotherapy use and survival among young and middle-aged patients with colon cancer. JAMA Surg 2017; 152(5):452–9.

137. Archambault AN, Su YR, Jeon J, et al. Cumulative burden of colorectal cancer-associated genetic variants is more strongly associated with early-onset vs late-onset cancer. Gastroenterology 2020;158(5):1274–86.

138. Chang SH, Patel N, Du M, et al. Trends in early-onset vs late-onset colorectal cancer incidence by race/ethnicity in the United States cancer statistics database. Clin Gastroenterol Hepatol 2021;26:S1542–3565 (21)00817-X. Online ahead of print.

139. Demb J, Liu L, Murphy CC, et al. Young-onset colorectal cancer risk among individuals with iron-deficiency anaemia and haematochezia. Gut 2020;70(8): 1529–37.

140. Wolf AMD, Fontham ETH, Church TR, et al. Colorectal cancer screening for average-risk adults: 2018 guideline update from the American Cancer Society. CA Cancer J Clin 2018;68(4):250–81.

141. Enwerem N, Cho MY, Demb J, et al. Systematic review of prevalence, risk factors, and risk for metachronous advanced neoplasia in atients with young-onset colorectal adenoma. Clin Gastroenterol Hepatol 2021;19(4):680–9.

142. Anderson JC, Robinson CM, Butterly LF. Young adults and metachronous neoplasia: Risks for future advanced adenomas and large serrated polyps compared with older adults. Gastrointest Endosc 2020;91(3):669–75.

143. Shaukat A, Kahi CJ, Burke CA, et al. ACG clinical guidelines: Colorectal cancer screening 2021. Am J Gastroenterol 2021;116(3):458–79.

Risk Factors for Colorectal Polyps and Cancer

Jared A. Sninsky, MD[a], Brandon M. Shore, MD[b], Gabriel V. Lupu, MD[b], Seth D. Crockett, MD, MPH[a],*

KEYWORDS

- Risk factors • Polyps • Adenomas • Colorectal cancer • Serrated polyps
- Epidemiology

KEY POINTS

- The primary nonmodifiable risk factors for colorectal adenomas are age, sex, and family history.
- Modifiable risk factors consist of alcohol, obesity, physical activity, and diet.
- Obscure risk factors for colorectal adenomas include acromegaly, hereditary hemochromatosis, and patients who have had ureterosigmoidostomy.
- Serrated class polyps have different risk factors than conventional adenomas.

INTRODUCTION

Colorectal cancer (CRC) is among the most highly incident and deadly cancers in the United States and worldwide, resulting in nearly 1 million deaths per year across the globe.[1–6] Most CRCs arise from precursor adenomatous or serrated polyps, presenting the opportunity for CRC prevention via the detection and removal of precancerous lesions before they progress to malignancy and metastasis. A rich literature on the epidemiology of CRC and colorectal polyps has been published in the past 30 years that demonstrates that risk factors for sporadic CRC and its precursor polyps are largely similar. There are important differences in risk factors for adenomatous and serrated class polyps, however. Herein, the authors review this literature, with particular focus on nonmodifiable, modifiable, and certain unusual or overlooked factors that are of importance to gastroenterologists, patients, and public health professionals.

Colorectal polyps are defined as aberrant growths that typically arise from the mucosal layer of the large intestine and extend into the lumen. Colon polyps are

[a] Division of Gastroenterology and Hepatology, University of North Carolina School of Medicine, CB 7080, 130 Mason Farm Road, Chapel Hill, NC 27599-7555, USA; [b] Department of Medicine, University of North Carolina School of Medicine, CB 7080, 130 Mason Farm Road, Chapel Hill, NC 27599-7555, USA
* Corresponding author. Bioinformatics Building, CB 7080, 130 Mason Farm Road, Chapel Hill, NC 27599-7555.
E-mail address: sethc@med.unc.edu

Gastrointest Endoscopy Clin N Am 32 (2022) 195–213
https://doi.org/10.1016/j.giec.2021.12.008
giendo.theclinics.com

subdivided into neoplastic and nonneoplastic lesions. The predominant nonneoplastic polyps are inflammatory polyps, hamartomas, lymphoid polyps, mucosal prolapse polyps, and hyperplastic polyps. Neoplastic polyps, meanwhile, are characterized based on their potential to undergo malignant transformation and include primarily adenomatous and serrated polyps. Adenomatous polyps, the primary focus of this review, compose two-thirds of all colon polyps and are the most common precursor lesions to CRC. Histologically, conventional adenomas are categorized into tubular, tubulovillous or villous histologic subtypes. Neoplastic serrated polyps include traditional serrated adenomas and sessile serrated lesions (SSLs, also known as sessile serrated adenomas or polyps). SSLs are the most common premalignant serrated polyp type, and are predominately located in the right colon. As described in other chapters, conventional adenomas and serrated polyps exhibit different mutogenic pathways to invasive CRC.

NONMODIFIABLE RISK FACTORS

Nonmodifiable risk factors for adenomatous polyps include age, sex, race/ethnicity, genetic polyposis syndromes, and family history. Although these characteristics are generally immutable, identification of high-risk individuals can lead to improved screening and surveillance of precancerous lesions.

Age

Age is the predominant nonmodifiable risk factor in the development of colon adenomas. A large body of research has shown that the prevalence of adenomas increases predictably with age, rising 10% to 15% from individuals aged 50 to 55 years to the oldest age stratum at 70 to 75 years.[7,8] This effect of age on colon polyp risk holds true despite stratification by sex and ethnicity. Serial epidemiologic necropsies conducted in patients 20 to 89 years corroborate the increasing prevalence of polyps with age, noting a risk inflection point at age 50 years.[9] Recent data from a large US endoscopy quality improvement database clearly demonstrate this pattern (**Fig. 1**).[7] Likewise, age increases one's risk of large polyps, and the Clinical Outcome Research Initiative (CORI) revealed that patients older than 69 years have an odds ratio (OR) of 2.7 for polyps greater than 9 mm compared with patients younger than 50 years.[10,11]

Because of longstanding guidelines that (until recently) recommended initiating CRC screening at age 50 years, there is a paucity of colon polyp epidemiologic data on patients less than 50 years; however, the concerning increase in incidence of CRC in younger patients prompts investigation into colon polyps within these younger cohorts. A study by Dave and colleagues[12] comprising data from patients 20 to 49 years of age undergoing colonoscopy between 2016 and 2019 found that 20% of patients had neoplastic polyps, with 24% of patients in the 30- to 40-years age group and 37% in the 40- to 49-years age group. An increasing incidence of advanced polyps in younger patients correlates with the higher rates of CRC in patients under 50 years.[13–15] These data support the recent recommendation of the US Preventive Services Task Force to lower the age of initiation of CRC screening from 50 to 45 years.[16] Nevertheless, colorectal polyps and CRC are much more common in older individuals than they are in patients less than 50 years.

Sex

The prevalence of colon adenomas is consistently higher in men than women; however, despite this risk discrepancy, lifetime incidence is approximately equal between

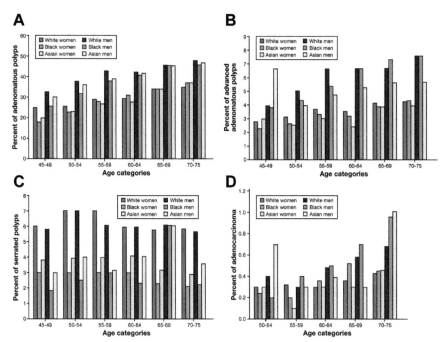

Fig. 1. Polyp and CRC data from a large sample of average risk screening colonoscopies in the United States from the GI Quality Improvement Consortium (GIQuIC), showing prevalence of adenomatous polyps (*A*), advanced adenomas (*B*), serrated polyps (*C*), and colorectal adenocarcinoma (*D*), stratified by age, sex, and race. Graphs demonstrate that (1) men are at higher risk of adenomatous polyps and CRC compared with women; (2) prevalence increases by age for adenomas, advanced adenomas, and CRC, but not for serrated polyps; and (3) white race is associated with a higher risk of serrated polyps than other races. (*From* Peery AF, Crockett SD, Murphy CC, Lund JL, Dellon ES, Williams JL, Jensen ET, Shaheen NJ, Barritt AS, Lieber SR, Kochar B, Barnes EL, Fan YC, Pate V, Galanko J, Baron TH, Sandler RS. Burden and Cost of Gastrointestinal, Liver, and Pancreatic Diseases in the United States: Update 2018. Gastroenterology. 2019 Jan;156(1):254-272.e11.)

the sexes, as women tend to live longer. One cross-sectional study reported that men have 1.77 times the risk of adenomas on screening colonoscopy compared with women.[8] The CORI database revealed that men also had a 50% increased risk of large polyps (>9 mm) compared with women (OR, 1.5; 95% confidence interval [CI], 1.42–164).[17] Men also appear to have increased risk of polyps on surveillance colonoscopy compared with women.[11] The higher prevalence of colon polyps in men versus women is reflected in the Gastroenterology Society guidelines for adenoma detection rate targets, of 25% for women and 30% for men.[18] It is important to note that this sex discrepancy in adenoma prevalence is not true of sessile serrated polyps, which are equally prevalent among men and women (see **Fig. 1**).[19] The reduced risk of adenomatous polyps in women has been hypothesized to be related to estrogen receptor genes, decreased insulin-like growth factors, and/or reduced bile acid production.[17,20–22]

Race and Ethnicity

Epidemiologic studies demonstrate that there are minor differences in risk of adenomas based on race and ethnicity.[8] In particular, proximal adenoma risk is around

25% higher in blacks than whites, and this risk is reflected in proximal colon cancer rates as well.[23,24] African Americans also have a higher risk of large polyps (>9 mm) on screening colonoscopy until age 65 years at which point the prevalence between blacks and whites is equivalent. However, it is well known that African Americans have a higher incidence and mortality of CRC compared with other racial groups. A Department of Veterans Affairs cohort of 4038 veterans revealed that 24% of African American patients on screening colonoscopy had villous pathologic condition compared with only 16% of Caucasians.[25] This indicates that despite equitable health care access, African Americans could have higher rates of more aggressive polyp histology. Particularly concerning, the incidence and mortality of CRC in Alaskan Natives are double that of the African American population.[26] Meanwhile, Hispanic persons have a 25% lower risk of large adenomas than non-Hispanic whites from 50 to 79 years,[27,28] and Asian Americans appear to have an adenoma prevalence similar to whites.[8]

Racial and ethnic differences are difficult to study because of heterogeneity within groups and the inability to disentangle lifestyle factors from genetics. For example, although native Japanese populations have a low prevalence of adenomatous polyps, Hawaiian ethnic Japanese have a higher adenoma prevalence at around 61%.[29] This is further illustrated by differing risk of large polyps observed in Hispanic persons from Mexican-predominant states and non-Mexican-predominant states.[30] Overall, there appears to be subtle differences between ethnic groups in polyp risk that may largely be driven by lifestyle exposures or other factors.

High-Risk Genetic Syndromes

There are several well-described hereditary polyposis syndromes, including familial adenomatous polyposis, serrated polyposis syndrome, MYH-associated polyposis, polymerase proofreading associated polyposis, juvenile polyposis syndrome, and Peutz-Jeghers syndrome.[31] Hereditary nonpolyposis CRC syndrome, or Lynch syndrome, is associated with an increased risk of malignancy that can occur with or without precursor polyps.[32] Further discussion of these genetic syndromes is beyond the scope of this review, which focuses primarily on sporadic colorectal polyps, but is outlined clearly within recent guidelines.[33]

Family History of Colorectal Cancer

Having a first-degree relative with a history of CRC increases one's risk of colon cancer substantially. In fact, the risk of CRC increases by a factor of 1.76 (CI, 1.59–1.94) in patients who have a first-degree family member diagnosed with CRC, even after age 80 years.[34] Patients who have a first-degree relative with CRC also have an increased risk of adenomas in general (OR, 1.82; 95% CI, 1.66–2.00) as well as a higher risk of advanced adenomas (OR, 2.43; 95% CI, 1.66–2.00).[35,36] This body of research has prompted the US Multi-Society Task Force on Colorectal Cancer to recommend that patients with a first-degree family member with CRC or advanced polyp start screening colonoscopy at age 40 or 10 years before the age of youngest affected relative, and that patients with a first-degree relative with CRC under the age of 60 years undergo closest surveillance.[37,38]

Family History of Polyps

A recent Swedish case-control study reported that patients with a first-degree relative with a colorectal polyp had a 40% higher risk of polyps themselves.[39] Interestingly, the investigators reported that the risk of colorectal polyps increases with each additional first-degree relative with polyps as well as a decreasing age at diagnosis of polyps in family members. Similarly, Ahsan and colleagues[40] found that having a family member diagnosed with polyps at age less than 50 years increases one's own risk of polyps by 4 times compared with having a family member diagnosed with polyps after age 60 years. However, despite the findings above, given that roughly half of average risk persons undergoing screening colonoscopy harbor at least 1 adenomatous polyp, having a first-degree relative with small or diminutive polyps is unlikely to be associated with an appreciably elevated risk of CRC. In addition, the difficulty of ascertaining an accurate family history of polyps limits the clinical applicability of these findings.

Personal History of Polyps or Colorectal Cancer

Both the number and the size of adenomatous polyps on one's baseline examination increase the risk of developing both future advanced adenomas and CRC. Martínez and colleagues,[41] in a pooled prospective analysis, found that having greater than 5 adenomas at baseline colonoscopy or having at least 1 adenoma greater than 19 mm in size increased absolute risk of metachronous advanced adenoma by approximately 20% to 25%. In addition, patients with a history of CRC also have a risk of metachronous CRC that is at least 70% higher than the expected population rate.[42]

Inflammatory Bowel Disease

Patients with IBD with colonic involvement (ulcerative colitis [UC] and Crohn colitis involving at least 30% of the colon) are at a higher risk of CRC than the general population.[43] For this reason, colonoscopy surveillance is recommended starting 8 to 10 years after the onset of colitis symptoms.[44,45] Compared with expected population incidence, patients with UC with proctitis have an OR of 1.7 for CRC, patients with left-sided colitis have an OR of 2.8, and patients with pancolitis have an OR of 14.8.[46] However, most CRC in IBD bypasses the traditional sporadic adenoma-to-carcinoma sequence and is instead defined by nonpolypoid dysplasia with late APC mutations.[47] Patients with primary sclerosing cholangitis with UC have an exceedingly high risk of CRC, with an OR of 4.79 for developing CRC compared with patients with UC without primary sclerosing cholangitis.[48,49]

Despite the higher risk of CRC in UC, patients with UC are at roughly equivalent risk of colon adenomas compared with the general population.[47,50] A prospective surveillance study by Rutter and colleagues[51] found that CRC incidence in UC has dropped substantially from 1970 to 2000, likely attributable to newer IBD therapies and increased use of surveillance colonoscopy. It has also been hypothesized that mesalamine has a chemoprotective effect, and it has been shown to induce apoptosis and curb mucosal proliferation in patients with sporadic polyps.[52] Interestingly, patients with IBD that do have adenomas have a greater risk of developing advanced neoplasia than patients with matched adenoma without IBD.[53]

Diabetes

Diabetes has been noted to increase the risk of colorectal adenomas within younger age groups. Patients with diabetes aged 40 to 49 years have a 3 times greater risk of polyps than nondiabetic patients within the same age group. In fact, patients with diabetes aged 40 to 49 years had just as many polyps as nondiabetic patients in the 50- to 59-years age group.[54] Among all age groups, diabetes increases polyp risk by 50%. Although hyperglycemia is associated with CRC risk, it is unclear if hyperglycemia or hyperinsulinemia specifically is the dominant driver of polyp risk.[55,56]

MODIFIABLE RISK FACTORS

Although there are several nonmodifiable risk factors for precancerous polyps and CRC, such as age, sex, and family history,[57,58] as discussed above, several modifiable risk factors and protective factors have also been identified (**Table 1**). Identification and management of these risk factors are important in assessing and potentially decreasing patients' risk for CRC. Indeed, it is hypothesized that upwards of two-thirds of CRC cases are attributable to modifiable risk factors.[59] Given the relatively long latency period from adenoma to invasive cancer,[60,61] modification of such risk factors has the potential to mitigate CRC risk in some patients.

Smoking

Tobacco smoking is an important risk factor for the development of CRC and colonic polyps.[57] The mechanism for this association is via oxidative stress and damage to cellular DNA.[62] Specifically, carcinogens in smoke diffuse passively through the circulatory system into the colonic mucosa, interrupting cellular replication and hindering the DNA repair process.[62] In addition, the carbon monoxide in cigarette smoke indirectly leads to DNA mutations and cellular hypoxia.[62] In fact, compared with nonsmokers, both current (OR, 1.29; 95% CI, 1.11–1.49) and former smokers (OR, 1.18; 95% CI, 1.05–1.32) have an increased risk of adenomatous polyps.[63] Smoking also increases the risk of serrated polyps. In a meta-analysis examining this association, there was an increased risk of the development of SSLs in smokers in comparison to nonsmokers (relative risk [RR], 2.47; 95% CI, 2.12–2.87).[59,64] Some studies suggest that smoking increases the risk of serrated polyps primarily within the distal colon.[65] Smoking also increases the risk of CRC in a dose-dependent manner.[66] Recent studies have shown that the risk of CRC decreases after 25 years of smoking cessation, underpinning the importance of counseling for smoking cessation.[67]

Alcohol Use

Alcohol use is common with a prevalence of 60% of adults in the United States.[68] Numerous studies confirm that consuming greater than 1 alcoholic beverage per day has been shown to have a clear relationship with the development of both colon polyps and CRC.[69] One Korean study found that significant alcohol consumption increased the risk of adenomas on surveillance colonoscopy by approximately 86% compared with nondrinkers.[70] Another study, by Bardou and colleagues,[71] similarly demonstrated an increased risk of large adenomas (>10 mm) in heavy drinkers (OR, 1.8; 95% CI, 1.2–2.7) compared with control patients. With respect to serrated polyps, a 2015 meta-analysis demonstrated a 24% increase in risk of serrated polyps in subjects who drank alcohol daily compared with nondrinkers. More specifically, there was a dose-dependent relationship with alcohol and serrated polyp risk, with an RR of 1.19 (95% CI, 1.02–1.40) for moderate drinkers (8–36 g/d) and 1.60 (95% CI, 1.35–1.91) for heavy drinkers (>36 g) compared with nondrinkers.[72] A recent analysis using pooled data from the Nurses' Health Study and the Health Professions Follow-up Study (n = 141,143) found that heavy alcohol drinkers had a higher risk of both conventional adenomas (OR, 1.17; 95% CI, 1.10–1.25) and serrated polyps (OR, 1.33; 95% CI, 1.24–1.43) compared with never drinkers.[64,73]

Obesity

Obesity accounts for nearly 3 million deaths per year.[74] One explanation for excess mortality in this group is an increased risk of malignancy, including CRC.[57] It is hypothesized that those who are obese have higher levels of chronic inflammation because of

Table 1
Risk factors associated with adenomatous polyps, serrated polyps, and colorectal cancer

Risk Factor	Adenomatous Polyps	Serrated Polyps	Colorectal Cancer
Nonmodifiable			
Older age	Increased risk ⬆	Minimal or no increased risk ⬌	Increased risk ⬆
Male sex	Increased risk ⬆	No increased risk ⬌	Increased risk ⬆
Family history of CRC	Increased risk ⬆	Minimal or no increased risk ⬌	Increased risk ⬆
Modifiable			
Smoking	Increased risk ⬆	Increased risk ⬆	Increased risk ⬆
Alcohol	Increased risk ⬆	Increased risk ⬆	Increased risk ⬆
Red meat	Increased risk ⬆	Increased risk ⬆	Increased risk ⬆
Calcium/vitamin D/folate	Decreased risk ⬇	Increased risk ⬆	Decreased risk ⬇
NSAIDs/aspirin	Decreased risk ⬇	Decreased risk ⬇	Decreased risk ⬇
Rare			
Acromegaly	Increased risk ⬆	Unknown	Increased risk ⬆
Hereditary hemochromatosis	Unknown	Unknown	Increased risk ⬆
Ureterosigmoidostomy	Increased risk ⬆	Unknown	Increased risk ⬆

the release of proinflammatory cytokines (tumor necrosis factor, interleukin-6) from adipose tissue.[62,75] One meta-analysis found that a 5-unit increase in body mass index (BMI) was associated with a 19% higher risk of a colorectal adenomas.[75] This was supported in another study that noted a 2% to 3% increase in CRC risk with each increase in BMI unit.[57] Patients with high waist circumference also appear to have an increased risk of metachronous neoplasia.[76]

Physical Activity and Exercise

Physical activity decreases the risk of both CRC and adenomas. A meta-analysis found a 16% decrease in risk of adenomas in the most active men and women compared with sedentary participants.[77] In men, the most physically active quartile had a significantly lower risk of adenomatous polyp recurrence and those in the least physically active quartile.[78]

Diet

Red meat has been implicated with an increased risk of CRC as well as colorectal adenomas.[57,62] One study found this risk of adenoma recurrence was increased (OR, 1.85; 95% CI, 1.10–3.13) in those who consumed cooked red meat when compared with those who did not.[79] The pathogenesis is thought to be related to the production of heterocyclic amines, which have a direct effect on the DNA production/mutation process.[62] One study found that for every 100 g of red meat consumed daily, there was a 1.16 times (95% CI, 1.04–1.30) elevated risk of CRC.[57,80] Indeed, the American Cancer Society guidelines recommend limiting red meat in order to mitigate the risks of CRC.[64]

In contrast, there is evidence to suggest that the consumption of a Mediterranean diet (defined as low in saturated fats, meat, and dairy, and high in vegetables, fruits, and nuts[81]) or vegetarian diet decreases risk of CRC (OR, 0.86; 95% CI, 0.80–0.92).[69] The additive effects of a healthy balanced diet, including higher quantities of whole grains, dairy, fruits, and vegetables, and lower content of saturated fat content (specifically red meat), are thought to be responsible for the reduced risk of CRC.[69]

Several epidemiologic studies have found that both dietary calcium intake and vitamin D intake are associated with decreased risk of CRC.[82,83] The mechanisms of both are hypothesized to regulate cell proliferation and apoptosis.[84] Milk intake has a similar level of evidence, as it contains both calcium and vitamin D.

Fiber has convincing evidence to support a lower risk of CRC (RR, 0.84; 95% CI, 0.78–0.89) and recurrence rate of colorectal polyps.[39,84,85] The mechanism by which fiber mitigates CRC risk is uncertain, but may be due to its effects on stool transmit time, diluting carcinogenic colonic contents, and forming fatty acids that can regulate apoptosis.[62,80,84] Specifically, whole grain intake is also associated with decreased CRC risk (RR, 0.88; 95% CI, 0.83–0.94).[80,86]

Fruits are thought to have anticarcinogenic properties, and there is limited evidence that high fruit intake is associated with a decreased risk of CRC.[80,84,86] There is no clear evidence that vitamin B6, A, C, and E, methionine, coffee, and caffeine affect CRC risk.[80] A healthy and balanced diet may also influence the gut microbiome in a beneficial manner, and in doing so, decrease the production of certain bacterial metabolites that can be carcinogenic.[87]

Medications

Many different compounds have been studied for their chemopreventive properties with respect to CRC over the past 40 years. A detailed discussion of these agents is beyond the scope of this review but can be found elsewhere.[88,89] Suffice to say that several medications have been found to affect the risk of CRC, most notably aspirin, nonsteroidal anti-inflammatory drugs (NSAIDs), and hormone replacement therapy. In a study published in 2020 from data collected from 1980 to 2014 involving more than 94,000 participants, those who used aspirin on a daily basis had a decreased risk of CRC compared with those who did not (hazard ratio [HR], 0.80;

95% CI, 0.72–0.90).[90] Importantly, this risk was only applicable to those 70 years old or older who had initiated aspirin use before the age of 70. There was no benefit to initiating aspirin after the age of 70.[90] Furthermore, it was found in multiple studies that this protective effect may be stronger in the proximal colon.[59,60] Accordingly, a recent Clinical Practice Update from the American Gastroenterological Association recommended use of aspirin for prevention of CRC in certain persons based on their age and cardiovascular risk profile.[89]

In patients with diabetes, metformin use is associated with a decreased risk of CRC (OR, 0.73; 95% CI, 0.62–0.86) compared with diabetics not taking metformin.[91] Hormone replacement therapy for postmenopausal women has also been studied and shown to mitigate the risk of CRC. Specifically, those who take estrogen on a daily basis were found to have up to a 40% decreased risk of CRC compared with women who did not.[92] The estrogen receptor gene hypothesis is supported by findings from the Nurses' Heath Study, which demonstrated that postmenopausal women on hormone replacement therapy had a decreased risk for large adenomas.[93,94]

Despite the reduced risk of CRC observed with aspirin, NSAIDs, and hormone replacement therapies, the inherent risks of these medications, including bleeding, heart disease, and other malignancies, limit their broad application in chemoprevention.

RARE OR UNUSUAL RISK FACTORS FOR COLORECTAL CANCER

Additional rare factors have been linked to developing CRC, such as acromegaly, hereditary hemochromatosis, ureterosigmoidostomy, and history of childhood cancer.

Acromegaly

Acromegaly poses increased risk of CRC because of excess growth hormone and insulin-like growth factor 1, which cause colonic epithelial cell proliferation, diminished cellular apoptosis, slowed intestinal transit, and redundant bowel.[95]

A study by Rokkas and colleagues[96] involving 701 patients with acromegaly demonstrated increased risk of both adenomatous polyps (OR, 2.54; 95% CI, 1.91–3.26), and CRC (OR, 4.35; 95% CI, 1.53–12.35).[95] A more recent meta-analysis involving 529 patients with acromegaly found a standard incidence ratio (SIR) of 2.6 (95% CI, 1.7–4.0) for CRC.[95,97] Similarly, another study (n = 700) found that patients with acromegaly have a 2.4-fold increased risk of colonic adenomas and a 7.4-fold greater risk of CRC.[95] However, a separate meta-analysis in 2017 (n = 3896) revealed contradictory findings from multiple retrospective analyses, suggesting that the data regarding CRC risk in acromegaly are insufficient.[98,99] Furthermore, the impact on mortality remains unclear.[95]

Hereditary Hemochromatosis

HH is an inherited genetic disorder of iron overload with increased iron absorption and possible risk for CRC. Iron can be carcinogenic via forming hydroxyl free radicals, dampening immune response, and being a nutrient for carcinogenesis.[100] Both HFE gene mutations are common and estimated to be approximately 15% of the US population.[101] A Melbourne cohort study (n = 28,509) found that C282Y homozygotes were at a 2-fold increased risk of CRC (HR, 2.28; 95% CI, 1.22–4.25).[100] However, heterozygotes were not at an increased risk in this study.[100] Shaheen and colleagues[101] in a case-control study (n = 1308) found that subjects with any HFE gene mutation were significantly more likely to have CRC than subjects with no HFE gene mutations (OR, 1.40; 95% CI, 1.07–1.87). Other studies that support an association between HH and CRC include a Swedish cohort study (n = 6849) that reported that patients with HH had a 40% increased for colon adenocarcinoma (SIR, 1.4; 95% CI, 1.1–1.9), and Nelson and colleagues (n = 1950),[102,103] which showed a small increased risk for CRC among patients heterozygous for HH (RR, 1.28; CI, 1.07–1.53). Some studies found an association with CRC in only male *HFE* C282Y homozygotes, and one study found no association.[104,105] Overall, the evidence is compelling that special attention to risk for CRC be attributed to patients with the HFE gene and HH especially in homozygotes.

Childhood Cancer Survivors

Childhood cancer survivors are at risk for gastrointestinal subsequent malignant neoplasms. The British Childhood Cancer Survivor Study (n = 17,981) demonstrated an SIR of 4.6 for digestive malignancies, with the greatest SIR observed following Wilm's tumor and heritable retinoblastoma.[106] Henderson et al. showed at 22.8-year median follow up (n=14,358) an increased risk of subsequent gastrointestinal cancer that was 4.6-fold higher than the general population.[107] Abdominopelvic radiation posed the highest risk (SIR = 11.2; 95% CI 7.6-16.4), followed by previous receipt of procarbazine or platinum drugs.[107] Nottage et al. found that among childhood cancer survivors (n = 13,048), the 40-year cumulative incidence of secondary CRC was 1.4%, with a SIR of 10.9 (95% CI, 6.6 to 17.0) compared to the general population.[108] The same authors also reported that abdominopelvic radiation (dose-dependent) and alkylating agents increased the risk.

These findings were further corroborated by Daniel et al., who demonstrated that children exposed to abdominopelvic radiotherapy had a 4- to 11-fold greater risk of CRC.[109]

Despite these findings, the appropriate screening strategy remains unclear.[110] The Children's Oncology Group recommends colonoscopy every 5 years or stool testing every 3 years following abdominopelvic radiation beginning either at age 30 or 5 years after radiation exposure.[111]

Ureterosigmoidostomy

Ureterosigmoidostomy is a procedure where the ureters are inserted into the sigmoid colon, typically following cystectomy for bladder cancer. Ureterosigmoidostomy increases the risk of CRC with an incidence of 2-15%.[112] The mean latency times from surgery to adenoma and CRC are estimated to be 20 years and 26 years respectively.[112,113] Carcinogenesis is proposed to involve colonic exposure to urinary amines and amides that undergo N-nitrosation with colonic bacteria.[114] Ureterosigmoidostomy is a less favored operation in the current era because of multiple complications, including malignancy, and thus is now rarely performed, having been replaced by newer techniques of urinary diversion procedures. However, clinicians should be aware that patients who did have this surgery performed should undergo yearly colonoscopy starting 3-10 years post-operatively.[112,115]

DIFFERENCES IN RISK FACTORS FOR ADENOMATOUS VERSUS SERRATED POLYPS

There are important differences in the epidemiology of serrated class polyps and adenomatous polyps. Precancerous subtypes of serrated polyps (SSLs and traditional serrated adenomas [TSAs]) are less common than conventional adenomas. TSAs are quite rare, found in less than 1% of patients undergoing colonoscopy.[116] SSLs occur in roughly 15% of average-risk patients undergoing colonoscopy, when examinations are performed by high-detecting endoscopists.[116,117] In terms of nonmodifiable risk factors, neither age nor male sex appears to be strongly related to prevalence of serrated lesions, in contrast to adenomatous polyps (see **Fig. 1**).[118]

However, white race is a risk factor for serrated polyps, particularly SSLs and microvesicular hyperplastic polyps.[65,118,119] With respect to modifiable risk factors, both smoking and alcohol intake appear to be more strongly associated with increased risk of serrated polyps compared with conventional adenomas.[59,120,121] Whereas supplemental calcium, vitamin D, and folate use have all been linked to decreased risk of conventional adenomas, some evidence suggests that these agents may actually increase the risk of serrated class polyps.[122,123] However, similar to conventional adenomas, both aspirin use and NSAID use are associated with decreased risk of serrated polyps.[65,89,123]

SUMMARY

The strongest nonmodifiable risk factors for CRC and precancerous polyps are age, male sex, and family history of CRC. Current evidence indicates that smoking, obesity, and diet are key modifiable risk factors for sporadic CRC. Unusual or uncommon CRC risk factors include acromegaly, HH, childhood cancer survivors, and patients who have undergone ureterosigmoidostomy. In contrast to adenomatous polyps, serrated polyp prevalence does not seem to vary much by age, and men and women appear to be at roughly equivalent risk. White race and smoking are stronger risk factors for serrated polyps than adenomatous polyps.

These data can be used to construct risk scores to identify persons at higher risk of advanced colorectal neoplasia and/or those who may benefit more from colonoscopy versus noninvasive CRC screening tests. Better knowledge of the epidemiology of colorectal polyps and cancer can also be useful in patient care, particularly when counseling patients regarding modifiable risk factors.

CLINICS CARE POINTS

- There is a 10% to 15% higher risk of adenomas in patients 70 to 75 years of age compared with the 50- to 55-year age group.

- Persons of black race and Alaskan native ethnicity have higher incidence of colorectal cancer compared with other races and ethnicities.

- Family history of colorectal cancer in first-degree relatives, particularly if family members are diagnosed under the age of 60 years, increases one's risk of both polyps and cancer.

- Diets high in red meat are associated with increased risk of precancerous polyps and colorectal cancer, whereas diets rich in intake of calcium, fiber, and fruits and vegetables are associated with lower risk.

- Patients with a history of childhood cancer (particularly with abdominopelvic radiation exposure), acromegaly, hereditary hemochromatosis, primary sclerosing cholangitis, and prior ureterosigmoidostomy surgery are at increased risk of colorectal cancer and therefore merit more frequent screening.

- The risk factor profile for serrated class polyps differs somewhat from that of adenomatous polyps, reflecting etiologic heterogeneity of colorectal cancer.

DISCLOSURE

Dr S.D. Crockett has received research funding (clinical trial agreements) from Freenome, Guardant, and Exact Sciences. None of the other authors have financial, professional, or personal conflicts of interest.

FUNDING

This research was supported, in part, by a grant from the National Institutes of Health T32 DK007634.

REFERENCES

1. Sung H, Ferlay J, Siegel RL, et al. Global cancer statistics 2020: GLOBOCAN estimates of incidence and mortality worldwide for 36 cancers in 185 countries. CA Cancer J sClin 2021;71(3):209–49. https://doi.org/10.3322/caac.21660.

2. Carlsson G, Petrelli NJ, Nava H, et al. The value of colonoscopic surveillance after curative resection for colorectal cancer or synchronous adenomatous polyps. Arch Surg 1987;122(11):1261–3. https://doi.org/10.1001/archsurg. 1987.01400230047008.

3. Rex DK, Hassan C, Bourke MJ. The colonoscopist's guide to the vocabulary of colorectal neoplasia: histology, morphology, and management. Gastrointest Endosc 2017;86(2):253–63. https://doi.org/10.1016/j.gie.2017.03.1546.

4. Fearon ER, Vogelstein B. A genetic model for colorectal tumorigenesis. Cell 1990;61(5):759–67. https://doi.org/10.1016/0092-8674(90)90186-I.

5. Smit WL, Spaan CN, Johannes de Boer R, et al. Driver mutations of the adenoma-carcinoma sequence govern the intestinal epithelial global translational capacity. Proc Natl Acad Sci 2020;117(41):25560. https://doi.org/10. 1073/pnas.1912772117.

6. Snover DC, Jass JR, Fenoglio-Preiser C, et al. Serrated polyps of the large intestine: a morphologic and molecular review of an evolving concept. Am J Clin Pathol 2005;124(3):380–91.

7. Peery AF, Crockett SD, Murphy CC, et al. Burden and cost of gastrointestinal, liver, and pancreatic diseases in the United States: update 2018. Gastroenterology 2019;156(1):254–72.e11. https://doi.org/10.1053/j.gastro.2018.08.063.

8. Corley DA, Jensen CD, Marks AR, et al. Variation of adenoma prevalence by age, sex, race, and colon location in a large population: implications for screening and quality programs. Clin Gastroenterol Hepatol 2013;11(2): 172–80. https://doi.org/10.1016/j.cgh.2012.09.010.

9. Pendergrass CJ, Edelstein DL, Hylind LM, et al. Occurrence of colorectal adenomas in younger adults: an epidemiologic necropsy study. Clin Gastroenterol Hepatol 2008;6(9):1011–5. https://doi.org/10.1016/j.cgh.2008.03.022.

10. McCashland TM, Brand R, Lyden E, et al. Gender differences in colorectal polyps and tumors. Am J Gastroenterol 2001;96(3):882–6. https://doi.org/10. 1111/j.1572-0241.2001.3638_a.x.

11. Noshirwani KC, van Stolk RU, Rybicki LA, et al. Adenoma size and number are predictive of adenoma recurrence: implications for surveillance colonoscopy. Gastrointest Endosc 2000;51(4, Part 1):433–7. https://doi.org/10.1016/S0016-5107(00)70444-5.

12. Dave D, Lu R, Klair JS, et al. 128 Prevalence and predictors of adenomas in young adults undergoing diagnostic colonoscopy in a multicenter midwest U.S. cohort. J Am Coll Gastroenterol 2019;114.

13. Lam T-J, Wong BCY, Mulder CJJ, et al. Increasing prevalence of advanced colonic polyps in young patients undergoing colonoscopy in a referral academic hospital in Hong Kong. World J Gastroenterol 2007;13(28):3873–7. https://doi.org/10.3748/wjg.v13.i28.3873.

14. Lee SE, Jo HB, Kwack WG, et al. Characteristics of and risk factors for colorectal neoplasms in young adults in a screening population. World J Gastroenterol 2016;22(10):2981–92. https://doi.org/10.3748/wjg.v22.i10.2981.
15. Bailey CE, Hu C-Y, You YN, et al. Increasing disparities in the age-related incidences of colon and rectal cancers in the United States, 1975-2010. JAMA Surg 2015;150(1):17–22. https://doi.org/10.1001/jamasurg.2014.1756.
16. Davidson KW, Barry MJ, Mangione CM, et al. Screening for colorectal cancer: US Preventive Services Task Force recommendation statement. JAMA 2021; 325(19):1965–77. https://doi.org/10.1001/jama.2021.6238.
17. McCashland TM, Brand R, Lyden E, et al. Gender differences in colorectal polyps and tumors. Am J Gastroenterol 2001;96(3):882–6. https://doi.org/10.1016/S0002-9270(00)02431-X.
18. Rex DK, Schoenfeld PS, Cohen J, et al. Quality indicators for colonoscopy. Am J Gastroenterol 2015;110(1):72–90. https://doi.org/10.1038/ajg.2014.385.
19. Parikh MP, Muthukuru S, Jobanputra Y, et al. Proximal sessile serrated adenomas are more prevalent in Caucasians, and gastroenterologists are better than nongastroenterologists at their detection. Gastroenterol Res Pract 2017; 2017:6710931. https://doi.org/10.1155/2017/6710931.
20. Issa JP, Ottaviano YL, Celano P, et al. Methylation of the oestrogen receptor CpG island links ageing and neoplasia in human colon. Nat Genet 1994;7(4):536–40. https://doi.org/10.1038/ng0894-536.
21. Everson GT, McKinley C, Kern F Jr. Mechanisms of gallstone formation in women. Effects of exogenous estrogen (Premarin) and dietary cholesterol on hepatic lipid metabolism. J Clin Invest 1991;87(1):237–46. https://doi.org/10.1172/jci114977.
22. Campagnoli C, Biglia N, Altare F, et al. Differential effects of oral conjugated estrogens and transdermal estradiol on insulin-like growth factor 1, growth hormone and sex hormone binding globulin serum levels. Gynecol Endocrinol 1993;7(4):251–8. https://doi.org/10.3109/09513599309152509.
23. Demb J, Earles A, Martínez ME, et al. Risk factors for colorectal cancer significantly vary by anatomic site. BMJ Open Gastroenterol 2019;6(1):e000313. https://doi.org/10.1136/bmjgast-2019-000313.
24. Shavers VL. Racial/ethnic variation in the anatomic subsite location of in situ and invasive cancers of the colon. J Natl Med Assoc 2007;99(7):733–48.
25. Jackson CS, Vega KJ. Higher prevalence of proximal colon polyps and villous histology in African-Americans undergoing colonoscopy at a single equal access center. J Gastrointest Oncol 2015;6(6):638–43. https://doi.org/10.3978/j.issn.2078-6891.2015.096.
26. Siegel RL, Miller KD, Goding Sauer A, et al. Colorectal cancer statistics, 2020. CA Cancer J Clin 2020;70(3):145–64. https://doi.org/10.3322/caac.21601.
27. Lieberman DA, Williams JL, Holub JL, et al. Race, ethnicity, and sex affect risk for polyps >9 mm in average-risk individuals. Gastroenterology 2014;147(2): 351. https://doi.org/10.1053/j.gastro.2014.04.037, e14–5.
28. Orsak G, Allen CM, Sorensen W, et al. Risk of colorectal polyps and malignancies among predominantly rural hispanics. J Immigr Minor Health 2019; 21(5):931–7. https://doi.org/10.1007/s10903-018-0802-x.
29. Stemmermann GN, Yatani R. Diverticulosis and polyps of the large intestine. A necropsy study of Hawaii Japanese. Cancer 1973;31(5):1260–70. https://doi.org/10.1002/1097-0142(197305)31:5<1260::aid-cncr2820310535>3.0.co;2-n.
30. Avalos DJ, Zuckerman MJ, Dwivedi A, et al. Differences in prevalence of large polyps between Hispanic Americans from Mexican- and non-Mexican-

predominant states. Dig Dis Sci 2019;64(1):232–40. https://doi.org/10.1007/s10620-018-5304-0.

31. Stoffel EM, Mangu PB, Gruber SB, et al. Hereditary colorectal cancer syndromes: American Society of Clinical Oncology clinical practice guideline endorsement of the familial risk–colorectal cancer: European Society for Medical Oncology clinical practice guidelines. J Clin Oncol 2014;33(2):209–17. https://doi.org/10.1200/JCO.2014.58.1322.

32. Macaron C, Leach BH, Burke CA. Hereditary colorectal cancer syndromes and genetic testing. J Surg Oncol 2015;111(1):103–11. https://doi.org/10.1002/jso.23706.

33. Monahan KJ, Bradshaw N, Dolwani S, et al. Guidelines for the management of hereditary colorectal cancer from the British Society of Gastroenterology (BSG)/Association of Coloproctology of Great Britain and Ireland (ACPGBI)/United Kingdom Cancer Genetics Group (UKCGG). Gut 2020;69(3):411. https://doi.org/10.1136/gutjnl-2019-319915.

34. Samadder NJ, Smith KR, Hanson H, et al. Increased risk of colorectal cancer among family members of all ages, regardless of age of index case at diagnosis. Clin Gastroenterol Hepatol 2015;13(13):2305–11.e1. https://doi.org/10.1016/j.cgh.2015.06.040.

35. Samadder NJ, Curtin K, Tuohy TM, et al. Increased risk of colorectal neoplasia among family members of patients with colorectal cancer: a population-based study in Utah. Gastroenterology 2014;147(4):814–21.e5. https://doi.org/10.1053/j.gastro.2014.07.006 [quiz e15–6].

36. Abou Khalil M, Boutros M, Nedjar H, et al. Incidence rates and predictors of colectomy for ulcerative colitis in the era of biologics: results from a provincial database. J Gastrointest Surg 2018;22(1):124–32. https://doi.org/10.1007/s11605-017-3530-y.

37. Shaukat A, Kahi CJ, Burke CA, et al. ACG clinical guidelines: colorectal cancer screening 2021. Am J Gastroenterol 2021;116(3):458–79.

38. Rex DK, Boland CR, Dominitz JA, et al. Colorectal cancer screening: recommendations for physicians and patients from the U.S. Multi-Society Task Force on colorectal cancer. Am J Gastroenterol 2017;112(7):1016–30. https://doi.org/10.1038/ajg.2017.174.

39. Song M, Emilsson L, Roelstraete B, et al. Risk of colorectal cancer in first degree relatives of patients with colorectal polyps: nationwide case-control study in Sweden. BMJ 2021;373:n877. https://doi.org/10.1136/bmj.n877.

40. Ahsan H, Neugut AI, Garbowski GC, et al. Family history of colorectal adenomatous polyps and increased risk for colorectal cancer. Ann Intern Med 1998;128(11):900–5. https://doi.org/10.7326/0003-4819-128-11-199806010-00006.

41. Martínez ME, Baron JA, Lieberman DA, et al. A pooled analysis of advanced colorectal neoplasia diagnoses after colonoscopic polypectomy. Gastroenterology 2009;136(3):832–41. https://doi.org/10.1053/j.gastro.2008.12.007.

42. Yang L, Xiong Z, Xie QK, et al. Second primary colorectal cancer after the initial primary colorectal cancer. BMC Cancer 2018;18(1):931. https://doi.org/10.1186/s12885-018-4823-6.

43. Cairns SR, Scholefield JH, Steele RJ, et al. Guidelines for colorectal cancer screening and surveillance in moderate and high risk groups (update from 2002). Gut 2010;59(5):666. https://doi.org/10.1136/gut.2009.179804.

44. Eaden JA, Mayberry JF, British Society for G, et al. Guidelines for screening and surveillance of asymptomatic colorectal cancer in patients with inflammatory

bowel disease. Gut 2002;51(Suppl 5):V10–2. https://doi.org/10.1136/gut.51. suppl_5.v10.

45. Clarke WT, Feuerstein JD. Colorectal cancer surveillance in inflammatory bowel disease: practice guidelines and recent developments. World J Gastroenterol 2019;25(30):4148–57. https://doi.org/10.3748/wjg.v25.i30.4148.

46. Ekbom A, Helmick C, Zack M, et al. Ulcerative colitis and colorectal cancer. A population-based study. N Engl J Med 1990;323(18):1228–33. https://doi.org/ 10.1056/nejm199011013231802.

47. Stidham RW, Higgins PDR. Colorectal cancer in inflammatory bowel disease. Clin Colon Rectal Surg 2018;31(3):168–78. https://doi.org/10.1055/s-0037-1602237.

48. Soetikno RM, Lin OS, Heidenreich PA, et al. Increased risk of colorectal neoplasia in patients with primary sclerosing cholangitis and ulcerative colitis: a meta-analysis. Gastrointest Endosc 2002;56(1):48–54. https://doi.org/10. 1067/mge.2002.125367.

49. Broomé U, Löfberg R, Veress B, et al. Primary sclerosing cholangitis and ulcer-ative colitis: evidence for increased neoplastic potential. Hepatology 1995; 22(5):1404–8. https://doi.org/10.1002/hep.1840220511.

50. Gordillo J, Zabana Y, Garcia-Planella E, et al. Prevalence and risk factors for colorectal adenomas in patients with ulcerative colitis. United Eur Gastroenterol J 2018;6(2):322–30. https://doi.org/10.1177/2050640617718720.

51. Rutter MD, Saunders BP, Wilkinson KH, et al. Thirty-year analysis of a colono-scopic surveillance program for neoplasia in ulcerative colitis. Gastroenterology 2006;130(4):1030–8. https://doi.org/10.1053/j.gastro.2005.12.035.

52. Reinacher-Schick A, Seidensticker F, Petrasch S, et al. Mesalazine changes apoptosis and proliferation in normal mucosa of patients with sporadic polyps of the large bowel. Endoscopy 2000;32(3):245–54. https://doi.org/10.1055/s-2000-135.

53. van Schaik FD, Mooiweer E, van der Have M, et al. Adenomas in patients with inflammatory bowel disease are associated with an increased risk of advanced neoplasia. Inflamm Bowel Dis 2013;19(2):342–9. https://doi.org/10.1097/MIB. 0b013e318286f771.

54. Vu HT, Ufere N, Yan Y, et al. Diabetes mellitus increases risk for colorectal ade-nomas in younger patients. World J Gastroenterol 2014;20(22):6946–52. https:// doi.org/10.3748/wjg.v20.i22.6946.

55. Ottaviano LF, Li X, Murray M, et al. Type 2 diabetes impacts colorectal adenoma detection in screening colonoscopy. Sci Rep 2020;10(1):7793. https://doi.org/ 10.1038/s41598-020-64344-2.

56. Vulcan A, Manjer J, Ohlsson B. High blood glucose levels are associated with higher risk of colon cancer in men: a cohort study. BMC Cancer 2017;17(1): 842. https://doi.org/10.1186/s12885-017-3874-4.

57. Kuipers EJ, Grady WM, Lieberman D, et al. Colorectal cancer. Nat Rev Dis Primers 2015;1:15065. https://doi.org/10.1038/nrdp.2015.65.

58. O'Sullivan DE, Sutherland RL, Town S, et al. Risk factors for early-onset colo-rectal cancer: a systematic review and meta-analysis. Clin Gastroenterol Hepa-tol 2021. https://doi.org/10.1016/j.cgh.2021.01.037.

59. Bailie L, Loughrey MB, Coleman HG. Lifestyle risk factors for serrated colorectal polyps: a systematic review and meta-analysis. Gastroenterology 2017;152(1): 92–104. https://doi.org/10.1053/j.gastro.2016.09.003.

60. Chapelle N, Martel M, Toes-Zoutendijk E, et al. Recent advances in clinical practice: colorectal cancer chemoprevention in the average-risk population. Gut 2020;69(12):2244–55. https://doi.org/10.1136/gutjnl-2020-320990.

61. Brenner H, Kloor M, Pox CP. Colorectal cancer. Lancet 2014;383(9927): 1490–502. https://doi.org/10.1016/s0140-6736(13)61649-9.

62. Hao Y, Wang Y, Qi M, et al. Risk factors for recurrent colorectal polyps. Gut Liver 2020;14(4):399–411. https://doi.org/10.5009/gnl19097.

63. Figueiredo JC, Crockett SD, Snover DC, et al. Smoking-associated risks of conventional adenomas and serrated polyps in the colorectum. Cancer Causes Control 2015;26(3):377–86. https://doi.org/10.1007/s10552-014-0513-0.

64. Øines M, Helsingen LM, Bretthauer M, et al. Epidemiology and risk factors of colorectal polyps. Best Pract Res Clin Gastroenterol 2017;31(4):419–24. https://doi.org/10.1016/j.bpg.2017.06.004.

65. Haque TR, Bradshaw PT, Crockett SD. Risk factors for serrated polyps of the colorectum. Dig Dis Sci 2014;59(12):2874–89. https://doi.org/10.1007/s10620-014-3277-1.

66. Botteri E, Borroni E, Sloan EK, et al. Smoking and colorectal cancer risk, overall and by molecular subtypes: a meta-analysis. Am J Gastroenterol 2020;115(12): 1940–9. https://doi.org/10.14309/ajg.0000000000000803.

67. Botteri E, Iodice S, Bagnardi V, et al. Smoking and colorectal cancer: a meta-analysis. JAMA 2008;300(23):2765–78. https://doi.org/10.1001/jama.2008.839.

68. Patel R, Mueller M, Doerr C. Alcoholic liver disease (nursing). In: StatPearls. Treasure Island (FL): StatPearls Publishing LLC; 2021.

69. Veettil SK, Wong TY, Loo YS, et al. Role of diet in colorectal cancer incidence: umbrella review of meta-analyses of prospective observational studies. JAMA Netw Open 2021;4(2):e2037341. https://doi.org/10.1001/jamanetworkopen. 2020.37341.

70. Yang YJ, Bang CS, Choi JH, et al. Alcohol consumption is associated with the risk of developing colorectal neoplasia: propensity score matching analysis. Sci Rep 2019;9(1):8253. https://doi.org/10.1038/s41598-019-44719-w.

71. Bardou M, Montembault S, Giraud V, et al. Excessive alcohol consumption favours high risk polyp or colorectal cancer occurrence among patients with adenomas: a case control study. Gut 2002;50(1):38–42. https://doi.org/10.1136/gut.50.1.38.

72. Wang YM, Zhou QY, Zhu JZ, et al. Systematic review with meta-analysis: alcohol consumption and risk of colorectal serrated polyp. Dig Dis Sci 2015;60(7): 1889–902. https://doi.org/10.1007/s10620-014-3518-3.

73. He X, Wu K, Ogino S, et al. Association between risk factors for colorectal cancer and risk of serrated polyps and conventional adenomas. Gastroenterology 2018;155(2):355–73.e18. https://doi.org/10.1053/j.gastro.2018.04.019.

74. Bardou M, Barkun AN, Martel M. Obesity and colorectal cancer. Gut 2013;62(6): 933–47. https://doi.org/10.1136/gutjnl-2013-304701.

75. Ben Q, An W, Jiang Y, et al. Body mass index increases risk for colorectal adenomas based on meta-analysis. Gastroenterology 2012;142(4):762–72. https://doi.org/10.1053/j.gastro.2011.12.050.

76. Ashbeck EL, Jacobs ET, Martínez ME, et al. Components of metabolic syndrome and metachronous colorectal neoplasia. Cancer Epidemiol Biomarkers Prev 2009;18(4):1134–43. https://doi.org/10.1158/1055-9965.Epi-08-1015.

77. Wolin KY, Yan Y, Colditz GA. Physical activity and risk of colon adenoma: a meta-analysis. Br J Cancer 2011;104(5):882–5. https://doi.org/10.1038/sj.bjc. 6606045.

78. Molmenti CLS, Hibler EA, Ashbeck EL, et al. Sedentary behavior is associated with colorectal adenoma recurrence in men. Cancer Causes Control 2014; 25(10):1387–95. https://doi.org/10.1007/s10552-014-0444-9.
79. Martínez ME, Jacobs ET, Ashbeck EL, et al. Meat intake, preparation methods, mutagens and colorectal adenoma recurrence. Carcinogenesis 2007;28(9): 2019–27. https://doi.org/10.1093/carcin/bgm179.
80. Song M, Garrett WS, Chan AT. Nutrients, foods, and colorectal cancer prevention. Gastroenterology 2015;148(6):1244–60.e16. https://doi.org/10.1053/j. gastro.2014.12.035.
81. Davis C, Bryan J, Hodgson J, et al. Definition of the Mediterranean diet; a literature review. Nutrients 2015;7(11):9139–53. https://doi.org/10.3390/nu7115459.
82. Meng Y, Sun J, Yu J, et al. Dietary intakes of calcium, iron, magnesium, and potassium elements and the risk of colorectal cancer: a meta-analysis. Biol Trace Elem Res 2019;189(2):325–35. https://doi.org/10.1007/s12011-018-1474-z.
83. Liu Y, Yu Q, Zhu Z, et al. Vitamin and multiple-vitamin supplement intake and incidence of colorectal cancer: a meta-analysis of cohort studies. Med Oncol 2015;32(1):434. https://doi.org/10.1007/s12032-014-0434-5.
84. Song M, Chan AT, Sun J. Influence of the gut microbiome, diet, and environment on risk of colorectal cancer. Gastroenterology 2020;158(2):322–40. https://doi. org/10.1053/j.gastro.2019.06.048.
85. Reynolds A, Mann J, Cummings J, et al. Carbohydrate quality and human health: a series of systematic reviews and meta-analyses. Lancet 2019; 393(10170):434–45. https://doi.org/10.1016/s0140-6736(18)31809-9.
86. Schwingshackl L, Schwedhelm C, Hoffmann G, et al. Food groups and risk of colorectal cancer. Int J Cancer 2018;142(9):1748–58. https://doi.org/10.1002/ ijc.31198.
87. O'Keefe SJ. Diet, microorganisms and their metabolites, and colon cancer. Nat Rev Gastroenterol Hepatol 2016;13(12):691–706. https://doi.org/10.1038/ nrgastro.2016.165.
88. Katona BW, Weiss JM. Chemoprevention of colorectal cancer. Gastroenterology 2020;158(2):368–88. https://doi.org/10.1053/j.gastro.2019.06.047.
89. Liang PS, Shaukat A, Crockett SD. AGA clinical practice update on chemoprevention for colorectal neoplasia: expert review. Clin Gastroenterol Hepatol 2021; 19(7):1327–36. https://doi.org/10.1016/j.cgh.2021.02.014.
90. Guo C-G, Ma W, Drew DA, et al. Aspirin use and risk of colorectal cancer among older adults. JAMA Oncol 2021;7(3):428–35. https://doi.org/10.1001/jamaoncol. 2020.7338.
91. Liu F, Yan L, Wang Z, et al. Metformin therapy and risk of colorectal adenomas and colorectal cancer in type 2 diabetes mellitus patients: a systematic review and meta-analysis. Oncotarget 2017;8(9):16017–26. https://doi.org/10.18632/ oncotarget.13762.
92. Giovannucci E. Modifiable risk factors for colon cancer. Gastroenterol Clin North Am 2002;31(4):925–43. https://doi.org/10.1016/s0889-8553(02)00057-2.
93. Grodstein F, Martinez ME, Platz EA, et al. Postmenopausal hormone use and risk for colorectal cancer and adenoma. Ann Intern Med 1998;128(9):705–12. https://doi.org/10.7326/0003-4819-128-9-199805010-00001.
94. Foley EF, Jazaeri AA, Shupnik MA, et al. Selective loss of estrogen receptor beta in malignant human colon. Cancer Res 2000;60(2):245–8.
95. Dworakowska D, Grossman AB. Colonic cancer and acromegaly. Front Endocrinol (Lausanne) 2019;10:390. https://doi.org/10.3389/fendo.2019.00390.

96. Rokkas T, Pistiolas D, Sechopoulos P, et al. Risk of colorectal neoplasm in patients with acromegaly: a meta-analysis. World J Gastroenterol 2008;14(22): 3484–9. https://doi.org/10.3748/wjg.14.3484.

97. Terzolo M, Puglisi S, Reimondo G, et al. Thyroid and colorectal cancer screening in acromegaly patients: should it be different from that in the general population? Eur J Endocrinol 2020;183(4):D1–13. https://doi.org/10.1530/eje-19-1009.

98. Tirosh A, Shimon I. Complications of acromegaly: thyroid and colon. Pituitary 2017;20(1):70–5. https://doi.org/10.1007/s11102-016-0744-z.

99. Jenkins PJ, Fairclough PD. Screening guidelines for colorectal cancer and polyps in patients with acromegaly. Gut 2002;51(Suppl 5):V13–4. https://doi.org/10.1136/gut.51.suppl_5.v13.

100. Osborne NJ, Gurrin LC, Allen KJ, et al. HFE C282Y homozygotes are at increased risk of breast and colorectal cancer. Hepatology 2010;51(4): 1311–8. https://doi.org/10.1002/hep.23448.

101. Shaheen NJ, Silverman LM, Keku T, et al. Association between hemochromatosis (HFE) gene mutation carrier status and the risk of colon cancer. J Natl Cancer Inst 2003;95(2):154–9. https://doi.org/10.1093/jnci/95.2.154.

102. Lagergren K, Wahlin K, Mattsson F, et al. Haemochromatosis and gastrointestinal cancer. Int J Cancer 2016;139(8):1740–3. https://doi.org/10.1002/ijc.30229.

103. Nelson RL, Davis FG, Persky V, et al. Risk of neoplastic and other diseases among people with heterozygosity for hereditary hemochromatosis. Cancer 1995;76(5):875–9. https://doi.org/10.1002/1097-0142(19950901)76:5<875::aid-cncr2820760523>3.0.co;2-q.

104. Asberg A, Thorstensen K, Irgens W, et al. Cancer risk in HFE C282Y homozygotes: results from the HUNT 2 study. Scand J Gastroenterol 2013;48(2): 189–95. https://doi.org/10.3109/00365521.2012.752028.

105. Hagström H, Ndegwa N, Jalmeus M, et al. Morbidity, risk of cancer and mortality in 3645 HFE mutations carriers. Liver Int 2021;41(3):545–53. https://doi.org/10.1111/liv.14792.

106. Reulen RC, Frobisher C, Winter DL, et al. Long-term risks of subsequent primary neoplasms among survivors of childhood cancer. JAMA 2011;305(22):2311–9. https://doi.org/10.1001/jama.2011.747.

107. Henderson TO, Oeffinger KC, Whitton J, et al. Secondary gastrointestinal cancer in childhood cancer survivors: a cohort study. Ann Intern Med 2012; 156(11):757–66. https://doi.org/10.7326/0003-4819-156-11-201206050-00002, w-260.

108. Nottage K, McFarlane J, Krasin MJ, et al. Secondary colorectal carcinoma after childhood cancer. J Clin Oncol 2012;30(20):2552–8. https://doi.org/10.1200/jco.2011.37.8760.

109. Daniel CL, Kohler CL, Stratton KL, et al. Predictors of colorectal cancer surveillance among survivors of childhood cancer treated with radiation: a report from the Childhood Cancer Survivor Study. Cancer 2015;121(11):1856–63. https://doi.org/10.1002/cncr.29265.

110. Teepen JC, Ronckers CM, Kremer LCM. Colorectal cancer screening in childhood cancer survivors. J Natl Cancer Inst 2019;111(11):1114–5. https://doi.org/10.1093/jnci/djz063.

111. Hudson MM, Bhatia S, Casillas J, et al. Long-term follow-up care for childhood, adolescent, and young adult cancer survivors. Pediatrics 2021;148(3). https://doi.org/10.1542/peds.2021-053127. e2021053127.

112. Przydacz M, Corcos J. Revisiting ureterosigmoidostomy, a useful technique of urinary diversion in functional urology. Urology 2018;115:14–20. https://doi.org/10.1016/j.urology.2018.01.003.
113. Stewart M, Macrae FA, Williams CB. Neoplasia and ureterosigmoidostomy: a colonoscopy survey. Br J Surg 1982;69(7):414–6. https://doi.org/10.1002/bjs.1800690720.
114. Stewart M. Urinary diversion and bowel cancer. Ann R Coll Surg Engl 1986; 68(2):98–102.
115. Khan MN, Naqvi AH, Lee RE. Carcinoma of sigmoid colon following urinary diversion: a case report and review of literature. World J Surg Oncol 2004;2: 20. https://doi.org/10.1186/1477-7819-2-20.
116. Crockett SD, Nagtegaal I. Terminology, molecular features, epidemiology, and management of serrated colorectal neoplasia. Gastroenterology 2019;157(4): 949–66. https://doi.org/10.1053/j.gastro.2019.06.041.
117. Crockett SD, Gourevitch RA, Morris M, et al. Endoscopist factors that influence serrated polyp detection: a multicenter study. Endoscopy 2018;50(10):984–92. https://doi.org/10.1055/a-0597-1740.
118. Peery AF, Crockett SD, Murphy CC, et al. Burden and cost of gastrointestinal, liver, and pancreatic diseases in the United States: update 2018. Gastroenterology 2018;156(1):254–72. https://doi.org/10.1053/j.gastro.2018.08.063.
119. Qazi TM, O'Brien MJ, Farraye FA, et al. Epidemiology of goblet cell and microvesicular hyperplastic polyps. Am J Gastroenterol 2014;109(12):1922–32. https://doi.org/10.1038/ajg.2014.325.
120. Figueiredo JC, Crockett SD, Snover DC, et al. Smoking-associated risks of conventional adenomas and serrated polyps in the colorectum. Cancer Causes Control 2015;26(3):377–86. https://doi.org/10.1007/s10552-014-0513-0.
121. He X, Wu K, Ogino S, et al. Association between risk factors for colorectal cancer and risk of serrated polyps and conventional adenomas. Gastroenterology 2018;155(2):355–73.e18. https://doi.org/10.1053/j.gastro.2018.04.019.
122. Crockett SD, Barry EL, Mott LA, et al. Calcium and vitamin D supplementation and increased risk of serrated polyps: results from a randomised clinical trial. Gut 2018. https://doi.org/10.1136/gutjnl-2017-315242.
123. Wallace K, Grau MV, Ahnen D, et al. The association of lifestyle and dietary factors with the risk for serrated polyps of the colorectum. Cancer Epidemiol Biomarkers Prev 2009;18(8):2310–7.

Effectiveness and Harms of Colorectal Cancer Screening Strategies

Briton Lee, MD[a], Kevin Lin, MD[a], Peter S. Liang, MD, MPH[a,b,]*

KEYWORDS

- Colorectal cancer • Screening • Effectiveness • Harm • Adenoma • Endoscopy
- Imaging • Cost

KEY POINTS

- Screening tests with evidence that show a reduction in CRC mortality include gFOBT, FIT, sigmoidoscopy, and colonoscopy.
- Harms related to CRC screening occur infrequently, although colonoscopy and sigmoidoscopy are associated with a risk of major bleeding and perforation.
- The USPSTF currently recommends 6 screening tests: gFOBT, FIT, mt-sDNA, CTC, sigmoidoscopy, and colonoscopy.
- Medicare currently reimburses 5 screening tests: gFOBT, FIT, mt-sDNA, sigmoidoscopy, and colonoscopy.

INTRODUCTION

Colorectal cancer (CRC) remains the third most common malignancy for both women and men, but the incidence has declined for several decades.[1] This trend is partly driven by screening, which allows the detection and removal of precancerous polyps. The United States Preventive Service Task Force (USPSTF) recommends CRC screening in adults aged 45 to 75 years using any of several modalities, including stool-based, endoscopic, and radiographic tests.[2] In this review, we compare the effectiveness, harms, and costs of the various screening strategies. Given the large variation in cost for tests based on location and insurance, we have provided 2021 Medicare reimbursement amounts when possible.[58,59]

a Department of Medicine, NYU Langone Health, 550 First Avenue, NBV 16 North 30, New York, NY 10016, USA; b Department of Medicine, VA New York Harbor Health Care System, 423 E 23rd Street, 11N, GI, New York, NY 10010, USA
* Corresponding author. Department of Medicine, VA New York Harbor Health Care System, 423 E 23rd Street, 11N, GI, New York, NY 10010.
E-mail address: Peter.Liang@nyulangone.org

Gastrointest Endoscopy Clin N Am 32 (2022) 215–226
https://doi.org/10.1016/j.giec.2021.12.002
1052-5157/22/Published by Elsevier Inc.
giendo.theclinics.com

Stool Tests

Guaiac-based fecal occult blood test

Guaiac-based fecal occult blood tests (gFOBT) use the pseudoperoxidase activity of heme to detect blood products in the stool, which is a potential marker of neoplasia. The test requires stool samples from 3 separate bowel movements. The high-sensitivity version of gFOBT has a sensitivity range of 50% to 75% for CRC, with a specificity of 96% to 98%.[3] Medicare reimbursed gFOBT at $4 in 2021.

Several randomized controlled trials (RCTs) have shown that compared with no screening, biennial gFOBT reduces CRC mortality by 9% to 22% with 11 to 30 years of follow-up.[4–8] One RCT found that annual screening led to an even greater reduction in CRC mortality (32%) as well as lower CRC incidence.[4] Adherence to gFOBT in community-based screening programs ranges from 41% to 66%.[9,10]

Fecal immunochemical test

The fecal immunochemical test (FIT) uses an antibody specific to the globin component of hemoglobin to detect occult blood in the stool. FIT requires only one sample and no dietary restrictions before testing, and it is approximately 8% to 19% more sensitive than gFOBT for advanced neoplasia.[11] It has a pooled sensitivity of 79% and specificity of 94% for CRC.[12] Given FIT's improved test characteristics and ease of use, it has largely replaced gFOBT in most screening programs.

Fecal hemoglobin detection is associated with adenoma size, number, and histology.[13] FIT sensitivity for advanced neoplasia also varies by site, and in one study the sensitivity was 23% for distal lesions and 9% for proximal lesions.[14] Accordingly, a national screening program found FIT screening was more effective in reducing incidence and mortality of CRC in the distal colon compared with the proximal colon.[15]

Despite its advantages over gFOBT, FIT has less long-term data and no RCTs that demonstrate CRC mortality reduction. However, given the similar mechanism of testing with improved test characteristics, mortality benefits are expected to be equivalent if not better.[16] The Taiwanese national screening program compared organized biennial screening over 5 years with 10 years of follow-up and found a 34% reduction in the incidence of advanced-stage CRC and 40% reduction in CRC mortality in the screening group.[15] Another study comparing FIT in an organized screening program to historical controls found increased screening rates were associated with a 25% and 52% reduction in CRC incidence and mortality.[17]

Medicare reimbursed FIT at $16 in 2021. Overall participation for FIT has been shown to be higher than for gFOBT (43% vs 33%),[18] and this seems durable over multiple rounds of screening.[19]

For both gFBOT and FIT, the main harms are associated with false positives (leading to unnecessary colonoscopy and its associated risks) and false negatives (leading to missed cancer). False positives are more common for gFOBT as the test is not specific for human heme and can be affected by certain foods. Though there is potential psychological harm from false positives, these results have not been shown to increase levels of anxiety or depression.[20] False negatives can occur with delays in returning test samples to the laboratory as hemoglobin degrades over time.[21]

Multitarget stool DNA

Similar to FIT, the multitarget stool DNA test (mt-sDNA; Cologuard, Exact Sciences) uses a single stool sample and includes a hemoglobin immunoassay. It also tests for 10 additional biomarkers, including KRAS mutations and aberrant methylation of NDRG4 and BMP3.[22] A unique feature of this product is proactive and on-demand patient navigation services provided by the manufacturer.

The mt-sDNA test has higher sensitivity (92% vs 74%) than FIT for CRC but lower specificity (87% vs 95%) for advanced neoplasia.[22] It also possesses greater sensitivity than FIT for sessile serrated lesions measuring 10 mm or greater (42% vs 5%). Cost has been a limiting factor in the widespread adoption of the test. The Centers for Medicare and Medicaid Services (CMS) reimbursed mt-sDNA at $509 in 2021, but modeling suggests screening with mt-sDNA may only be cost-effective at a much lower $40 to $60 per test.[23] Overall cross-sectional adherence to mt-sDNA was 71% in a Medicare population, and higher adherence was seen when ordered by a gastroenterologist (78%).[24] The optimal screening interval for mt-sDNA remains unclear and the USPSTF currently recommends testing every 1 to 3 years.[2]

All the harms of gFOBT and FIT mentioned above also apply to mt-sDNA. Moreover, there is a concern that false positives may indicate neoplastic lesions not detectable on colonoscopy or arising elsewhere in the gastrointestinal tract. However, individuals with false-positive mt-sDNA results had similar incidence of aerodigestive cancers as the general population with a median of 5.3 years of follow-up.[25] Therefore, those with false-positive mt-sDNA do not seem to require additional workup.

Blood Test

Methylated septin9

Methylated septin9 DNA (mSEPT9) is associated with tumorigenesis and has been shown to be increased in the presence of CRC and adenomas compared with normal or inflamed colonic mucosa.[26] The US Food and Drug Administration (FDA) has approved one mSEPT9 assay (Epi proColon, Epigenomics), but it is not currently recommended by major US guidelines. Testing interval has not been established empirically, although annual testing was found to be optimal in a modeling study.[27] The proposed Medicare reimbursement for mSEPT9 was $192,[27] but ultimately CMS declined to cover the test. Community adherence to mSEPT9 has not yet been reported, but in an observational study of individuals who declined colonoscopy and were offered mSEPT9 or FIT, 83% chose the blood test.[28] In an RCT of individuals who were overdue for screening, 99.5% completed the blood test within 6 weeks, compared with 88.1% for FIT.[29]

Using samples from a large prospective study and the current version of the assay, the measured sensitivity and specificity for CRC were 68% and 79%.[30]

Similar to stool tests, there are limited direct harms of undergoing the mSEPT9 test. Given the lower sensitivity and specificity of mSEPT9 compared with available stool tests, the main risk is the higher rate of false-positive and false-negative results.

Endoscopy

Flexible sigmoidoscopy

Flexible sigmoidoscopy is usually performed without sedation and allows direct visualization of the distal colon. The USPSTF recommends a 5-year screening interval for sigmoidoscopy or a 10-year interval if performed with FIT.[2] Medicare reimbursed screening sigmoidoscopy at $794 in 2021. A 2011 systematic review and meta-analysis found that one-time participation in sigmoidoscopy alone was 35% based on 18 studies, while participation increased to 41% for sigmoidoscopy combined with gFOBT/FIT based on 9 studies.[31]

Performance characteristics of sigmoidoscopy have not been directly assessed compared with colonoscopy, but studies generally assume that proximal polyps are detected with the same sensitivity as colonoscopy. In a 2017 meta-analysis and modeling study, the sensitivity of sigmoidoscopy for CRC was estimated to be 67%.[32] With the addition of FIT, sensitivity for CRC increased to 89%. Based on 4

RCTs with 11 to 17 years of follow-up, a 2021 meta-analysis found sigmoidoscopy reduced CRC incidence and mortality by 22% and 26%.[3] The protective benefit has been shown to be stronger for distal colon CRC in a previous meta-analysis, whereby incidence and mortality were reduced by 31% and 46%.[33]

Colonoscopy

Colonoscopy allows for the evaluation of the entire colon and is usually performed with moderate or deep sedation. The USPSTF recommends screening every 10 years with colonoscopy, but in individuals with a history of neoplasia the surveillance interval varies depending on the number, size, and histology of the lesions.[34] In 2021, Medicare reimbursed $794 for a screening colonoscopy and $1037 for a colonoscopy with polypectomy. One-time adherence to colonoscopy was found to be 28% based on a meta-analysis of 4 prospective screening studies.[31]

Based on 3 studies that used colonoscopy and CT colonography as the reference, the sensitivity of colonoscopy for adenomas ≥10 mm and ≥6 mm ranged from 89% to 95% and 75% to 93%.[3] These studies were not powered to measure the sensitivity for CRC. In a single study, the specificity of colonoscopy was 89% for adenomas ≥10 mm and 94% for adenomas ≥6 mm.[35] A 2019 meta-analysis of 43 tandem colonoscopy studies found that the miss rate for adenomas ≤ 5 mm, 6 to 9 mm, and ≥10 mm in size were 28%, 17%, and 6%.[36] Sessile and flat adenomas also had higher miss rates of 30% and 34%. In a prospective cohort study with 22 years of follow-up, screening colonoscopy was associated with a 68% reduction in CRC mortality and 43% to 56% reduction in CRC incidence.[37]

The primary harms of endoscopic screening are perforation and major bleeding events. Risk is lower for sigmoidoscopy compared with colonoscopy, as would be expected given the shorter and less complex procedure. In a large pooled analysis, the risk of perforation was 0.2 per 10,000 procedures for sigmoidoscopy and 3.1 per 10,000 procedures for colonoscopy.[3] Perforation risk increases with age and presence of other comorbidities.[38] Major bleeding risk was 0.5 per 10,000 procedures for sigmoidoscopy and 14.6 per 10,000 procedures for colonoscopy.[3] Both perforation and bleeding risk are higher for diagnostic colonoscopies following abnormal stool tests or sigmoidoscopies. Transient bacteremia occurs in 4% of colonoscopy and 0.5% of sigmoidoscopy, although clinical infection is rarely reported.[39]

Imaging

Computed tomography colonography

Computed tomography colonography (CTC) requires patients to undergo a full bowel preparation, after which a rectal balloon catheter is used to insufflate the colon, the CT is performed, and 2- and 3-dimensional reconstructions are used to identify colonic lesions. Intravenous contrast can be used to augment imaging. The USPSTF recommends repeat screening every 5 years.[2] A meta-analysis of 3 prospective screening studies found one-time adherence to CTC was 22%.[31] The adoption of CTC as a screening modality has been limited by its noncoverage by CMS. The proposed Medicare reimbursement for CTC was $236.[27]

In a meta-analysis of 7 studies, CTC sensitivity and specificity for adenomas ≥10 mm were 89% and 94%.[3] Sensitivity and specificity for adenomas ≥6 mm were 86% and 88%. Test characteristics are similar across age groups, as patients aged 50 to 65 years compared with greater than 65 years had the same sensitivity in CRC detection.[40] Data from an RCT showed that CTC had a significantly lower detection rate than colonoscopy for high-risk sessile serrated lesions (0.4% vs 3.1%).[41]

CTC is relatively safe, with little to no risk of serious adverse events following screening.[3] Exposure to low-dose radiation (1–5 mSv per examination) may increase the risk of malignancy. Additionally, CTC detects potentially important incidental extracolonic findings in 1% to 11% of examinations that require additional follow-up[42]

Colon capsule endoscopy

Colon capsule endoscopy (CCE) uses an ingestible camera that is wirelessly connected to a data recorder. The only commercially available CCE (PillCam COLON 2, Medtronic) has received FDA approval for CRC screening in individuals with prior incomplete colonoscopy as well as those with lower gastrointestinal bleeding.

CCE generally requires a sodium phosphate booster in addition to a full bowel preparation to increase small bowel transit of the capsule.[43] The proposed Medicare reimbursement of CCE was $939,[27] but it is currently not covered for screening. The 2021 USPSTF guidelines did not address CCE because of insufficient evidence, and adherence to CCE is unclear.

In a prospective study of 884 average-risk individuals, sensitivity and specificity of CCE for adenomas ≥10 mm were 92% and 95%.[44] For adenomas ≥6 mm, the sensitivity and specificity were 88% and 82%. Sensitivity for sessile serrated lesions was substantially lower than for adenomas, at 33% and 29% for polyps ≥10 mm and ≥6 mm.[44]

Potential harms associated with CCE include the small risk of kidney injury due to the sodium phosphate booster, and alternative boosters such as magnesium citrate and oral sulfate solution have been tried.[44,45] The significant bowel preparation needed results in technical failure in 1.4% of cases.[46] There is also a 0.8% risk of capsule retention,[46] and therefore, CCE is contraindicated in patients with swallowing disorders as well as bowel stricture or obstruction.[43] CCE is also contraindicated in pregnancy because of the microwave transmission from the capsule.[43]

DISCUSSION

A variety of factors including benefits, harms, costs, invasiveness, screening interval, patient preferences, and test availability should be taken into account when determining which CRC screening modality to use. Decisions should be individualized to optimize screening adherence. For this reason, the USPSTF no longer ranks tests in its current guideline.

The lack of head-to-head, long-term studies comparing screening strategies makes establishing which test is most effective difficult. Given that FIT and colonoscopy are the 2 predominant screening modalities worldwide, most of the discussion will focus on these 2 tests. **Table 1** provides a comparison of the various screening tests.

Adherence and Effectiveness

In a Dutch study comparing the diagnostic yield of one-time colonoscopy to 4 rounds of mailed FIT, the cumulative participation rate was higher for FIT (73%) than colonoscopy (24%).[47] In the intention-to-treat analysis, the cumulative diagnostic yield of advanced neoplasia was higher for FIT than colonoscopy (4.5% vs 2.2%), highlighting the importance of the participation rate on a population level. The baseline report of a large Spanish RCT comparing biennial FIT to colonoscopy also found those in the FIT group had higher participation and similar rates of CRC detection, but lower advanced adenoma detection.[48] Similarly, an Italian RCT comparing biennial FIT, sigmoidoscopy, and colonoscopy showed increased adherence with FIT, but a higher number of cancers and advanced adenomas detected with colonoscopy.[49] Taken together, these findings show that one-time screening is higher for stool-based tests, but this may not necessarily reflect long-term screening adherence and CRC outcomes.

Table 1
Comparison of colorectal cancer screening methods

	Test Characteristics	Screening Interval	Approximate Cost[a]	Advantages/Effectiveness	Disadvantages/Harms
Stool tests					
gFOBT	50%–75% sens, 96%–98% spec for CRC	1 y	$	• Reduces CRC mortality • Noninvasive	• Three stool samples • Lowest sensitivity of all stool tests • Need dietary restrictions
FIT	79% sens, 94% spec for CRC	1 y	$	• Reduces CRC mortality • Noninvasive • One stool sample • More sensitive than gFOBT	• Less sensitive than mt-sDNA
mt-sDNA	92% sens for CRC, 87% spec for advanced neoplasia	1–3 y	$$	• Noninvasive • More sensitive than FIT • One stool sample • Built-in patient navigation • Longer screening interval	• Mortality benefit not demonstrated • Less specific than FIT • Screening interval not based on clinical data
Blood test					
mSEPT9	68% sens, 79% spec for CRC	1 y	$$	• Noninvasive • High patient adherence	• Mortality benefit not demonstrated • Less sensitive and specific than FIT • Not recommended by USPSTF • Not covered by Medicare
Endoscopy					
Flexible Sigmoidoscopy	67% sens for CRC (model)	Every 5 y Every 10 y w/FIT	$$$	• Reduces CRC mortality • No sedation	• Invasive • Small risk of bleeding and perforation

	Test performance	Interval	Cost[a]	Benefits	Harms
				• Does not require bowel prep	
Colonoscopy	89%–95% sens, 89% spec for adenomas ≥10 mm	Every 10 y	$$$	• Reduces CRC mortality • Longest screening interval	• Requires bowel prep • Invasive • Higher bleeding and perforation risk than sigmoidoscopy • Requires sedation
Imaging					
CT Colonography	89% sens, 94% spec for adenomas ≥10 mm	Every 5 y	$$	• Noninvasive	• Mortality benefit not demonstrated • Requires bowel prep • Radiation exposure • Incidental extracolonic findings • Not covered by Medicare
Capsule Endoscopy	sens 92%, spec 95% for adenomas ≥10 mm	Every 5–10 y	$$$	• Noninvasive	• Mortality benefit not demonstrated • Requires bowel prep • Risk with NaPhos booster • Risk of retention • Not covered by Medicare

[a] Cost estimates are based on current or proposed Medicare reimbursement. $: 0 to 100, $$: 100 to 600, $$$: 600+.

Currently, there are multiple ongoing RCTs comparing the effect of FIT and colonoscopy on CRC mortality over 10 to 15 years.[48,50,51]

CRC screening programs and outreach have been evaluated to systematically increase participation rates. One pragmatic RCT that randomized approximately 6000 patients to mailed FIT outreach, mailed colonoscopy outreach, or usual care in a safety net setting found screening was significantly higher for FIT than for colonoscopy outreach over 1 year (41% vs 25%).[52] However, a similarly-designed RCT that also randomized approximately 6000 patients to the same interventions found screening completion over 3 years was significantly higher in the colonoscopy outreach group compared with the FIT outreach group (38% vs 28%).[53]

In comparing CTC with colonoscopy, one RCT found participation for CTC was higher than for colonoscopy (34% vs 22%), but CTC also detected significantly fewer advanced neoplasia (6.1 vs 8.7 per 100 patients).[54] When compared with mt-sDNA, one study found CTC had similar detection rates for CRC, though CTC had a significantly higher detection rate for advanced neoplasia (5.0% vs 2.7%).[55]

Cost-Effectiveness

Multiple studies evaluating the cost-effectiveness of CRC screening have concluded that compared with no screening, all modalities are cost-effective.[56,57] A recent modeling study compared the cost-effectiveness of six tests, with an emphasis on alternatives to FIT and colonoscopy.[27] When considering all 6 tests (FIT, colonoscopy, CTC, mSEPT9, CCE, and mt-sDNA) relative to no screening, FIT was cost-saving, colonoscopy was cost-effective at a $100,000 quality-adjusted life-year gained (QALYG) threshold, and the other modalities were dominated. When excluding FIT and colonoscopy, CTC every 5 years and annual mSEPT9 were the only cost-effective strategies. In the setting of perfect adherence to screening, follow-up, and surveillance, annual mSEPT9 had more QALYG and prevented more CRC cases and deaths than annual FIT. Based on this, the authors concluded annual mSEPT9 should be the preferred screening test if individuals decline FIT and colonoscopy.[27]

SUMMARY

We have provided an overview of the effectiveness and harms of various CRC screening tests. A reduction in CRC mortality has only been shown for colonoscopy, sigmoidoscopy, gFOBT, and FIT. Noninvasive tests have minimal harms, while major bleeding and perforation occur infrequently with colonoscopy and sigmoidoscopy. Colonoscopy and FIT are the 2 predominant screening modalities, and several ongoing RCTs comparing the 2 may help determine which is the optimal population-level screening strategy. Regardless of what the "best" test may be, long-term adherence to any form of screening is essential to reducing CRC incidence and mortality. Patient buy-in and participation are keys to success, and shared decision-making should take into account the benefits, harms, costs, test availability, and patient preferences to determine the best screening test.

CLINICS CARE POINTS

- Colorectal cancer screening falls into several categories: stool-based (gFOBT, FIT, mt-SDNA), blood-based (mSEPT9), imaging-based (CTC, CCE), and endoscopic (flexible sigmoidoscopy, colonoscopy).

- FIT is an improvement over gFOBT in terms of test performance and ease of use, and there is robust evidence supporting using these tests every 1 to 2 years.
- The mt-sDNA test includes several quantitative molecular assays as well as a FIT. It is more sensitive but less specific than FIT.
- Blood-based tests have a strong potential for improving screening adherence. However, the only currently FDA-approved test, mSEPT9, has a relatively low sensitivity and specificity and is not recommended by major guidelines.
- Imaging tests (CTC and CCE) still require full bowel preparation. CTC is recommended by major guidelines, but neither CTC nor CCE are covered by Medicare as a screening test.
- Sigmoidoscopy and colonoscopy both have robust evidence for effectiveness. Observational studies suggest colonoscopy offers greater protection against CRC and CRC mortality than sigmoidoscopy.

DISCLOSURE

P.S. Liang has received research funding from Epigenomics and Freenome and is a consultant for Guardant Health. The other authors have no disclosures.

REFERENCES

1. Islami F, Ward EM, Sung H, et al. Annual Report to the Nation on the Status of Cancer, Part 1: National Cancer Statistics. J Natl Cancer Inst 2021. https://doi.org/10.1093/jnci/djab131. djab131.
2. US Preventive Services Task Force, Davidson KW, Barry MJ, et al. Screening for Colorectal Cancer: US Preventive Services Task Force Recommendation Statement. JAMA 2021;325(19):1965.
3. Lin JS, Perdue LA, Henrikson NB, et al. Screening for colorectal cancer: updated evidence report and systematic review for the US preventive services task force. JAMA 2021;325(19):1978.
4. Shaukat A, Mongin SJ, Geisser MS, et al. Long-term mortality after screening for colorectal cancer. N Engl J Med 2013;369(12):1106–14.
5. Faivre J, Dancourt V, Lejeune C, et al. Reduction in colorectal cancer mortality by fecal occult blood screening in a French controlled study. Gastroenterology 2004;126(7):1674–80.
6. Kronborg O, Jørgensen OD, Fenger C, et al. Randomized study of biennial screening with a faecal occult blood test: results after nine screening rounds. Scand J Gastroenterol 2004;39(9):846–51.
7. Lindholm E, Brevinge H, Haglind E. Survival benefit in a randomized clinical trial of faecal occult blood screening for colorectal cancer. Br J Surg 2008;95(8):1029–36.
8. Scholefield JH, Moss SM, Mangham CM, et al. Nottingham trial of faecal occult blood testing for colorectal cancer: a 20-year follow-up. Gut 2012;61(7):1036–40.
9. Stokamer CL, Tenner CT, Chaudhuri J, et al. Randomized controlled trial of the impact of intensive patient education on compliance with fecal occult blood testing. J Gen Intern Med 2005;20(3):278–82.
10. Grazzini G, Castiglione G, Ciabattoni C, et al. Colorectal cancer screening programme by faecal occult blood test in Tuscany: first round results. Eur J Cancer Prev 2004;13(1):19–26.

11. Shapiro JA, Bobo JK, Church TR, et al. A comparison of fecal immunochemical and high-sensitivity guaiac tests for colorectal cancer screening. Am J Gastroenterol 2017;112(11):1728–35.

12. Lee JK, Liles EG, Bent S, et al. Accuracy of fecal immunochemical tests for colorectal cancer: systematic review and meta-analysis. Ann Intern Med 2014; 160(3):171.

13. Rozen P, Levi Z, Hazazi R, et al. Identification of colorectal adenomas by a quantitative immunochemical faecal occult blood screening test depends on adenoma characteristics, development threshold used and number of tests performed. Aliment Pharmacol Ther 2009;29(8):906–17.

14. Levy BT, Bay C, Xu Y, et al. Test Characteristics of fecal immunochemical tests (FIT) compared with optical colonoscopy revised JMS-14-003.R2. J Med Screen 2014;21(3):133–43.

15. Chiu H-M, Jen GH-H, Wang Y-W, et al. Long-term effectiveness of faecal immunochemical test screening for proximal and distal colorectal cancers. Gut 2021. https://doi.org/10.1136/gutjnl-2020-322545.

16. Lord SJ, Irwig L, Simes RJ. When is measuring sensitivity and specificity sufficient to evaluate a diagnostic test, and when do we need randomized trials? Ann Intern Med 2006;144(11):850–5.

17. Levin TR, Corley DA, Jensen CD, et al. Effects of organized colorectal cancer screening on cancer incidence and mortality in a large community-based population. Gastroenterology 2018;155(5):1383–91.e5.

18. Akram A, Juang D, Bustamante R, et al. Replacing the guaiac fecal occult blood test with the fecal immunochemical test increases proportion of individuals screened in a large healthcare setting. Clin Gastroenterol Hepatol 2017;15(8): 1265–70.e1.

19. Benito L, Travier N, Binefa G, et al. Longitudinal adherence to immunochemical fecal occult blood testing vs guaiac-based FOBT in an Organized Colorectal Cancer Screening Program. Cancer Prev Res (Phila) 2019;12(5):327–34.

20. Kirkøen B, Berstad P, Botteri E, et al. Do no harm: no psychological harm from colorectal cancer screening. Br J Cancer 2016;114(5):497–504.

21. van Rossum LGM, van Rijn AF, van Oijen MGH, et al. False negative fecal occult blood tests due to delayed sample return in colorectal cancer screening. Int J Cancer 2009;125(4):746–50.

22. Imperiale TF, Ransohoff DF, Itzkowitz SH, et al. Multitarget Stool DNA Testing for Colorectal-Cancer Screening. N Engl J Med 2014;370(14):1287–97.

23. Zauber AG, Lansdorp-Vogelaar I, Wilschut J, et al. Cost-effectiveness of DNA stool testing to screen for colorectal cancer. Agency for Healthcare Research and Quality (US); 2007. Available at: http://www.ncbi.nlm.nih.gov/books/NBK285164/. Accessed July 7, 2021.

24. Weiser E, Parks PD, Swartz RK, et al. Cross-sectional adherence with the multitarget stool DNA test for colorectal cancer screening: real-world data from a large cohort of older adults. J Med Screen 2021;28(1):18–24.

25. Berger BM, Kisiel JB, Imperiale TF, et al. Low incidence of aerodigestive cancers in patients with negative results from colonoscopies, regardless of findings from multitarget stool DNA Tests. Clin Gastroenterol Hepatol 2020;18(4):864–71.

26. Semaan A, van Ellen A, Meller S, et al. SEPT9 and SHOX2 DNA methylation status and its utility in the diagnosis of colonic adenomas and colorectal adenocarcinomas. Clin Epigenetics 2016;8:100.

27. Peterse EFP, Meester RGS, de Jonge L, et al. Comparing the cost-effectiveness of innovative colorectal cancer screening tests. J Natl Cancer Inst 2021;113(2): 154–61.

28. Adler A, Geiger S, Keil A, et al. Improving compliance to colorectal cancer screening using blood and stool based tests in patients refusing screening colonoscopy in Germany. BMC Gastroenterol 2014;14(1):183.

29. Liles EG, Coronado GD, Perrin N, et al. Uptake of a colorectal cancer screening blood test is higher than of a fecal test offered in clinic: A randomized trial. Cancer Treat Res Commun 2017;10:27–31.

30. Potter NT, Hurban P, White MN, et al. Validation of a real-time PCR-based qualitative assay for the detection of methylated SEPT9 DNA in human plasma. Clin Chem 2014;60(9):1183–91.

31. Khalid-de Bakker C, Jonkers D, Smits K, et al. Participation in colorectal cancer screening trials after first-time invitation: a systematic review. Endoscopy 2011; 43(12):1059–86.

32. Niedermaier T, Weigl K, Hoffmeister M, et al. Diagnostic performance of flexible sigmoidoscopy combined with fecal immunochemical test in colorectal cancer screening: meta-analysis and modeling. Eur J Epidemiol 2017;32(6):481–93.

33. Brenner H, Stock C, Hoffmeister M. Effect of screening sigmoidoscopy and screening colonoscopy on colorectal cancer incidence and mortality: systematic review and meta-analysis of randomised controlled trials and observational studies. BMJ 2014;348:g2467.

34. Gupta S, Lieberman D, Anderson JC, et al. Recommendations for follow-up after colonoscopy and polypectomy: a consensus update by the US Multi-Society task force on colorectal cancer. Gastroenterology 2020. https://doi.org/10.1053/j. gastro.2019.10.026.

35. Zalis ME, Blake MA, Cai W, et al. Diagnostic accuracy of laxative-free computed tomographic colonography for detection of adenomatous polyps in asymptomatic adults: a prospective evaluation. Ann Intern Med 2012;156(10):692.

36. Zhao S, Wang S, Pan P, et al. Magnitude, risk factors, and factors associated with adenoma miss rate of tandem colonoscopy: a systematic review and meta-analysis. Gastroenterology 2019;156(6):1661–74.e11.

37. Nishihara R, Wu K, Lochhead P, et al. Long-Term Colorectal-Cancer Incidence and Mortality after Lower Endoscopy. N Engl J Med 2013;369(12):1095–105.

38. Gatto NM, Frucht H, Sundararajan V, et al. Risk of perforation after colonoscopy and sigmoidoscopy: a population-based study. J Natl Cancer Inst 2003;95(3): 230–6.

39. Nelson DB. Infectious disease complications of GI endoscopy: Part I, endogenous infections. Gastrointest Endosc 2003;57(4):546–56.

40. Pickhardt PJ, Correale L, Delsanto S, et al. CT Colonography performance for the detection of polyps and cancer in adults ≥ 65 years old: systematic review and meta-analysis. AJR Am J Roentgenol 2018;211(1):40–51.

41. IJspeert JEG, Tutein Nolthenius CJ, Kuipers EJ, et al. CT-Colonography vs. colonoscopy for detection of high-risk sessile serrated polyps. Am J Gastroenterol 2016;111(4):516–22.

42. Lin JS, Perdue LA, Henrikson NB, et al. Screening for colorectal cancer: an evidence update for the u.s. preventive services task force. Agency for Healthcare Research and Quality (US); 2021. Available at: http://www.ncbi.nlm.nih.gov/ books/NBK570913/. Accessed July 1, 2021.

43. Han YM, Im JP. Colon capsule endoscopy: where are we and where are we going. Clin Endosc 2016;49(5):449–53.

44. Rex DK, Adler SN, Aisenberg J, et al. Accuracy of capsule colonoscopy in detecting colorectal polyps in a screening population. Gastroenterology 2015; 148(5):948–57.e2.
45. Kakugawa Y, Saito Y, Saito S, et al. New reduced volume preparation regimen in colon capsule endoscopy. World J Gastroenterol 2012;18(17):2092–8.
46. Palimaka S, Blackhouse G, Goeree R. Colon capsule endoscopy for the detection of colorectal polyps: an economic analysis. Ont Health Technol Assess Ser 2015; 15(15):1–43.
47. Grobbee EJ, van der Vlugt M, van Vuuren AJ, et al. Diagnostic yield of one-time colonoscopy vs one-time flexible sigmoidoscopy vs multiple rounds of mailed fecal immunohistochemical tests in colorectal cancer screening. Clin Gastroenterol Hepatol 2020;18(3):667–75.e1.
48. Quintero E, Castells A, Bujanda L, et al. Colonoscopy versus fecal immunochemical testing in colorectal-cancer screening. N Engl J Med 2012;366(8):697–706.
49. Segnan N, Senore C, Andreoni B, et al. Comparing attendance and detection rate of colonoscopy with sigmoidoscopy and FIT for colorectal cancer screening. Gastroenterology 2007;132(7):2304–12.
50. Dominitz JA, Robertson DJ, Ahnen DJ, et al. Colonoscopy vs. fecal immunochemical test in reducing mortality from colorectal cancer (CONFIRM): Rationale for Study Design. Am J Gastroenterol 2017;112(11):1736–46.
51. SCREESCO - Screening of Swedish Colons. Available at: https://clinicaltrials.gov/ct2/show/NCT02078804. Accessed May 4, 2018.
52. Gupta S, Halm EA, Rockey DC, et al. Comparative effectiveness of fecal immunochemical test outreach, colonoscopy outreach, and usual care for boosting colorectal cancer screening among the underserved: a randomized clinical trial. JAMA Intern Med 2013;173(18):1725–32.
53. Singal AG, Gupta S, Skinner CS, et al. Effect of colonoscopy outreach vs fecal immunochemical test outreach on colorectal cancer screening completion: a randomized clinical trial. JAMA 2017;318(9):806–15.
54. Stoop EM, de Haan MC, de Wijkerslooth TR, et al. Participation and yield of colonoscopy versus non-cathartic CT colonography in population-based screening for colorectal cancer: a randomised controlled trial. Lancet Oncol 2012;13(1): 55–64.
55. Pickhardt PJ, Graffy PM, Weigman B, et al. Diagnostic Performance of Multitarget Stool DNA and CT Colonography for Noninvasive Colorectal Cancer Screening. Radiology 2020;297(1):120–9.
56. Ran T, Cheng C-Y, Misselwitz B, et al. Cost-effectiveness of colorectal cancer screening Strategies-A systematic review. Clin Gastroenterol Hepatol 2019; 17(10):1969–81.e15.
57. Patel SS, Kilgore ML. Cost effectiveness of colorectal cancer screening strategies. Cancer Control 2015;22(2):248–58.
58. https://www.cms.gov/medicaremedicare-fee-service-paymentclinicallabfeeschedclinical-laboratory-fee-schedule-files/21clabq3 (Accessed 29 Dec 2021), 2021.
59. https://www.cms.gov/license/ama?file=/files/zip/procedure-price-lookup-comparison-file.zip (Accessed 12 Dec 2021), 2021.

Endoscopic Recognition and Classification of Colorectal Polyps

Karl Mareth, MD[a,b], Hashroop Gurm, MD[a,b],
Mohammad F. Madhoun, MD, MS[a,b],*

KEYWORDS

- Polyps • Classifications • Recognition

KEY POINTS

- An essential component of colon lesion evaluation is an accurate classification based on features such as size, location, morphology, surface pattern, and response to interventions
- Intraprocedural lesion classification informs the decision of when and how to apply endoscopic therapy
- Multiple classification schemes have been established as a way of standardizing this evaluation process

BACKGROUND

When properly applied, colonoscopy has been shown to be a powerful tool to screen for and ultimately remove neoplastic colon lesions, thereby reducing the risk of colon cancer.[1] An essential component of colon lesion evaluation is an accurate classification based on features such as size, location, morphology, surface pattern, and response to interventions, such as lifting, which are suggestive of the depth of tissue involvement and likelihood of benignity.[2] In this way, intraprocedural lesion classification informs the decision of when and how to apply endoscopic therapy. Multiple classification schemes have been established and subsequently endorsed in society

Grant support: None.
Writing assistance: None.
[a] Veterans Affairs Medical Center, 921 NE 13th St, Oklahoma City, OK 73104, USA;
[b] Gastroenterology and Hepatology, Division of Digestive Diseases and Nutrition, University of Oklahoma Health Sciences Center, 800 Stanton L. Young Boulevard, COMD 7400, Oklahoma City, OK 73104, USA
* Corresponding author. Gastroenterology and Hepatology, Division of Digestive Diseases and Nutrition, University of Oklahoma Health Sciences Center, 800 Stanton L. Young Boulevard, COMD 7400, Oklahoma City, OK 73104.
E-mail address: mohammad-madhoun@ouhsc.edu

guidelines as a way of standardizing this evaluation process and aiding in intraprocedural decision-making.[3,4]

Polyp Characterization (Size)

There is a strong positive correlation between polyp size and the presence of advanced histology, such as villous features or high-grade dysplasia, as well as adenocarcinoma. Diminutive (<5 mm) and small (6–9 mm) polyps account for more than 80% of polyps encountered during colonoscopy, and these polyps carry very little overall risk both in terms of advanced histology (0.8%–1.6%) and malignancy (0%–0.1%).[5] Conversely, lesions greater than 10 mm had a 22.9% likelihood of advanced pathology, while those lesions ≥30 mm carried a 60% likelihood.[6] Cancer rates in larger polyps are also significantly higher, accounting for 0.5% of 10-to-19-mm polyps and 2.2% of 20-to-50-mm polyps.[5] While for practical purposes a polyp's size is often estimated by careful visual inspection by the endoscopist, this is inherently subjective given the frequent lack of comparative reference, a problem compounded by the technological limitations of the monocular objective lens, which distorts objects in the periphery relative to the central part of the image. Consequently, accurate sizing within 10% margin of error is only achieved 25% of the time.[7] Multiple strategies have been implemented to provide a standard visual reference for aid in size estimation, including the introduction of open biopsy forceps or snares with known diameter, ruled catheters, and virtual tape measures, among others.[8–11] Ultimately, polyp size determination remains imprecise, and the ideal method for its estimation is an area of active research.

Polyp Characterization (Location)

The role of the endoscopists in reporting neoplastic lesions is important, and a systemic approach is necessary. The description of the location of the lesion is paramount. Lesions located in the proximal colon are associated with an increased risk of complications during endoscopic resection.[12] The colonic cecal wall is the thinnest and has the highest risk or postpolypectomy complications, that is, bleeding or perforation.[12] Meanwhile, the distal colon has the thickest colonic wall; thus, lesions in the rectum are easier and safer to excise. In some situations, such as lesions with ileocecal valve involvement, polyps tend to be more difficult to remove endoscopically and increase the risk for incomplete removal.[12] Polyps in the distal rectum that extends downward near the dentate line are very challenging due to the sensory nerve supply and vascular network that can cause patient discomfort and intraprocedural bleeding.[13] Although rare, polyps that are peri-appendiceal may extend into the appendix, thereby complicating endoscopic resection due to high risk of perforation.[13] Thus, once these complex lesions in locations that are not ideal for endoscopic resection are identified, proper systemic reporting of location is necessary with referral to an expert center for further optimal treatment.

Polyp Characterization (Endoscopic Surface Pattern Classification)

In recent years, there have been many technological developments in endoscopic imaging that have allowed for *in vivo* characterization of colonic polyps. It is important to characterize polyps based on histologic class (adenoma vs serrated) and to be able to identify features associated with deep submucosal invasion, as it determines the optimal treatment approach.

In the past, chromoendoscopy was performed using indigo carmine dye to yield better characterization of the vascular and surface morphology of the polyps. This approach has now largely been replaced by an advanced imaging system that applies optic digital methods (eg, narrow-band imaging [NBI]; Olympus, Center Valley, PA and Fujinon Blue

Light Imaging; Fujinon, Valhalla, NY) or by postprocessing modifications with real-time mapping technology (eg, Fujinon Linked Color Imaging and PENTAX i-SCAN; Pentax Medical, Montvale, NJ). Optical magnification, when available, may allow for more detailed characterization. Later in discussion, we will discuss some of the common endoscopic classification systems that have been used and validated (**Fig. 1**).

Narrow-Band Imaging International Colorectal Endoscopic Classification

The NICE classification is an international endoscopic classification of colorectal polyps using NBI (**Table 1**). A narrowband spectrum functions via filtering illumination lights with the use of a spectral narrow band instead of the optical filter.[14] NBI use during high-resolution colonoscopy provides a detailed description of the colonic tissue to characterize polyps, with or without the need for optical magnification. The characterization of a lesion occurs based on color change compared with the background, vascular, and surface patterns.[15] NICE classification has been validated and shown to have a good diagnostic ability when classifying polyps as type 1 (hyperplastic or sessile serrated polyp), type 2 (conventional adenoma), or type 3 (deep submucosal invasion).[16,17] Two limitations of the NICE classification are (1) the inability to differentiate sessile serrated lesions (SSLs) in type 1 and 2 lesions and (2) inability to distinguish low-grade dysplasia, high-grade dysplasia, and superficial mucosal invasion in type 2 lesions.

Workgroup serrAted polypS and Polyposis

The Workgroup serrAted polypS and polyposis (WASP) classification combines the NICE classification (Type I and II) with at least 2 of the following 4 typical sessile

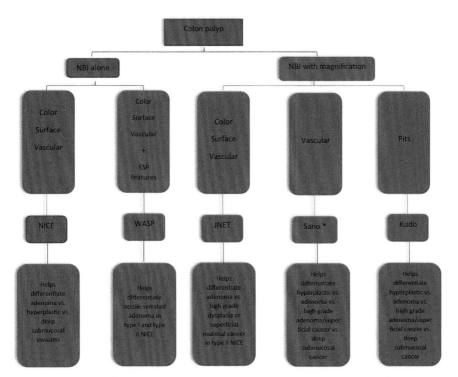

Fig. 1. Comparison of the various polyp evaluation systems' major criteria and utility.

Table 1			
NICE classification			
Narrow-Band Imaging International Colorectal Endoscopic (NICE) Classification			
	Color	Vessels	Surface
Type 1- hyperplastic lesions	Same or lighter	None or isolated lacy, no recognizable pattern	Dark or white uniform spots
Type II-adenomas	Brown	Brown vessels surround white pits	Tubular or branched
Type III-invasive tumors, that is, deep submucosal or cancer	Brown or dark brown	Disrupted vessels	Amorphous or absent pattern

serrated features: clouded surface, indistinctive border, irregular shape, and dark spots inside crypts for the differentiation of SSLs[18] (**Fig. 2**). Ijspreert and colleagues[19] integrated the WASP classification system, which showed accuracy of optical diagnosis after 6 months, increasing to 0.84 (95% CI [0.81, 0.88]) from 0.76 (95% CI [0.72, 0.80]).[19]

Japanese Narrow-Band Imaging Expert Team Classification
Japanese narrow-band imaging expert team classification (JNET) classification (**Fig. 3**) further subdivided NICE type II lesions into Type IIA (adenoma) or type IIB (high-grade intramucosal neoplasia/superficial submucosal invasive cancer).[20,21] Kobayashi and colleagues performed a retrospective study that demonstrated the high diagnostic performance of the JNET classification in a clinical setting for expert and nonexpert endoscopists. The study found that greater than 87% accuracy is achieved in differentiating neoplastic and nonneoplastic lesions and in diagnosing low-grade intramucosal neoplasia, high-grade intramucosal neoplasia/shallow submucosal invasive cancer, and deep submucosal invasive cancer. Nonexpert endoscopists had higher sensitivity, positive predictive value, and accuracy for JNET type 2A. There was no significant difference between the expert and nonexpert endoscopists for JNET types 2B or 3. The researchers found 100% specificity of JNET type 3 for deep SM invasive cancer for both expert and nonexpert endoscopists.[20]

Kudo Pit Pattern Classification
The Kudo pit pattern highlighted by Kudo and colleagues[22] describes "pit patterns" to identify neoplastic and nonneoplastic polyps with the use of magnifying endoscopy with (chromoendoscopy) or without (NBI) dye spray. Pits, which are openings of crypts, are classified based on appearance, structure, and staining patterns (**Fig. 4**).[23,24] The Kudo pit pattern distinguishes nonneoplastic (Type I/II) versus neoplastic (Type III/IV) adenomas with high sensitivity and specificity.[25] A type II-O (open) pit has been proposed for SSLs as a modification of the Kudo pit pattern.[26]

Sano and Modified Sano Classification
In 2006, after the development of NBI, the Sano classification was the first to be used for polyp characterization based on vascular findings only.[27] The addition of color and surface patterns allows modified Sano to have higher predictability for the invasive potential of colorectal polyps.[28] (**Table 2**).

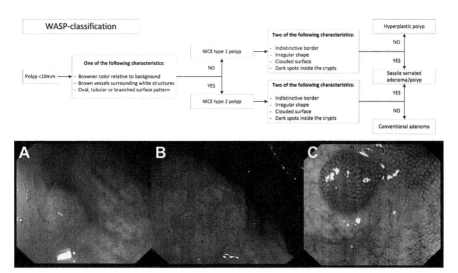

Fig. 2. WASP classification. *(From* Vleugels JL, IJspeert JE, Dekker E. Serrated lesions of the colon and rectum: the role of advanced endoscopic imaging. Best Pract Res Clin Gastroenterol. 2015 Aug;29(4):675-86.)

Japanese NBI Expert Team (JNET) classification

NBI	Type 1	Type 2A	Type 2B	Type 3
Vessel pattern	• Invisible [*1]	• Regular caliber • Regular distribution [*2] (meshed/spiral pattern)	• Variable caliber • Irregular distribution	• Loose vessel areas • Interruption of thick vessels
Surface pattern	• Regular dark or white spots • Similar to surrounding normal mucosa	• Regular (tubular/branched/papillary)	• Irregular or obscure	• Amorphous areas
Most likely histology	Hyperplastic polyp/ Sessile serrated polyp	Low-grade intramucosal [*4] neoplasia	High-grade intramucosal [*5] neoplasia/ Superficial [*3] submucosal invasive cancer	Deep submucosal invasive cancer
Examples				

* 1. If visible, the caliber in the lesion is similar to surrounding normal mucosa.
* 2. Microvessels are often distributed in a punctate pattern and well-ordered reticular or spiral vessels may not be observed in depressed lesions.
* 3. Deep submucosal invasive cancer may be included.
* 4. Low-grade intramucosal neoplasia: low-grade dysplasia.
* 5. High-grade intramucosal neoplasia: high-grade dysplasia.

Fig. 3. JNET classification. *(From* Sumimoto K, Tanaka S, Shigita K, Hayashi N, Hirano D, Tamaru Y, Ninomiya Y, Oka S, Arihiro K, Shimamoto F, Yoshihara M, Chayama K. Diagnostic performance of Japan NBI Expert Team classification for differentiation among noninvasive, superficially invasive, and deeply invasive colorectal neoplasia. Gastrointest Endosc. 2017 Oct;86(4):700-709.)

Type	Schematic	Endoscopic	Description	Suggested Pathology	Ideal Treatment
I	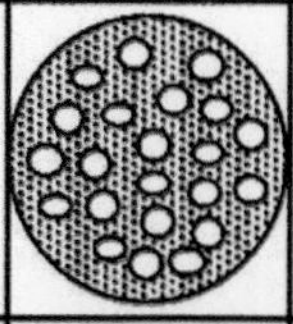	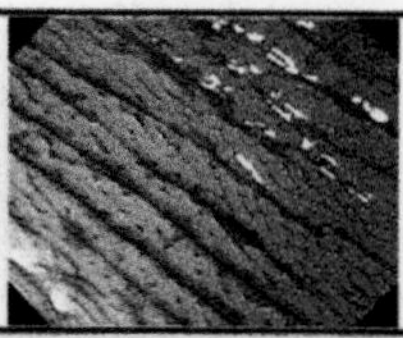	Round pits.	Non-neoplastic.	Endoscopic or none.
II	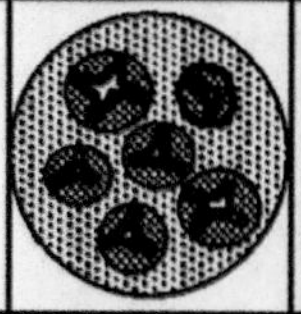	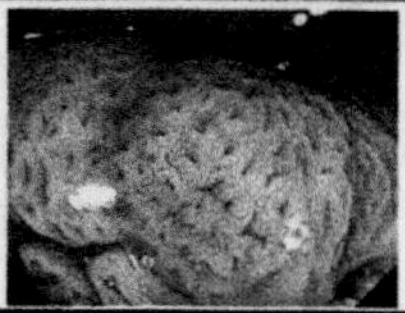	Stellar or papillary pits.	Non-neoplastic.	Endoscopic or none.
IIIs	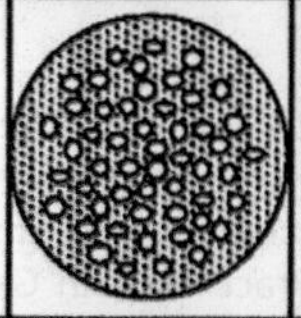	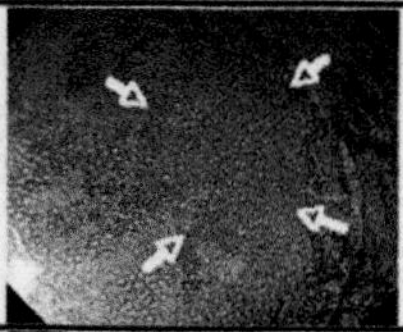	Small tubular or round pits that are smaller than the normal pit	Neoplastic.	Endoscopic.
IIIL	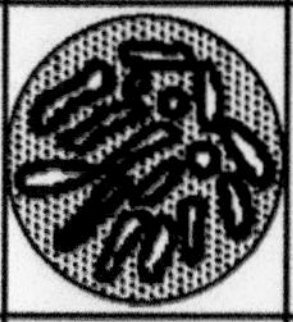	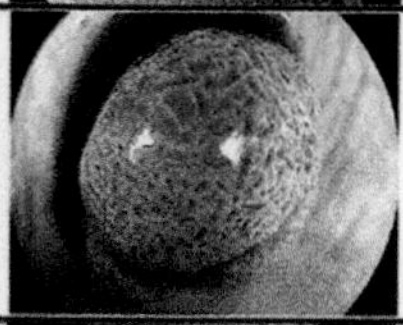	Tubular or roundish pits that are larger than the normal pits.	Neoplastic.	Endoscopic.
IV	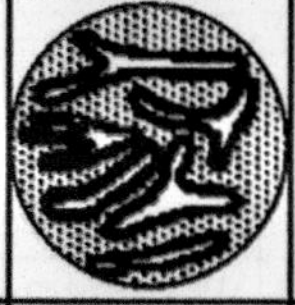	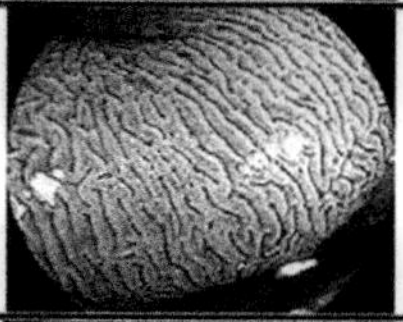	Branch-like or gyrus-like pits.	Neoplastic.	Endoscopic.
VI	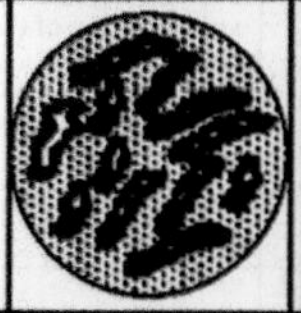		Irregularly arranged pits with type IIIs, IIIL, IV type pit patterns.	Neoplastic (invasive).	Endoscopic or surgical.
VN	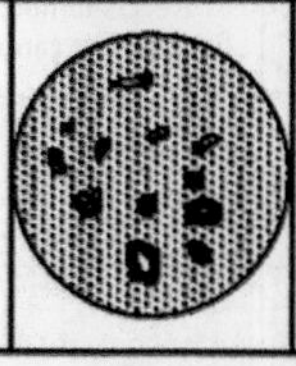	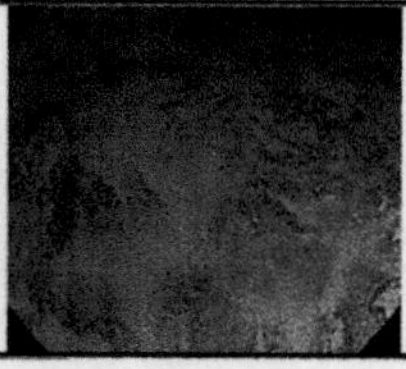	Non-structural pits.	Neoplastic (massive submucosal invasive).	Surgical.

Fig. 4. The Kudo pit pattern classification. *(From* Tanaka S, Kaltenbach T, Chayama K, Soetikno R. High-magnification colonoscopy (with videos). Gastrointest Endosc. 2006 Oct;64(4):604-13.)

Polyp Characterization (Endoscopic Morphologic Classification Systems)

The Paris classification system was the product of an international workshop held with the goal of promoting systematic evaluation and classification of neoplastic lesions in the esophagus, stomach, and colon. Superficial lesions, termed Type 0 lesions,

Table 2
Modified Sano classification

	Color	Vessels	Pits
MS I (hyperplastic polyp)	Pale color	Minute capillaries	Round pits with central brown star-like dots or bland appearance
MS II[a] (Tubular adenoma with low-grade dysplasia)	Light dark or dark color	Linear or oval regular capillary network	Linear or oval pits
MS IIIa (Tubular adenoma with high-grade dysplasia, tubulovillous, or superficial cancer)	Light dark or dark color	Tortuous/branched mildly regular capillary network surrounding pits	White villous/cerebriform pits
MS IIIB (Invasive cancer)	Dark surrounding with pale central area	Loss of vascular pattern	Loss of pit pattern

[a] MS IIo for sessile serrated polyps; pale or light-dark color ± open pits ± 3 out of 5: cloud-like surface, inconspicuous margins, mucus cap, irregular shape, and varicose microvascular vessels.

grossly seem confined to the mucosa and submucosa and are considered separately from Type I–IV lesions, which represent advanced cancers.[2] The basis of the Paris classification lies in the observation in prior Japanese studies that certain morphologic subtypes of type 0 lesions were associated with a greater likelihood of submucosal invasion and metastatic spread to local lymph nodes. The clinical utility of the classification system is primarily through its impact on treatment decisions, as invasion into the colonic submucosa is associated with nodal metastasis rates as high as 15%, thus representing a contraindication to most endoscopic interventions.[2]

Neoplasms are broadly defined in the Paris classification system as protruding/polypoid (0-Ip, 0-Is) or nonpolypoid, depending on whether they are raised 2.5 mm relative to the surrounding mucosa, a measure that can be compared intraprocedurally to the height of closed biopsy forceps. The distinction between 0-Ip lesions and 0-Is lesions lies in the thickness of the lesion base, which is relatively narrow compared with the upper portion of the lesion in the former and uniform in the latter. Nonprotruding lesions can be further stratified as 0-IIa (slightly elevated), 0-IIb (flat), 0-IIc (slightly depressed without ulceration), and 0-III (excavated or ulcerated) (**Fig. 5**). The distinction between 0-IIc and 0-III lesions is apparent in the pathologic specimen and is characterized by sharp interruption of the mucosa to include the disruption of the muscularis mucosae (**Fig. 6**). There also exist multiple mixed types of lesions associated with their own risk of submucosal involvement, although clinically it is often sensible to classify lesions according to the above strata. It is worth noting that raised lesions with central depression are classified as absolutely depressed if that depression is lower than the mucosa surrounding the lesion, and relatively depressed if the central depression in the lesion is still higher than the mucosa surrounding the lesion itself. The initial study of 3680 colon specimens presented in support of the model showed that for 0-Ip, 0-Is, 0-IIa, 0-IIb, and 0-IIc lesions, involvement in the submucosa was found in 5%, 34%, 4%, 0%, and 61%, respectively. This finding clearly

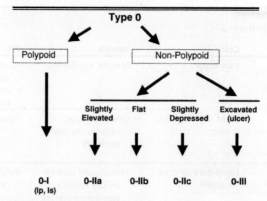

Fig. 5. The Paris classification. *(From* The Paris endoscopic classification of superficial neoplastic lesions: esophagus, stomach, and colon: November 30 to December 1, 2002. Gastrointest Endosc. 2003 Dec;58(6 Suppl):S3-43.)

demonstrated that 0-Is and especially 0-IIc lesions are more likely to involve the submucosa with respect to the other lesions evaluated, as can be assumed for 0-III lesions, which are defined by deeper tissue involvement. The data also showed a positive correlation with lesion size and likelihood of submucosal invasion, a trend more pronounced for 0-I and 0-IIc lesions than 0-IIa and 0-IIb lesions. Thus, both lesion diameter and morphologic classification must be considered together in determining the likelihood of submucosal invasion. It should be noted that although accepted in clinical and research settings, the Paris criteria are subject to variable interobserver agreement, which was found to be only moderate even among international experts.[29]

Lateral Spreading Tumors
A superficial neoplasm at least 10 mm in diameter that spreads laterally rather than extending significantly into the lumen is said to be a laterally spreading tumor (LST). By the Paris classification, these tumors may often be described as 0-IIa, 0-IIb, or 0-IIc. However, they are typically described by their own classification system based on surface morphology (**Fig. 7**).[30] These lesions are broadly categorized into granular (LST-G) and nongranular (LST-NG) lesions based on the dense nodular surface

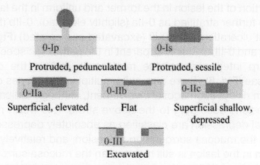

Fig. 6. The Paris classification. *(From* The Paris endoscopic classification of superficial neoplastic lesions: esophagus, stomach, and colon: November 30 to December 1, 2002. Gastrointest Endosc. 2003 Dec;58(6 Suppl):S3-43.)

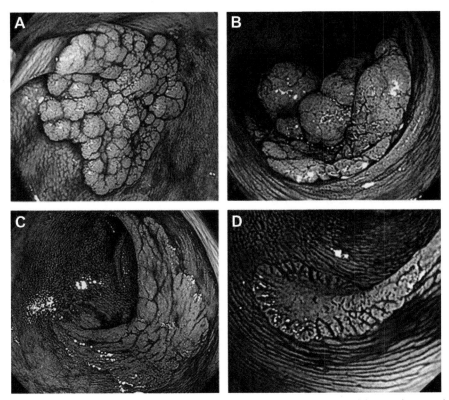

Fig. 7. Lateral Spreading Polyp Morphologies. (*A*) Granular homogenous (*B*) Granular Mixed (*C*) Nongranular Flat Elevated (*D*) Nongranular pseudodepressed. *(From Ishigaki T, Kudo SE, Miyachi H, Hayashi T, Minegishi Y, Toyoshima N, Misawa M, Mori Y, Kudo T, Wakamura K, Baba T, Sawada N, Ishida F, Hamatani S. Treatment policy for colonic laterally spreading tumors based on each clinicopathologic feature of 4 subtypes: actual status of pseudo-depressed type. Gastrointest Endosc. 2020 Nov;92(5):1083-1094.e6.)*

pattern seen in the former but not the latter during endoscopy, and particularly with the application of chromoendoscopy. LST-G lesions may be further subcategorized by homogenous and nodular mixed types (LST-GM) based on the presence of a so-called dominant nodule, while LST-NG lesions are subcategorized into elevated and pseudodepressed types. Homogenous granular-type lesions carry a very low risk of harboring submucosal invasive cancer (0.5%) versus nongranular LSTs, which carry a risk of 10.5% with the flat elevated morphology and 31.6% in pseudodepressed morphology.[31] Size is a major determinant of risk. In pseudodepressed lesions, the risk of submucosal invasion increases to 83% in lesions greater than 3 cm.[32] LST-GM lesions have an intermediate risk of submucosal invasive cancer of approximately 10%, with size greater than 4 cm and rectal location as independent risk factors.[33]

Malignant Polyps

The term "carcinoma in situ" is used by pathologists to characterize carcinoma that is confined to the epithelial layer without invasion into the lamina propria.[34] A "mucosal carcinoma" is distinguished by invasion into the lamina propria.[34] A malignant polyp is defined a lesion (polypoid, flat, or depressed) with submucosal invasion, but without invasion into the muscularis propria.[35] When a polyp becomes malignant, it has the potential to spread to lymph nodes or distant sites.[34] Recognition of a malignant polyp is crucial for optimal management via endoscopic (endoscopic submucosal dissection [ESD]/endoscopic mucosal resection [EMR]) or surgical resection. The depth of submucosal invasion of superficial lesions, as described by the Kikuchi classification system, has a significant impact on the likelihood of nodal metastasis.[36] Pathology specimens are assessed for maximal depth of invasion and categorized accordingly. Lesions in the upper third (sm1), the middle third (sm2), and the lower third (sm3) of the submucosa are associated with nodal metastases in less than 1%, 6%, and 14% of cases, respectively.[2]

Surface Pattern (NICE 3, Kudo VN)

During endoscopy, the assessment and identification of a lesion as having submucosal invasion is important to determine a treatment strategy.[12] We will further discuss the accuracy of the NICE Type III classification and Kudo VN pit pattern. Hayashi and colleagues performed a study to validate NICE Type III classification for the characterization of deep submucosal invasive carcinoma (SM-d). The negative predictive values for diagnosis of SM-d carcinoma were 76.2% (color), 88.5% (vessels), and 79.1% (surface pattern) with a sensitivity of 94.9%, and high-confidence prediction of SM-d carcinoma of 92%.[37] Meanwhile, Kudo VN pit pattern classification in a metanalysis study by Li and colleagues showed that all of the studies of mucosal patterns with magnification resulted in a sensitivity of 89.0% (95% CI [85.2, 91.9]) and specificity of 85.7% (95% CI [81.3, 89.2]). The researchers concluded that Kudo's pit pattern classification is an accurate diagnostic tool during endoscopy.[23] Burgess and colleagues performed a large prospective cohort study that assessed 2277 lesions in 2106 patients and found that the accuracy of large colorectal invasive lesions using Kudo VN was 93.2% (95% CI [92.1,94.2]) and specificity for cancer prediction was 97.5% (95% CI [96.7, 98.1]) with a sensitivity of 40.4% (95% CI [33.3, 47.8]).[38] If lesions that exhibit a Kudo Type VN pit pattern or NICE Type III are identified, it is suggested the patient be referred to an expert center for optimal resection technique and that resection not be attempted in regular practice[12] (see **Fig. 6**).

Nonlifting Sign

Submucosal injection of saline or a lifting agent may be performed in preparation for the endoscopic resection of lesions that are large or have a difficult orientation along the bowel wall. A uniform elevation of the lesion is expected with continued submucosal expansion. However, the so-called "nonlifting sign" is present when the tissue surrounding the lesion elevates, but the lesion itself elevates partly or not at all (**Fig. 8**).[39] This finding may represent submucosal fibrosis and/or invasive neoplasia that tethers the lesion to the deep submucosa and impedes uniform lift during the expansion of the fluid bleb. Indeed, this nonlifting sign is present more commonly in submucosal cancer (45%) than in adenomas (12%).[40] When initially described, the nonlifting sign was reported to have a sensitivity of 100% and a specificity of 99% for invasive carcinoma.[39] Subsequent studies have also shown similar results for sm3 lesions with deep submucosal invasion[41] and a positive predictive value of 80% for at least sm2 infiltration.[42] However, this sign has lower sensitivity and accuracy in predicting deep invasion when compared with other lesion features apparent during endoscopy.[42] The results must also be taken in the context of any prior biopsy, partial polypectomy, thermal therapy, or local tattoo, which has also been known to induce submucosal fibrosis.

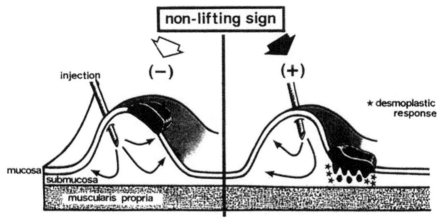

Fig. 8. Nonlifting sign. *(From* Uno Y, Munakata A. The non-lifting sign of invasive colon cancer. Gastrointest Endosc. 1994 Jul-Aug;40(4):485-9.)

CLINICS CARE POINTS

- When colon polyps encountered:
- Document location and size of polyp
- Classify polyp based on endoscopic morphology
- Classify polyp based on endoscopic surface pattern
- Identify the presence or absence of high-risk features for deep submucosal invasion
- Know your limitations; when to resect, biopsy, or refer to the specialized center

CONFLICT OF INTEREST

The authors of this article report no conflicts of interest, including consulting fees, paid expert testimony, employment, grants, honoraria, patents, royalties, stocks, or other financial or material gains that may involve the subject matter.

REFERENCES

1. Corley DA, Jensen CD, Marks AR, et al. Adenoma detection rate and risk of colorectal cancer and death. N Engl J Med 2014;370(14):1298–306.
2. The Paris endoscopic classification of superficial neoplastic lesions: esophagus, stomach, and colon: November 30 to December 1, 2002. Gastrointest Endosc 2003;58(6 Suppl):S3–43.
3. Kaltenbach T, Anderson JC, Burke CA, et al. Endoscopic removal of colorectal lesions-recommendations by the US Multi-Society Task Force on Colorectal Cancer. Gastroenterology 2020;158(4):1095–129.
4. Rutter MD, Chattree A, Barbour JA, et al. British Society of Gastroenterology/Association of Coloproctologists of Great Britain and Ireland guidelines for the management of large non-pedunculated colorectal polyps. Gut 2015;64(12): 1847–73.

5. Turner KO, Genta RM, Sonnenberg A. Lesions of All Types Exist in Colon Polyps of All Sizes. Off J Am Coll Gastroenterol ACG 2018;113(2):303–6.

6. Gupta N, Bansal A, Rao D, et al. Prevalence of advanced histological features in diminutive and small colon polyps. Gastrointest Endosc 2012;75(5): 1022–30.

7. Shamsi N, Shaukat A, Halperin-Goldstein S, et al. Sizing of Polyp Illustrations Differs by Endoscopists' gender and improves with a measurement reference. Eval Health Prof 2020;43(4):270–3.

8. Kim JH, Park SJ, Lee JH, et al. Is forceps more useful than visualization for measurement of colon polyp size? World J Gastroenterol 2016;22(11):3220–6.

9. Kaz AM, Anwar A, O'Neill DR, et al. Use of a novel polyp "ruler snare" improves estimation of colon polyp size. Gastrointest Endosc 2016;83(4):812–6.

10. Gopalswamy N, Shenoy VN, Choudhry U, et al. Is in vivo measurement of size of polyps during colonoscopy accurate? Gastrointest Endosc 1997;46(6):497–502.

11. Goldstein O, Segol O, Gross SA, et al. Novel device for measuring polyp size: an ex vivo animal study. Gut 2018;67(10):1755–6.

12. Vleugels JLA, Hazewinkel Y, Dekker E. Morphological classifications of gastrointestinal lesions. Best Pract Res Clin Gastroenterol 2017;31(4). https://doi.org/10.1016/j.bpg.2017.05.005.

13. Tholoor S, Tsagkournis O, Basford P, et al. Managing difficult polyps: techniques and pitfalls. Ann Gastroenterol Q Publ Hell Soc Gastroenterol 2013;26(2):114–21.

14. Gono K, Obi T, Yamaguchi M, et al. Appearance of enhanced tissue features in narrow-band endoscopic imaging. J Biomed Opt 2004;9(3):568–77.

15. Patrun J, Okreša L, Iveković H, et al. Diagnostic accuracy of NICE classification system for optical recognition of predictive morphology of colorectal polyps. Gastroenterol Res Pract 2018;2018:7531368.

16. Hewett DG, Kaltenbach T, Sano Y, et al. Validation of a simple classification system for endoscopic diagnosis of small colorectal polyps using narrow-band imaging. Gastroenterology 2012;143(3):599–607.e1.

17. Hamada Y, Tanaka K, Katsurahara M, et al. Utility of the narrow-band imaging international colorectal endoscopic classification for optical diagnosis of colorectal polyp histology in clinical practice: a retrospective study. BMC Gastroenterol 2021;21(1):336.

18. Vleugels JLA, IJspeert JEG, Dekker E. Serrated lesions of the colon and rectum: the role of advanced endoscopic imaging. Best Pract Res Clin Gastroenterol 2015;29(4):675–86.

19. IJspeert JEG, Bastiaansen BAJ, van Leerdam ME, et al. Development and validation of the WASP classification system for optical diagnosis of adenomas, hyperplastic polyps and sessile serrated adenomas/polyps. Gut 2016;65(6).

20. Kobayashi S, Yamada M, Takamaru H, et al. Diagnostic yield of the Japan NBI Expert Team (JNET) classification for endoscopic diagnosis of superficial colorectal neoplasms in a large-scale clinical practice database. United Eur Gastroenterol J 2019;7(7):914–23.

21. Sumimoto K, Tanaka S, Shigita K, et al. Diagnostic performance of Japan NBI Expert Team classification for differentiation among noninvasive, superficially invasive, and deeply invasive colorectal neoplasia. Gastrointest Endosc 2017; 86(4):700–9.

22. Kudo S, Tamura S, Nakajima T, et al. Diagnosis of colorectal tumorous lesions by magnifying endoscopy. Gastrointest Endosc 1996;44(1):8–14.

23. Li M, Ali SM, Umm-a-OmarahGilani S, et al. Kudo's pit pattern classification for colorectal neoplasms: a meta-analysis. World J Gastroenterol WJG 2014; 20(35):12649–56.

24. Tanaka S, Kaltenbach T, Chayama K, et al. High-magnification colonoscopy (with videos). Gastrointest Endosc 2006;64(4):604–13.

25. Moss A, Bourke MJ, Williams SJ, et al. Endoscopic mucosal resection outcomes and prediction of submucosal cancer from advanced colonic mucosal neoplasia. Gastroenterology 2011;140(7):1909–18.

26. Kimura T, Yamamoto E, Yamano H-O, et al. A novel pit pattern identifies the precursor of colorectal cancer derived from sessile serrated adenoma. Am J Gastroenterol 2012;107(3):460–9.

27. Sano Y, Tanaka S, Kudo S-E, et al. Narrow-band imaging (NBI) magnifying endoscopic classification of colorectal tumors proposed by the Japan NBI Expert Team. Dig Endosc Off J Jpn Gastroenterol Endosc Soc 2016;28(5):526–33.

28. Pu LZCT, Cheong KL, Koay DSC, et al. Randomised controlled trial comparing modified Sano's and narrow band imaging international colorectal endoscopic classifications for colorectal lesions. World J Gastrointest Endosc 2018;10(9): 210–8.

29. van Doorn SC, Hazewinkel Y, East JE, et al. Polyp morphology: an interobserver evaluation for the Paris classification among international experts. Am J Gastroenterol 2015;110(1):180–7.

30. Ishigaki T, Kudo S-E, Miyachi H, et al. Treatment policy for colonic laterally spreading tumors based on each clinicopathologic feature of 4 subtypes: actual status of pseudo-depressed type. Gastrointest Endosc 2020;92(5):1083–94, e6.

31. Bogie RMM, Veldman MHJ, Snijders LARS, et al. Endoscopic subtypes of colorectal laterally spreading tumors (LSTs) and the risk of submucosal invasion: a meta-analysis. Endoscopy 2018;50(3):263–82.

32. Kudo S ei, Lambert R, Allen JI, et al. Nonpolypoid neoplastic lesions of the colorectal mucosa. Gastrointest Endosc 2008;68(4 Suppl):S3–47.

33. D'Amico F, Amato A, Iannone A, et al. Risk of Covert Submucosal Cancer in Patients With Granular Mixed Laterally Spreading Tumors. Clin Gastroenterol Hepatol Off Clin Pract J Am Gastroenterol Assoc 2021;19(7):1395–401.

34. Bujanda L, Cosme A. Malignant colorectal polyps. World J Gastroenterol 2010; 16(25). https://doi.org/10.3748/wjg.v16.i25.3103.

35. Rex DK, Shaukat A, Wallace MB. Optimal management of malignant polyps, from endoscopic assessment and resection to decisions about surgery. Clin Gastroenterol Hepatol Off Clin Pract J Am Gastroenterol Assoc 2019;17(8):1428–37.

36. Kikuchi R, Takano M, Takagi K, et al. Management of early invasive colorectal cancer. Risk of recurrence and clinical guidelines. Dis Colon Rectum 1995; 38(12):1286–95.

37. Hayashi N, Tanaka S, Hewett DG, et al. Endoscopic prediction of deep submucosal invasive carcinoma: validation of the narrow-band imaging international colorectal endoscopic (NICE) classification. Gastrointest Endosc 2013;78(4):625–32.

38. Burgess NG, Hourigan LF, Zanati SA, et al. Risk stratification for covert invasive cancer among patients referred for colonic endoscopic mucosal resection: a large multicenter cohort. Gastroenterology 2017;153(3):732–42.e1.

39. Uno Y, Munakata A. The non-lifting sign of invasive colon cancer. Gastrointest Endosc 1994;40(4):485–9.

40. Park W, Kim B, Park SJ, et al. Conventional endoscopic features are not sufficient to differentiate small, early colorectal cancer. World J Gastroenterol WJG 2014; 20(21):6586–93.

41. Ishiguro A, Uno Y, Ishiguro Y, et al. Correlation of lifting versus non-lifting and microscopic depth of invasion in early colorectal cancer. Gastrointest Endosc 1999;50(3):329–33.

42. Kobayashi N, Saito Y, Sano Y, et al. Determining the treatment strategy for colorectal neoplastic lesions: endoscopic assessment or the non-lifting sign for diagnosing invasion depth? Endoscopy 2007;39(8):701–5.

Polypectomy for Diminutive and Small Colorectal Polyps

Melissa Zarandi-Nowroozi, MD, Roupen Djinbachian, MD, Daniel von Renteln, MD*

KEYWORDS

- Colorectal polyp • Colorectal cancer • Snare polypectomy
- Cold snare polypectomy • Hot snare polypectomy • Postpolypectomy bleeding
- Resect and discard • Diagnose and leave

KEY POINTS

- Diminutive and small colorectal polyps are frequently encountered during colonoscopy. Removing them contributes to colorectal cancer prevention.
- Cold snare polypectomy is recommended for the resection of diminutive and small polyps because studies report shorter procedure times, and a comparable safety profile and similar incomplete resection rates to hot snare polypectomy.
- Current guidelines recommend discontinuing dual antiplatelet therapy (leaving aspirin monotherapy), warfarin, and direct anticoagulant agents before polypectomy for diminutive and small polyps, although recent studies report low postpolypectomy bleeding rates in patients on continuous therapy.
- Optical diagnosis using real-time endoscopic assessment of the histology of diminutive colorectal polyps is a paradigm shift in the assessment and management of diminutive polyps, which with the development of technology, such as artificial intelligence, might help replace histopathology assessment and reduce colonoscopy-associated costs.

INTRODUCTION

Colorectal cancer is the third most common cancer and the second leading cause of cancer death globally.[1–10] Carcinogenesis arises from a multistep process involving the accumulation of genetic, histologic, and morphologic changes within a colorectal polyp.

The main objective of polypectomy is the successful removal of all neoplastic tissue and the subsequent reduction in colorectal cancer incidence. Polypectomy techniques are described based on whether they are completed with or without cautery,

Funded by: CANADALETR
Department of Medicine, Division of Gastroenterology, Montreal University Hospital (CHUM) and Montreal University Hospital Research Center (CRCHUM), 900 Rue Saint-Denis, Montréal, QC H2X 0A9, Canada
* Corresponding author.
E-mail address: renteln@gmx.net

Abbreviations	
ADR	Adenoma detection rate
AGA	American Gastroenterological Association
ASGE	American Society for Gastrointestinal Endoscopy
CSP	Cold snare polypectomy
CFP	Cold forceps polypectomy
DOACs	Direct oral anticoagulants
ESGE	European Society of Gastrointestinal Endoscopy
HFP	Hot forceps polypectomy
HSP	Hot snare polypectomy
IPB	Intraprocedural bleeding
JSGE	Japanese Society of Gastroenterology
KSGE	Korean Society of Gastrointestinal Endoscopy
PIVI	Preservation and Incorporation of Valuable Endoscopic Innovations
PPB	Postprocedural bleeding
PDR	Polyp detection rate
RCT	Randomized control trial

submucosal injections, en bloc, or piecemeal. The inherent characteristics of the encountered polyp, such as its size and morphology, dictate the polypectomy approach used. Two major techniques are available for diminutive and small lesions: biopsy-forceps polypectomy and snare polypectomy. Both procedures are performed with the presence or absence of electrocoagulation, distinguishing them as hot or cold.

FORCEPS POLYPECTOMY
Hot Forceps Polypectomy

Hot forceps polypectomy involves the use of a high-frequency current to simultaneously biopsy and electrocoagulate tissue. Jumbo forceps may also be used and are more effective in lesion removal because of their larger size. This technique has been forsaken by many endoscopists because it is often incapable of removing the entire lesion and confers an increased risk of polypectomy syndrome, perforation, and delayed bleeding. Impaired histologic evaluation of the biopsy specimen has also played a role in the loss in popularity of this procedure.

Cold Forceps Polypectomy

Cold forceps polypectomy (CFP) is analogous to hot forceps polypectomy without electrocautery. CFP is the preferred technique for removal of diminutive polyps less than 3 mm in diameter among endoscopists, because cold forceps are immediately available in most endoscopy units, and allow for easy retrieval of the resected tissue. This procedure also requires less coordination between the endoscopist and assistant and is related to fewer postpolypectomy adverse events, such as perforation and bleeding. However, more than one bite is frequently required to remove even a diminutive polyp, and there is concern that oozing blood after the initial bite interferes with accurate aiming of the following bites.

SNARE POLYPECTOMY

There are currently many different types of snares, each with specific advantages that are chosen depending on the clinical situation. The most commonly used snares are oval and hexagonal and are used with or without electrocautery.[11] Traditionally, the snares used for hot polypectomy were also manipulated for cold resection, but nowadays specific snares have been developed for cold snare polypectomy (CSP) using a thin wire and stiff catheter, producing reliable tissue transection.[12]

Cold Snare Polypectomy

Cold snaring involves an en bloc or piecemeal resection of lesions using mechanical transection of the tissue. Because CSP uses a snare without electrical current, tissue cutting relies solely on the closure of the snare wire. Cold snaring may be considered useful for reducing the risk of delayed bleeding, postpolypectomy syndrome, and perforation because it avoids electrocautery-associated thermal injury. Cold snares differ from traditional snares in that they are composed of a thin wired monofilament where the technique focuses on securing a 2- to 4-mm clear margin of normal tissue so that complete histologic eradication of neoplastic is ensured. The polyp is to be positioned at a 5-o'clock position with the snare opened and lowered over the lesion. The tip of the snare catheter is anchored several millimeters distal to the lesion and is angled down into the colon wall as it is advanced. This ensures ensnaring a margin of normal and healthy tissue surrounding the polyp. The endoscopist then strangulates the targeted lesion by enclosing the snare all while applying continuous forward pressure and downright angulation of the colonoscope tip, and ensuring adequate gas insufflation because suction carries the potential of promoting submucosal tissue entrapment and preventing tissue transection. Immediate bleeding is assessed and managed using endoscopic hemostatic measures.

Hot Snare Polypectomy

HSP is similar to CSP because it involves snaring a polyp using an electric wire. Electrocautery is then delivered in a controlled fashion until complete closure is achieved and the polyp is guillotined. The polyp can then be suctioned and retrieved for histologic assessment. The main purpose of electrocautery in the context of polypectomy is to deliver additional strength when excising tissue and provide coagulation to prevent immediate bleeding. Snares and hot forceps use monopolar electrocautery, and energy deliverance is proportional to the time it is applied. Cautery probes can also use bipolar electrocautery, which means that the electrical circuit runs between two electrodes both located on the tip of the probe. The use of coagulation current may potentially minimize immediate postpolypectomy bleeding by coagulation, but could damage deeper vessels with increased risks of delayed bleeding and perforation.

CURRENT GUIDELINES FOR POLYPECTOMY

Evolving evidence summarized in the 2020 update of the American Gastroenterological Association (AGA) Clinical Practice Guidelines[13] and 2017 version of the European Society of Gastrointestinal Endoscopy Clinical Guidelines[14] has highlighted safe, complete, and effective resection practices, and the superiority of certain techniques when specific lesions are encountered. The Japanese Society of Gastroenterology[15] issued its own guidelines in 2015 and recently published in 2020 a revised version, alongside the Korean Society of Gastrointestinal Endoscopy,[16] which released their own set of recommendations in 2012 (**Table 1**).[17,18]

POLYPECTOMY FOR DIMINUTIVE AND SMALL COLORECTAL POLYPS

Cold techniques are now widely used for addressing diminutive small colorectal polyps and are currently recommended in current guidelines tackling optimal management options for specific lesions. A recent survey published by Willems and colleagues[19] internationally assessed 808 endoscopists' preferred approach to diminutive and small polyps. CSP was the predominant polypectomy technique for 4- to 5-mm polyps (67.0%; 95% confidence interval [CI], 63.7%–70.2%) and 6- to 10-mm polyps (55.2%; 95% CI, 51.8%–58.6%). For 1- to 3-mm polyps, cold forceps remained the preferred technique (78.4%; 95% CI, 75.6%–81.3%), whereas hot snare polypectomy (HSP) was mainly used for 10- to 20-mm polyps (92.5%; 95% CI, 90.7%–94.3%). Additionally, 87.5% (95% CI, 85.2%–89.8%) of endoscopists reported an increase in CSP use during the past 5 years.

Diminutive Colorectal Polyps

Most encountered colorectal lesions measure less than 5 mm and rarely harbor features of high-grade dysplasia. These lesions benefit nonetheless from complete resection to reduce the impact of interval cancer and cancer mortality. Forceps and snare polypectomy, hot and cold, have been used for the resection of diminutive lesions.

CFP has been associated with a much higher rate of incomplete resection, ranging from 9% to 61% especially for small polyps 6 to 9 mm in size, and its use in these circumstances is not generally recommended outside the smallest of diminutive polyps. A randomized control trial (RCT) including 145 polyps less than 7 mm in size demonstrated that CSP is more effective in complete eradication of polyps when compared with CFP (96.6% vs 82.6%; P = .011).[20] However, the complete resection rates for polyps less than 4 mm did not differ significantly between the CSP and CFP groups (100% vs 96.9%; P = 1.000). A prospective RCT comprising 117 polyps less than 5 mm found significantly higher complete resection rates in the CSP group compared with the CFP group (93.2% vs 75.9%; P = .009).[21] The duration of polypectomy was also significantly shorter in the CSP group (14.29 vs 22.03 seconds; P<.001). In a 2018 meta-analysis of seven studies with 968 polyps, complete histologic eradication was best achieved when CSP was used in comparison with forceps polypectomy.[22] Forceps polypectomy may nevertheless play a key role in the management of certain diminutive polyps when jumbo forceps are specifically used. The AGA guidelines recommend that if CSP poses a technical difficulty in removing diminutive lesions less than 2 mm, jumbo or large-capacity forceps polypectomy may be considered and generally to those when resection in a single bite is anticipated. A prospective cohort study including 361 patients with 573 adenomas demonstrated CFP using jumbo forceps for diminutive lesions was a safe and effective way to achieve an adenoma-free colon.[23] The one-bite resection rate with CFP peaked for lesions 3 mm or smaller (94.4%) and decreased significantly with increasing lesion size.

Hot biopsy forceps (HBF) is occasionally considered as an alternative method for the removal of diminutive colorectal polyps, but is generally not recommended. The AGA guidelines state that HBF for polypectomy of lesions less than 10 mm is not endorsed because of high incomplete resection margins, inadequate histopathologic specimens, and nonnegligible complication rates. A prospective RCT evaluated the efficacy and safety between CSP and HBF in 208 patients with a total of 283 evaluated polyps ranging from 3 to 5 mm.[24] CSP achieved a much higher complete resection rate (80.4% vs 47.4%; P<.0001). The intraprocedural bleeding (IPB) rate was similar in both groups (8.6% vs 8.1%). The rate of severe tissue injury to the pathologic specimen was greater in the HBF group (52.6% vs 1.3%; P<.0001). The use of HBF for addressing diminutive colorectal polyps is generally not favored because of unacceptably high risks of adverse events, inadequate tissue sampling for histopathology, and high incomplete resection rates (IRRs).[25]

The most current AGA guidelines suggest that when compared with HSP techniques, CSP is generally regarded as safe and effective at addressing diminutive colorectal polyps. However, studies comparing HSP and CSP for lesions less than 5 mm specifically in terms of effectiveness and safety are scarce, because most also include polyps 6 to 9 mm in size or use unconventional cutoff values for polyp size, which prevent drawing exact conclusions for diminutive and small lesions separately. Most meta-analyses do not distinguish between both subgroups and many studies are often retrospective in nature or hampered by poor study quality. A retrospective study of 461 lesions resected using HSP or CSP found a trend toward higher complete resection rates among polyps less than or equal to 5 mm (81.3% vs 53.4%; $P = .057$) and there was no significant difference in the incidence of adverse events between the two groups (0.7% vs 0.6%).[26] A pilot study comparing HSP, CSP, and CFP for diminutive lesions (6 mm) reported similar rates of incomplete resection among the three groups. No significant adverse events related to polypectomy were reported intraprocedurally or at the 30-day follow-up.[27]

Diminutive colorectal polyps have traditionally been managed with either forceps polypectomy or cold snaring. Several studies have deemed CSP to be the preferred method for removing diminutive lesions comparatively to forceps polypectomy. Trials demonstrating CSP's superiority over HSP for diminutive polyps have been few and far between. Therefore, although current guidelines recommend CSP over HSP for diminutive lesions, it seems that its overall safety and effectiveness for removal of diminutive polyps can be considered comparable with that of HSP. More RCTs comparing CSP and HSP are required.

Small Colorectal Polyps

CSP is an effective removal technique for colorectal polyps less than 10 mm and has been thought to provide a superior safety profile to HSP with decreased postpolypectomy bleeding and coagulation syndrome. Resection methods for small lesions remain highly variable among endoscopists possibly because of specific exposure during training, personal preference, but also variability in efficacy and safety outcomes reported in current literature. Although CSP requires a shorter procedural time, little data support its general superiority to HSP. Complete resection rates and the occurrence of adverse events seem to be comparable among both techniques.

RCTs reporting on complete resection rates yield similar results for CSP and HSP, averaging around 95%. The CRESCENT study analyzed 796 polyps 4 to 9 mm in size and reported complete resection rates for CSP of 98.2% compared with 97.4% for HSP (<0.0001).[28] Suzuki and colleagues[29] demonstrated that CSP has sufficient resection width and depth to allow complete lesion resection after reporting mean mucosal defect diameter immediately after HSP and CSP of 5.1 mm and 7.5 mm, respectively ($P<.001$), but decreased by 25% ($P<.001$) at Day 1 after resection for CSP. Although the resection depth after CSP was more superficial, muscularis mucosa was obtained at similar rates with HSP and CSP (96% vs 92%; $P = .603$). Another RCT reported shorter procedure time with cold polypectomy as opposed to conventional polypectomy (18 vs 25 minutes; $P<.0001$) and identical complete polyp retrieval rates of 96%.[30]

Although RCTs demonstrate better outcomes with CSP comparatively with HSP, current systematic reviews and meta-analysis comparing data from available trials highlight comparable outcomes between the two. An analysis of eight studies recommended CSP as the standard treatment for resecting small benign colorectal polyps, because this procedure conferred an advantage in terms of shorter procedural time.[31] Complete resection rate using HSP was similar to CSP (relative risk, 1.02; $P = .31$).

Polyp retrieval after HSP was also similar to CSP (relative risk, 1.00; $P = .60$). However, total colonoscopy time for HSP was significantly longer than CSP (mean difference, 7.13 minutes; $P<.001$), and polypectomy time (mean difference, 30.92 seconds; $P = .005$). A systematic review of 18 studies further confirmed the noninferiority of CSP to HSP by reporting no statistical difference on complete histologic eradication (risk difference, 0.08; $P>.05$), but also established significantly shorter time of procedure with CSP (risk difference, -5.92; P 0.05).[32] Overall, although resection rates remain similar between CSP and HSP, CSP is usually preferred across different endoscopists because it is shorter in duration compared with HSP.

It has also been suggested that CSP offers an improved safety profile over HSP. At least eight studies have directly compared CSP with HSP in terms of adverse events in small polyps (**Table 2**).[27,28,33–45] For IPB, two studies found statistically significantly lower IPB for CSP when compared with HSP, whereas three studies found no difference. For post-procedural bleeding (PPB), two studies (one in anticoagulated patients) found statistically significantly lower PPB for CSP when compared with HSP, whereas six studies did not (see **Table 2**). No perforation was reported in all studies for either CSP or HSP. Current studies therefore do not support the superiority of CSP over HSP in terms of safety for the general population for small polyp resection.

Resect and Discard Strategy

The American Society for Gastrointestinal Endoscopy (ASGE) Preservation and Incorporation of Valuable Endoscopic Innovations (PIVI) released in 2011 two statements supporting the resect and discard and diagnose and leave strategies using optical biopsy achieved by real-time endoscopic assessment of the histology of diminutive colorectal polyps using currently available endoscopic technologies.[46] These approaches may allow for a paradigm shift in the assessment and management of diminutive polyps and for a reduction in total colonoscopy cost without compromising efficacy in colorectal cancer risk reduction. The diagnose and leave strategy involves leaving in place diminutive rectosigmoid polyps that are diagnosed as hyperplastic with high confidence. The resect and discard method entails resection of diminutive polyps after endoscopic optical diagnosis and without submission for histopathologic evaluation.

The ASGE Technology Committee published in 2015 a systematic review evaluating the ASGE PIVI thresholds for adopting real-time endoscopic assessment of the histology of diminutive colorectal polyps.[47] The pooled negative predictive value of narrow-band imaging for adenomatous polyps was 91% (95% CI, 88–94) and was even greater in academic medical centers (91.8%; 95% CI, 89–94), for experts (93%; 95% CI, 91–96), and when the optical biopsy assessment was made with high confidence (93%; 95% CI, 90–96). Of note, heterogeneity was high in this study ($I^2 = 89\%$). This systematic review confirmed that the thresholds set by the ASGE PIVI for real-time endoscopic assessment of the histology of diminutive polyps could be met, supporting the diagnose and leave strategy for rectosigmoid diminutive polyps.

A recent survey published in 2020 assessed the uptake of the resect and discard strategy and identified potential barriers preventing the widespread implementation of this method.[48] Eight hundred and eight endoscopists were surveyed internationally and 84.2% report not using the resect and discard strategy and 59.9% report not believing this method to be possible for implementation, identifying several deterrent factors, such as fear of misdiagnosis, not establishing an incorrect surveillance interval, and medicolegal concerns. As for the diagnose and leave strategy, more than half of individuals scheduled for a routine colonoscopy would be compliant to deferring resection of diminutive polyps[49]; this survey interrogating 557 individuals found that

57% of participants would be agreeable to adjourning resection of diminutive polyps outside of a clinical trial, with 50% willing to participate in an RCT setting. Factors associated with agreement of deferral of polyp resection included higher education ($P = .001$), greater knowledge about cancer risk ($P = .002$), and a lower perception of cancer risk ($P<.001$), whereas age, sex, income, history of polyps, and first-degree family history of colorectal cancer were not.

Motives for encouraging such strategies aiming at optical diagnosis are mainly that complications associated with colonoscopy are not trivial and might offset the benefit of surveillance. The risk of malignant transformation of diminutive polyps is low. A recent systematic review dived into the risk of metachronous colorectal cancer among patients with no adenomas, low-risk adenomas,[50] and high-risk adenomas at index colonoscopy in more than 500,000 patients over a follow-up of 8.5 years.[51] Low-risk adenomas carried a slightly higher incidence of colorectal cancer per 10,000 person-years in comparison with those with no adenomas (odds ratio [OR], 1.26; 95% CI, 1.06–1.51); however, the colorectal cancer–related mortality per 10,000 person-years was not significantly different between both groups (OR, 1.15; 95% CI, 0.76–1.74). Progression to cancer has been proven to be a lengthy process within diminutive and small polyps, which inherently carry low risk of malignant transformation. This further supports cost-effective strategies that prioritize optical diagnosis and may ultimately loosen current surveillance intervals and reduce colonoscopy burden.[52]

Colonoscopy performance is also greatly operator dependent. Numerous studies from academic and nonacademic endoscopy centers revealed that correct optical diagnosis of diminutive polyps was easily less than 90% in nonacademic settings, which could be palliated by appropriate diagnosis training sometimes lacking in community settings.[53–56] Raghavendra and colleagues[57] demonstrated that high accuracy and good interobserver agreement on optical diagnosis could be achieved after endoscopists were adequately trained, with rates increasing significantly from 47.6% to 90.8% ($P = .001$).

Despite literature being in support of the diagnose and leave and resect and discard strategies as economical, quick, and improving patient safety, uptake is low among current endoscopists. Better training programs should be instituted to better acquaint and prepare endoscopists to these strategies because resection and histologic evaluation in pathology units are significant and are prone to increase further with artificial intelligence–assisted optical diagnosis permitting improved polyp and adenoma detection rates. Such technologies carry a high yield in increased costs and shorter surveillance intervals with marginal significant benefits on colorectal cancer prevention, equally carrying potential for cumulative risk of colon perforation, estimated at 1.4% with colonoscopy repeated every 3 years.[58] This may controversially lead toward an incentive to limit adenoma detection rate thresholds to constrain such complications from arising. Solutions include focusing on the detection of high-risk lesions within diminutive polyps, even if most are adenomas carrying limited clinical impact,[59] and increasing uptake to alternatives to pathology, such as artificial intelligence–assisted optical diagnosis.

Incomplete Resection Rate

The IRR has been an outcome of interest for polypectomy after several studies reported that 20% to 30% of interval colorectal cancer cases are attributable to incomplete resection of colorectal cancer precursor lesions and often occur at previous polypectomy sites.[60] A meta-analysis of three studies further confirmed that HSP and CSP techniques can be effectively used for the complete removal of polyps 4 to 10 mm in size with IRR (HSP vs CSP: 2.4% vs 4.7%; OR, 0.51; 95% CI, 0.13–

1.99; $P = .33$; $I^2 = 73\%$).[61] Djinbachian and colleagues pooled results from 32 studies and reported that IRR for hot snare removal of polyps 1 to 10 mm was comparable with CSP, respectively 14.2% (95% CI, 5.2–23.2) versus 17.3% (95% CI, 14.3–20.3).[62–64] There was a statistically significant lower snare IRR for polyps 1 to 20 mm in size when expert endoscopists performed polypectomy in contrast to colleagues with less experience (8.0% [95% CI, 4.8–11.3] vs 18.0% [95% CI, 11.8–24.3]). Quality metrics for colonoscopy may include polypectomy technique and photodocumentation of polypectomy site.

Submucosal Injection

The inject and cut technique, also known as submucosal injection polypectomy, has gained in popularity in recent years given its simplicity. The role of submucosal injection in reducing IRR in small and diminutive polyps is not clear. Current literature has not demonstrated much added benefit in targeting such lesions and decreasing IRR accordingly. Djinbachian and colleagues[62] found no statistically significant difference in IRR when submucosal injections were performed for polyps less than 10 mm. Snare IRR using submucosal injection was 14.2% (95% CI, 5.2–23.2) compared with 17.6% (95% CI, 13.1–22.1) when the technique was not used. A recent abstract that assessed IRR when submucosal injection was integrated in standard CSP for 98 nonpedunculated polyps 4 to 20 mm in size showed promising results because overall IRR was 4.35% and so much lower when compared with historical data not using this technique. RCTs are needed to further confirm these results.

Adverse Events

Different complications are associated with polypectomy despite the minimally invasive nature of this procedure. Bleeding is most frequently observed and may occur either during or after the procedure. IPB is defined as occurring during the procedure and persisting for more than 60 seconds or requiring endoscopic intervention. PPB can manifest up to 30 days postpolypectomy and may result in an unplanned emergency department visit; hospitalization; or interventions, such as repeat endoscopy, angiography, or surgery.[14] The reported rate of PPB ranges from 0.07% to 1.7%.[65–67] Several factors associated with PPB have been identified by previous studies, including polyp size, sessile morphology, number of polyps, right colon location, comorbidities, endoscopists' experience, number of polyps removed, and use of antiplatelet and anticoagulant drugs.[68]

Perforation is a more serious and feared complication of polypectomy and is associated with higher morbidity and mortality. The incidence of perforation ranges from 0.016% in all diagnostic colonoscopy procedures to 5% as seen in therapeutic colonoscopies.[69] The rectosigmoid colon remains the most common site of colonic perforation because of sharp angulation at either the rectosigmoid junction or the sigmoid-descending colon junction, and the great mobility of the sigmoid. Factors increasing the risk of perforation include patient-related characteristics, such as increasing age, female sex, right colon polyp removal, and other medical comorbidities.[70] Procedure-related risk factors consist of type of snare or resection tool used, usage of electrocautery, inadequacy of submucosal cushioning for removal of larger lesions, and inexperience of the endoscopist.[71]

Postpolypectomy syndrome is a much rarer consequence of polypectomy, resulting from electrocoagulation injury to the mucosa and the muscularis layers, resulting in transmural burn and inflammation of the peritoneum without colonic perforation. This lesser-known entity has a reported incidence varying from 0.003% to 1%.[72] A large multicenter study identified several risk factors associated with postpolypectomy electrocoagulation syndrome, such as nonpolypoidal lesions, large lesion size (>2 cm), location in the right colon (attributed to decreased wall thickness), and hypertension.[73]

SUMMARY

Diminutive and small polyps are frequently encountered and CSP is considered the preferred technique to address these lesions. Evidence for its safety and efficacy has been established, even in patients taking anticoagulants and antiplatelet therapy. More recent evidence shows patients receiving continuous anticoagulation may safely undergo polypectomy using cold snaring with minimal risks with regards to immediate and postpolypectomy bleeding, although current guidelines seem to lean toward a discontinuation of anticoagulants, such as warfarin and direct oral anticoagulants because sufficient high-quality studies are lacking. Although large-capacity cold forceps are used to remove tiny polyps ($\leq$2 mm) in a single piece, cold snaring is considered effective for the resection of diminutive ($\leq$5 mm) and small (6–9 mm) polyps. CSP remains noninferior in terms of safety and efficacy in comparison with HSP when incomplete resection and complications rates are contrasted, and may confer a slight advantage with its shorter procedural time. Recent guidelines lean toward optimizing uptake in CSP for small polyps; however, data supporting its superiority to HSP are sparse and available RCTs show comparable incomplete resection and delayed bleeding rates, perhaps even a higher risk of immediate IPB. Hot forceps and ablation are no longer recommended for small and diminutive polyps. Even though uptake of different strategies, such as the resect and discard and diagnose and leave, is low for diminutive rectosigmoid polyps, studies show they are safe and cost-effective and negative predictive values with optical diagnosis are met. IRRs are an essential outcome pertaining to effective polypectomy and correlating with interval colorectal cancer and should be made aware to endoscopists to further improve and standardize current accredited training programs.

CLINICS CARE POINTS

- Practice cold snare polypectomy for all small polyps less than 10mm in diameter, including cold forceps polypectomy for diminutive polyps less than 3 mm remaining as an accepted alternative, and avoid using hot biopsy forceps and ablation.

- Individualise peri-polypectomy anticoagulation management after careful assessment of patient comorbidities and bleeding versus thrombosis risk and withhold anticoagulation accordingly by adhering to current guidelines and after consultation with cardiology and/or internal medicine.

- Integrate optical diagnosis techniques such as resect and discard and diagnose and leave in routine clinical practice for addressing diminutive colorectal polyps as this approach promotes more efficient and cost-effective colonoscopies, prevents costly and cumbersome histopathologic analysis, and may ultimately loosen colonoscopy surveillance interval recommendations.

- Interval colorectal cancer has raised concerns about ineffective polypectomy in regards to either missed or incompletely resected small polyps and creates an incentive to acknowledge incomplete resection rates as a key outcome of interest even if small colorectal polyp progression is slow.

- There is a need to standardize polypectomy training programs and define benchmarks of competent polypectomy in all geographic centers where colonoscopy is practiced to amend complete polyp resection rates and reduce post-polypectomy complications and costly referral to surgery.

DISCLOSURE

R. Djinbachian is supported by an American College of Gastroenterology resident research grant. D. von Renteln is supported by the Fonds de Recherche du Québec Santé career development award; has received research funding from ERBE, Ventage, Pendopharm, and Pentax; and is a consultant for Boston Scientific and Pendopharm.

REFERENCES

1. Amersi F, Agustin M, Ko CY. Colorectal cancer: epidemiology, risk factors, and health services. Clin Colon Rectal Surg 2005;18:133–40.
2. Ponugoti PL, Cummings OW, Rex DK. Risk of cancer in small and diminutive colorectal polyps. Dig Liver Dis 2017;49:34–7.
3. Liu WN, Zhang YY, Bian XQ, et al. Study on detection rate of polyps and adenomas in artificial-intelligence-aided colonoscopy. Saudi J Gastroenterol 2020; 26:13–9.
4. Castaneda D, Popov VB, Verheyen E, et al. New technologies improve adenoma detection rate, adenoma miss rate, and polyp detection rate: a systematic review and meta-analysis. Gastrointest Endosc 2018;88:209–222 e11.
5. Klare P, Sander C, Prinzen M, et al. Automated polyp detection in the colorectum: a prospective study (with videos). Gastrointest Endosc 2019;89:576–582 e1.
6. Rex DK, Boland CR, Dominitz JA, et al. Colorectal cancer screening: recommendations for physicians and patients from the U.S. multi-society task force on colorectal cancer. Gastroenterology 2017;153:307–23.
7. Rex DK. Detection measures for colonoscopy: considerations on the adenoma detection rate, recommended detection thresholds, withdrawal times, and potential updates to measures. J Clin Gastroenterol 2020;54:130–5.
8. Wong JCT, Chiu HM, Kim HS, et al. Adenoma detection rates in colonoscopies for positive fecal immunochemical tests versus direct screening colonoscopies. Gastrointest Endosc 2019;89:607–613 e1.
9. Siegel RL, Miller KD, Fuchs HE, et al. Cancer statistics, 2021. CA Cancer J Clin 2021;71:7–33.
10. Weston AP, Campbell DR. Diminutive colonic polyps: histopathology, spatial distribution, concomitant significant lesions, and treatment complications. Am J Gastroenterol 1995;90:24–8.
11. Fyock CJ, Draganov PV. Colonoscopic polypectomy and associated techniques. World J Gastroenterol 2010;16:3630–7.
12. Hewett DG. Cold snare polypectomy: optimizing technique and technology (with videos). Gastrointest Endosc 2015;82:693–6.
13. Kaltenbach T, Anderson JC, Burke CA, et al. Endoscopic removal of colorectal lesions-recommendations by the US multi-society task force on colorectal cancer. Gastroenterology 2020;158:1095–129.
14. Ferlitsch M, Moss A, Hassan C, et al. Colorectal polypectomy and endoscopic mucosal resection (EMR): European Society of Gastrointestinal Endoscopy (ESGE) Clinical Guideline. Endoscopy 2017;49:270–97.
15. Tanaka S, Saitoh Y, Matsuda T, et al. Evidence-based clinical practice guidelines for management of colorectal polyps. J Gastroenterol 2021;56:323–35.
16. Lee SH, Shin SJ, Park DI, et al. Korean guideline for colonoscopic polypectomy. Clin Endosc 2012;45:11–24.

17. Kaltenbach T, Anderson JC, Burke CA, et al. Endoscopic removal of colorectal lesions: recommendations by the US multi-society task force on colorectal cancer. Am J Gastroenterol 2020;115:435–64.
18. Takeuchi Y, Mabe K, Shimodate Y, et al. Continuous anticoagulation and cold snare polypectomy versus heparin bridging and hot snare polypectomy in patients on anticoagulants with subcentimeter polyps. Ann Intern Med 2019;171: 229–37.
19. Willems P, Orkut S, Ditisheim S, et al. An international polypectomy practice survey. Scand J Gastroenterol 2020;55:497–502.
20. Kim JS, Lee BI, Choi H, et al. Cold snare polypectomy versus cold forceps polypectomy for diminutive and small colorectal polyps: a randomized controlled trial. Gastrointest Endosc 2015;81:741–7.
21. Lee CK, Shim JJ, Jang JY. Cold snare polypectomy vs. cold forceps polypectomy using double-biopsy technique for removal of diminutive colorectal polyps: a prospective randomized study. Am J Gastroenterol 2013;108:1593–600.
22. Jung YS, Park CH, Nam E, et al. Comparative efficacy of cold polypectomy techniques for diminutive colorectal polyps: a systematic review and network meta-analysis. Surg Endosc 2018;32:1149–59.
23. Hasegawa H, Bamba S, Takahashi K, et al. Efficacy and safety of cold forceps polypectomy utilizing the jumbo cup: a prospective study. Intest Res 2019;17: 265–72.
24. Komeda Y, Kashida H, Sakurai T, et al. Removal of diminutive colorectal polyps: a prospective randomized clinical trial between cold snare polypectomy and hot forceps biopsy. World J Gastroenterol 2017;23:328–35.
25. Panteris V, Vezakis A, Triantafillidis JK. Should hot biopsy forceps be abandoned for polypectomy of diminutive colorectal polyps? World J Gastroenterol 2018;24: 1579–82.
26. Yamamoto T, Suzuki S, Kusano C, et al. Histological outcomes between hot and cold snare polypectomy for small colorectal polyps. Saudi J Gastroenterol 2017; 23:246–52.
27. Gomez V, Badillo RJ, Crook JE, et al. Diminutive colorectal polyp resection comparing hot and cold snare and cold biopsy forceps polypectomy. Results of a pilot randomized, single-center study (with videos). Endosc Int Open 2015;3:E76–80.
28. Kawamura T, Takeuchi Y, Asai S, et al. A comparison of the resection rate for cold and hot snare polypectomy for 4-9 mm colorectal polyps: a multicentre randomised controlled trial (CRESCENT study). Gut 2018;67:1950–7.
29. Suzuki S, Gotoda T, Kusano C, et al. Width and depth of resection for small colorectal polyps: hot versus cold snare polypectomy. Gastrointest Endosc 2018;87: 1095–103.
30. Ichise Y, Horiuchi A, Nakayama Y, et al. Prospective randomized comparison of cold snare polypectomy and conventional polypectomy for small colorectal polyps. Digestion 2011;84:78–81.
31. Shinozaki S, Kobayashi Y, Hayashi Y, et al. Efficacy and safety of cold versus hot snare polypectomy for resecting small colorectal polyps: systematic review and meta-analysis. Dig Endosc 2018;30:592–9.
32. Tranquillini CV, Bernardo WM, Brunaldi VO, et al. Best polypectomy technique for small and diminutive colorectal polyps: a systematic review and meta-analysis. Arq Gastroenterol 2018;55:358–68.

33. Horiuchi A, Nakayama Y, Kajiyama M, et al. Removal of small colorectal polyps in anticoagulated patients: a prospective randomized comparison of cold snare and conventional polypectomy. Gastrointest Endosc 2014;79:417–23.

34. Aslan F, Camci M, Alper E, et al. Cold snare polypectomy versus hot snare polypectomy in endoscopic treatment of small polyps. Turk J Gastroenterol 2014;25:279–83.

35. Yamashina T, Fukuhara M, Maruo T, et al. Cold snare polypectomy reduced delayed postpolypectomy bleeding compared with conventional hot polypectomy: a propensity score-matching analysis. Endosc Int Open 2017;5:E587–94.

36. Zhang Q, Gao P, Han B, et al. Polypectomy for complete endoscopic resection of small colorectal polyps. Gastrointest Endosc 2018;87:733–40.

37. Papastergiou V, Paraskeva KD, Fragaki M, et al. Cold versus hot endoscopic mucosal resection for nonpedunculated colorectal polyps sized 6-10 mm: a randomized trial. Endoscopy 2018;50:403–11.

38. Takeuchi Y, Mabe K, Shimodate Y, et al. Continuous anticoagulation and cold snare polypectomy versus heparin bridging and hot snare polypectomy in patients on anticoagulants with subcentimeter polyps: a randomized controlled trial. Ann Intern Med 2019;171:229–37.

39. Levy I, Gralnek IM. Complications of diagnostic colonoscopy, upper endoscopy, and enteroscopy. Best Pract Res Clin Gastroenterol 2016;30:705–18.

40. Choung BS, Kim SH, Ahn DS, et al. Incidence and risk factors of delayed postpolypectomy bleeding: a retrospective cohort study. J Clin Gastroenterol 2014;48:784–9.

41. Abraham NS. Antiplatelets, anticoagulants, and colonoscopic polypectomy. Gastrointest Endosc 2020;91:257–65.

42. Veitch AM, Vanbiervliet G, Gershlick AH, et al. Endoscopy in patients on antiplatelet or anticoagulant therapy, including direct oral anticoagulants: British Society of Gastroenterology (BSG) and European Society of Gastrointestinal Endoscopy (ESGE) guidelines. Endoscopy 2016;48:c1.

43. Makino T, Horiuchi A, Kajiyama M, et al. Delayed bleeding following cold snare polypectomy for small colorectal polyps in patients taking antithrombotic agents. J Clin Gastroenterol 2018;52:502–7.

44. Arimoto J, Chiba H, Ashikari K, et al. Safety of cold snare polypectomy in patients receiving treatment with antithrombotic agents. Dig Dis Sci 2019;64:3247–55.

45. Won D, Kim JS, Ji JS, et al. Cold snare polypectomy in patients taking dual antiplatelet therapy: a randomized trial of discontinuation of thienopyridines. Clin Transl Gastroenterol 2019;10:e00091.

46. Rex DK, Kahi C, O'Brien M, et al. The American Society for Gastrointestinal Endoscopy PIVI (Preservation and Incorporation of Valuable Endoscopic Innovations) on real-time endoscopic assessment of the histology of diminutive colorectal polyps. Gastrointest Endosc 2011;73:419–22.

47. Committee AT, Abu Dayyeh BK, Thosani N, et al. ASGE Technology Committee systematic review and meta-analysis assessing the ASGE PIVI thresholds for adopting real-time endoscopic assessment of the histology of diminutive colorectal polyps. Gastrointest Endosc 2015;81:502.e1–16.

48. Willems P, Djinbachian R, Ditisheim S, et al. Uptake and barriers for implementation of the resect and discard strategy: an international survey. Endosc Int Open 2020;8:E684–92.

49. von Renteln D, Bouin M, Barkun AN, et al. Patients' willingness to defer resection of diminutive polyps: results of a multicenter survey. Endoscopy 2018;50:221–9.

50. Arya R, Gulati S, Kabra M, et al. Folic acid supplementation prevents phenytoin-induced gingival overgrowth in children. Neurology 2011;76:1338–43.

51. Duvvuri A, Chandrasekar VT, Srinivasan S, et al. Risk of colorectal cancer and cancer related mortality after detection of low-risk or high-risk adenomas, compared with no adenoma, at index colonoscopy: a systematic review and meta-analysis. Gastroenterology 2021;160:1986–96.e3.

52. Benard F, von Renteln D. Adenoma detection: the more the merrier? Endoscopy 2018;50:835–6.

53. Kuiper T, Marsman WA, Jansen JM, et al. Accuracy for optical diagnosis of small colorectal polyps in nonacademic settings. Clin Gastroenterol Hepatol 2012;10: 1016–20 [quiz e79].

54. Ladabaum U, Fioritto A, Mitani A, et al. Real-time optical biopsy of colon polyps with narrow band imaging in community practice does not yet meet key thresholds for clinical decisions. Gastroenterology 2013;144:81–91.

55. Paggi S, Rondonotti E, Amato A, et al. Resect and discard strategy in clinical practice: a prospective cohort study. Endoscopy 2012;44:899–904.

56. Murino A, Hassan C, Repici A. The diminutive colon polyp: biopsy, snare, leave alone? Curr Opin Gastroenterol 2016;32:38–43.

57. Raghavendra M, Hewett DG, Rex DK. Differentiating adenomas from hyperplastic colorectal polyps: narrow-band imaging can be learned in 20 minutes. Gastrointest Endosc 2010;72:572–6.

58. Ransohoff DF, Lang CA, Kuo HS. Colonoscopic surveillance after polypectomy: considerations of cost effectiveness. Ann Intern Med 1991;114:177–82.

59. von Renteln D, Barkun AN. Increasing detection rates for diminutive adenomas: are we on the right track? Gut 2016;65:1056–7.

60. Robertson DJ, Lieberman DA, Winawer SJ, et al. Colorectal cancers soon after colonoscopy: a pooled multicohort analysis. Gut 2014;63:949–56.

61. Jegadeesan R, Aziz M, Desai M, et al. Hot snare vs. cold snare polypectomy for endoscopic removal of 4 - 10 mm colorectal polyps during colonoscopy: a systematic review and meta-analysis of randomized controlled studies. Endosc Int Open 2019;7:E708–16.

62. Djinbachian R, Iratni R, Durand M, et al. Rates of incomplete resection of 1- to 20-mm colorectal polyps: a systematic review and meta-analysis. Gastroenterology 2020;159:904–14.e12.

63. Duloy AM, Keswani RN. Assessing the quality of polypectomy and teaching polypectomy. Gastrointest Endosc Clin North Am 2019;29:587–601.

64. Tufman A, Neumann J, Manapov F, et al. Prognostic and predictive value of PD-L1 expression and tumour infiltrating lymphocytes (TiLs) in locally advanced NSCLC treated with simultaneous radiochemotherapy in the randomized, multicenter, phase III German Intergroup lung Trial (GILT). Lung Cancer 2021;160: 17–27.

65. Wexner SD, Garbus JE, Singh JJ, et al. A prospective analysis of 13,580 colonoscopies. Reevaluation of credentialing guidelines. Surg Endosc 2001;15:251–61.

66. Bowles CJ, Leicester R, Romaya C, et al. A prospective study of colonoscopy practice in the UK today: are we adequately prepared for national colorectal cancer screening tomorrow? Gut 2004;53:277–83.

67. Sieg A, Hachmoeller-Eisenbach U, Eisenbach T. Prospective evaluation of complications in outpatient GI endoscopy: a survey among German gastroenterologists. Gastrointest Endosc 2001;53:620–7.

68. Pigo F, Bertani H, Manno M, et al. Colonic postpolypectomy bleeding is related to polyp size and heparin use. Clin Endosc 2017;50:287–92.

69. Lohsiriwat V. Colonoscopic perforation: incidence, risk factors, management and outcome. World J Gastroenterol 2010;16:425–30.

70. Gatto NM, Frucht H, Sundararajan V, et al. Risk of perforation after colonoscopy and sigmoidoscopy: a population-based study. J Natl Cancer Inst 2003;95: 230–6.

71. Lohsiriwat V, Sujarittanakarn S, Akaraviputh T, et al. What are the risk factors of colonoscopic perforation? BMC Gastroenterol 2009;9:71.

72. Jehangir A, Bennett KM, Rettew AC, et al. Post-polypectomy electrocoagulation syndrome: a rare cause of acute abdominal pain. J Community Hosp Intern Med Perspect 2015;5:29147.

73. Cha JM, Lim KS, Lee SH, et al. Clinical outcomes and risk factors of post-polypectomy coagulation syndrome: a multicenter, retrospective, case-control study. Endoscopy 2013;45:202–7.

APPENDIX

Table 1	
Guidelines on polypectomy for diminutive and small colorectal polyps	
AGE Clinical Practice Guidelines 2020[72]	Diminutive ($\leq$ 5mm) and small (6-9mm) lesions. a. We recommend cold snare polypectomy to remove diminutive ($\leq$ 5mm) and small (6–9mm) lesions due to high complete resection rates and safety profile. (Strong recommendation, high-quality evidence) b. We recommend against the use of cold forceps polypectomy to remove diminutive ($\leq$ 5mm) lesions due to high rates of incomplete resection. For diminutive lesions $\leq$ 2mm, if cold snare polypectomy is technically difficult, jumbo or large-capacity forceps polypectomy may be considered. (Strong recommendation, moderate-quality evidence) c. We recommend against the use of hot biopsy forceps for polypectomy of diminutive ($\leq$ 5mm) and small (6–9mm) lesions due to high incomplete resection rates, inadequate histopathologic specimens, and complication rates. (Strong recommendation, moderate-quality evidence)
ESGE Clinical Guidelines 2017[11]	Diminutive polyps ($\leq$ 5mm). a. ESGE recommends cold snare polypectomy (CSP) as the preferred technique for removal of diminutive polyps (size $\leq$ 5mm). This technique has high rates of complete resection, adequate tissue sampling for histology, and low complication rates. (High quality evidence, strong recommendation.) Small sessile polyps (6-9mm). b. ESGE suggests CSP for sessile polyps 6 – 9mm in size because of its superior safety profile, although evidence comparing efficacy with hot snare polypectomy (HSP) is lacking. (Moderate quality evidence, weak recommendation.)
JSGE Clinical Practice Guidelines 2020[24]	Indications for cold snare polypectomy. a. Cold snare polypectomy (CSP) is indicated for nonpedunculated benign adenomas < 10mm in size (recommendation weak [agreement rate 100%], level of evidence B). b. CSP is recommended for diminutive lesions $\leq$ 5 mm in size and is acceptable for 6–9-mm lesions (recommendation strong [agreement rate 100%], level of evidence B). c. CSP should be avoided for "flat and depressed-type" lesions and lesions suspected of being carcinoma on colonoscopy even if $\leq$ 5 mm in size (recommendation weak [agreement rate 100%], level of evidence B).
KSGE Guidelines for Colonoscopic Polypectomy 2012[25]	Diminutive polyps ($\leq$ 5mm). a. Considering its complete resection rate, safety, and histological quality, hot biopsy is not recommended method for removing diminutive polyps (low quality evidence, strong recommendation).

Table 2
Studies directly comparing efficacy and adverse events from CSP to HSP

Study	Polyp size (mm)	Polypectomy technique	IPB	PPB	Perforation
Horiuchi et al. 2014[a] [40]	1-10	CSP	5.7% (2/35)	0% (0/35)	0% (0/35)
		HSP	23% (8/35)[b]	14% (5/35)[b]	0% (0/35)
Aslan et al. 2014 [41]	5-9	CSP	–	1.4% (1/77)	0% (0/77)
		HSP	–	1.3% (1/71)	0% (0/71)
Gomez et al. 2015 [73]	2-5	CSP	0% (0/21)	0% (0/21)	0% (0/21)
		HSP	0% (0/18)	0% (0/18)	0% (0/18)
Yamashina et al. 2017	2-11	CSP	–	0% (0/231)	0% (0/231)
		HSP	–	2.2% (4/177)[b]	0% (0/177)
Zhang et al. 2018	6-9	CSP	2.5% (5/179)	0% (0/179)	0% (0/179)
		EMR	1.7% (3/179)	0% (0/179)	0% (0/179)
Kawamura et al. 2018 [35]	4-9	CSP	7.1% (28/394)	0% (0/394)	0% (0/394)
		HSP	3.5% (14/402)[b]	0.5% (2/402)	0% (0/402)
Papastergiou et al. 2018 [44]	6-10	Cold EMR	3.6% (3/83)	0% (0/77)	0% (0/77)
		Hot EMR	1.2% (1/81)	0% (0/78)	0% (0/78)
Takeuchi et al. 2019	1-9	CSP	0% (0/85)	4.7% (4/85)	0% (0/85)
		HSP	0% (0/83)	12.0% (10/83)	0% (0/83)

IPB : intra-procedural bleeding; PPB : post-polypectomy bleeding
[a] Patients on anticoagulation
[b] Statistically significant

Box 1
BSG and ESGE recommendations for endoscopy in patients on antiplatelet or anticoagulant therapy

High-risk Procedures

a. For high-risk endoscopic procedures in patients at low thrombotic risk, we recommend discontinuing P2Y12 receptor antagonists (e. g., clopidogrel) five days before the procedure (moderate quality evidence, strong recommendation). In patients on dual antiplatelet therapy, we suggest continuing aspirin (low quality evidence, weak recommendation).

b. For high-risk endoscopic procedures in patients at low thrombotic risk, we recommend discontinuing warfarin 5 days before the procedure (high quality evidence, strong recommendation). Check INR prior to the procedure to ensure this value is < 1.5 (low quality evidence, strong recommendation).

c. For high-risk endoscopic procedures in patients at high thrombotic risk, we recommend continuing aspirin and liaising with a cardiologist about the risk/benefit of discontinuing P2Y12 receptor antagonists (e. g., clopidogrel) (high quality evidence, strong recommendation).

d. For high-risk endoscopic procedures in patients at high thrombotic risk, we recommend that warfarin should be temporarily discontinued and substituted with low molecular weight heparin (low quality evidence, strong recommendation).

e. For all patients on warfarin we recommend advising that there is an increased risk of post-procedure bleeding compared to non-anticoagulated patients (low quality evidence, strong recommendation).

f. For high-risk endoscopic procedures in patients on DOACs, we recommend that the last dose of DOACs be taken at least 48 hours before the procedure (very low quality evidence, strong recommendation).

g. For patients on dabigatran with a CrCl (or eGFR) of 30–50mL/min recommend that the last dose be taken 72 hours prior to the procedure (very low quality evidence, strong recommendation). In any patient with rapidly deteriorating renal function a hematologist should be consulted (low quality evidence, strong recommendation).

h. bIf antiplatelet or anticoagulant therapy is discontinued, then we recommend this should be resumed up to 48 hours after the procedure depending on the perceived bleeding and thrombotic risks (moderate quality evidence, strong recommendation).

Adapted from Veitch AM, Vanbiervliet G, Gershlick AH, Boustiere C, Baglin TP, Smith LA, Radaelli F, Knight E, Gralnek IM, Hassan C, Dumonceau JM. Endoscopy in patients on antiplatelet or anticoagulant therapy, including direct oral anticoagulants: British Society of Gastroenterology (BSG) and European Society of Gastrointestinal Endoscopy (ESGE) guidelines. Gut. 2016 Mar;65(3):374-89.

Polypectomy for Large Polyps with Endoscopic Mucosal Resection

Karl Kwok, MD, FASGE[a],*, Tri Tran, MD[b], Daniel Lew, MD[c]

KEYWORDS

- EMR • Endoscopic mucosal resection • Wide-field EMR
- Comparative effectiveness data • Cap assisted EMR • Cold snare EMR
- Underwater EMR

KEY POINTS

- Most noncancerous colon polyps, regardless of size, can be safely and effectively managed with organ-preserving techniques such as endoscopic mucosal resection (EMR)
- The 4 contributors of success in an EMR procedure include time, team, tool, and techniques
- Proper preprocedural planning (including review of images beforehand, and proper bowel preparation) is essential for safe and efficient EMR

INTRODUCTION

The foundation of modern endoscopic mucosal resection (EMR) was laid in 1955 by a surgeon named Norman Rosenberg. In his quest to increase safety during the fulguration of rectosigmoid polyps, he realized that after a submucosal saline injection, even a 10-s colonic burn with an electrosurgical dissection knife did not injure the muscularis propria.[1] The reason this technique is safe and efficacious is that the submucosal saline cushion acts as a heat sink for electrical energy to prevent deep mural injury. This is critical given the fact that healthy colonic tissue has an average total thickness of only 2–4 mm.[2,3]

Nearly 20 years later, Peter Deyhle's group released 2 landmark papers describing successful endoscopic polypectomy in humans, first with the resection of proximal colon pedunculated polyps in 1971,[4] then with the saline-assisted resection of distal colon sessile polyps in 1973.[5] The importance of these 2 studies cannot be overstated

[a] Interventional Endoscopy, Division of Gastroenterology, Kaiser Permanente, Los Angeles Medical Center, 1526 North Edgemont Street, 7th Floor, Los Angeles, CA 90027, USA; [b] Department of Medicine, Kaiser Permanente, Los Angeles Medical Center, 4867 W Sunset Boulevard, Los Angeles, CA 90027, USA; [c] Division of Gastroenterology, Cedars Sinai Medical Center, 8700 Beverly Boulevard, Los Angeles, CA 90048, USA
* Corresponding author.
E-mail address: karl.k.kwok@kp.org

Gastrointest Endoscopy Clin N Am 32 (2022) 259–276
https://doi.org/10.1016/j.giec.2021.12.004
1052-5157/22/© 2021 Elsevier Inc. All rights reserved.

Abbreviations	
ADR	adenoma detection rate
AADR	advanced adenoma detection rate
BBPS	Boston Bowel Preparation Score
BBS	bowel bubble score
CI	confidence interval
cm	centimeter(s)
CPT	Current Procedural Terminology (R)
CRC	colorectal cancer
EGD	esophagogastroduodenoscopy
EMR	endoscopic mucosal resection
ESD	endoscopic submucosal dissection
ESGE	European Society of Gastrointestinal Endoscopy
FDA	Food and Drug Administration
FICE	Fujinon Intelligent Color Enhancement
IQR	interquartile range
JNET	Japanese NBI Expert Team classification
K	inter-observer agreement (Kappa statistic)
LR	laparoscopic resection
LSL	laterally spreading lesion
mm	millimeter(s)
NBI	Narrow Band Imaging
NICE	Narrow Band Imaging International Colorectal Endoscopic classification
OR	odds ratio
s	second(s)
SEER	Surveillance, Epidemiology, and End Results program

as it demonstrated the ability of colonoscopy to remove polyps painlessly, with most polypectomy sites healing in 7 days, thereby sparing the patient "both a laparotomy and a lengthy stay in the hospital."

The next advancement in the field was the realization by Inoue and colleagues that the fitment of a transparent distal attachment cap allowed sufficient suction, and therefore, larger-sized en-bloc resection, during EMR of sessile and flat lesions across the esophagus, stomach, and colon.[6,7] Despite the fundamental technique of EMR being known for several decades (under various names such as the "strip biopsy,"[8] "endoscopic resection with hypertonic saline and epinephrine,"[9] and "endoscopic mucosectomy"[10]), concerns persisted that polyps above a certain size were too dangerous to remove endoscopically. Indeed, 1 gastroenterology practice guideline in 2000 stated "[polyps >2 cm] cannot be completely or safely excised during colonoscopy, and the patient should be referred for primary surgical resection."[11] Nonetheless, interest in, and perfection of the technique continued unabated at medical centers worldwide, in line with a general medical trend to advance minimally invasive, outpatient treatments.

This article aims to provide the reader a compendium of what is known about this modality, technical considerations including how to manage the more common clinical scenarios, and new advances in the field.

COMPARATIVE EFFECTIVENESS DATA

Endoscopic polypectomy reduces not only the subsequent risk of colorectal cancer (CRC)[12] but also of CRC mortality.[13] However, surgical referrals for large colon polyps, even of nonmalignant polyps, continue to occur in the background of the referring physician's unawareness of endoscopic options. In a population-based study of more than 4000 patients from France, Le Roy and colleagues found that 4.1% of patients (175/4251) who underwent colonoscopy for fecal occult blood in stool were referred directly to surgery for nonmalignant polyps; disturbingly, none of these individuals were evaluated by a tertiary endoscopic center beforehand. Subgroup analysis surprisingly confirmed that the referring gastroenterologist was a risk factor for inappropriate surgical referral.[14]

Fortunately, there is increasing awareness that EMR, even complex wide-field EMR, is successful in expert hands. For instance, in a 5-year tertiary referral center study by Raju and colleagues, 76% of patients (155/203) underwent successful EMR as an alternative to surgery; the success rate conceivably could have been even higher, were it not for technical failure in 14 cases due to prior intervention or tattoo, thereby requiring salvage surgical resection.[15] Moss and colleagues were also able to achieve a remarkably EMR high technical success rate (1000/1134%, 88%) in a nationwide Australian cohort in lesions as large as 12 cm; even in instances of adenoma recurrence, almost all were successfully managed by repeat endoscopy (135/145%, 93%).[16]

As a result, EMR is now clinically accepted as a first-line treatment of most eligible colonic lesions, meaning those lesions without evidence of deep submucosal/transmural invasion of cancer.[8,17] Beginning in 2014, dedicated Current Procedural Terminology (CPT) codes were established for upper (43211 esophagoscopy, 43254 EGD) and lower (45349 flexible sigmoidoscopy, 44403 colonoscopy through stoma, 45390 colonoscopy) gastrointestinal EMR procedures.[18]

From a health economics perspective, several articles highlight the advantages of EMR over surgical resection. Jayanna and colleagues found that, among an Australian cohort of more than 1300 patients who underwent EMR between 2010 and 2013, the mean anticipated cost savings per patient was $7602 when compared with a cost model for comparable, complication-free colon surgeries. Additionally, the hospital length of stay per patient was significantly reduced with EMR versus surgery (2.81 nights, 95% confidence interval (CI): 2.69–2.94, $P < .001$).[19] Keswani and colleagues similarly analyzed the costs and adverse events between the surgical and endoscopic resection of nonmalignant colon polyps. They compared a historical cohort of patients undergoing surgical resection for nonmalignant colon polyps over a 10-year period (2003–2013) versus those undergoing EMR during a 3-year period (2011–2013) at a single-center academic medical center in the United States. Not only was there a trend for lower adverse events in the EMR group versus the surgical resection group (10% vs 18%, $P = .09$) but also the length of stay in the EMR group was significantly lower (0 vs 5 days, IQR 4,7, $P < .0001$). The overall costs of EMR (including rescue surgery whereby needed) were significantly lower than the costs of primary surgical resection ($2152 vs $15,264, $P < .0001$).[20] Likewise, a thought-provoking Markov model by Law and colleagues found that the only situation in which laparoscopic colon resection (LR) is economically superior to EMR requires that 3 conditions are met: (1) technical success of index EMR, less than 75.8% of cases, (2) the adverse event of EMR, greater than 12%, and (3) the cost of laparoscopic resection, <$14,000. In routine clinical practice, none of these conditions are typically met; therefore, EMR is a superior modality compared with LR.[21] There are also complications associated with surgery. In a retrospective cohort study of nearly 500 colon surgeries over a 5-year period (2013–2018) in a high-volume Australian academic medical center, Louis and colleagues found that, of the 181 surgeries undertaken for benign pathologies, over 75% (136/181) experienced some type of complication as defined by the Clavien–Dindo classification. Additionally, although over half of the complications in the study were minor (53.2% grade I and II), these were associated with a 15.8% and 36.8% increase in hospital costs, respectively ($P < .0001$).[22]

PREDICTORS OF SUCCESS – TIME AND TEAM

A successful EMR begins with proper planning at the outset. This includes reviewing high-resolution photos beforehand to help the endoscopist formulate a resection strategy. Furthermore, EMR requires a dedicated block time—it should not be booked in a high-throughput, open-access room. The endoscopist should not feel rushed during the key phases of an EMR procedure that may increase the risk of technical failure, or increase the risk of complications. Ability to review high-resolution photos beforehand can help the endoscopist formulate a resection strategy.

Another key determinant to the success and safety of any EMR procedure is proper bowel preparation. In a single-center, cross-sectional study, Guo and colleagues determined that both the Boston Bowel Preparation Scale (BBPS) and the bowel bubble score (BBS) impact both adenoma detection rate (ADR) and advanced adenoma detection rate (AADR). The authors found that a colon segment's ADR jumped to 10.8 versus 3.2% for a Boston Bowel Preparation Score (BBPS) of 3 versus 1; likewise, the AADR jumped from 1.6% to 4.5% ($P < .05$). There was a similar trend toward increased ADR/AADR with a lower BBS (ie, fewer bubbles in the lumen).[23] Similarly, a nearly 15-year observational study of more than 25,000 American patients found that a systematic approach to CRC prevention (named the "CLEAR" protocol for Clean the colon, Look Everywhere, and complete Abnormality Removal) resulted in a 67% reduction in CRC compared with the Surveillance, Epidemiology, and End Results program (SEER-18) population.[24]d

Next, the importance of a highly skilled team cannot be understated—not just the nursing staff, but also other members of the multidisciplinary team such as the radiologist and the anesthesiologist. For instance, a nurse highly skilled in EMR can function similar to a professional golf caddie, highlighting a more optimal resection technique or even alerting the endoscopist to impending danger. Additionally, a skilled anesthesiologist can help optimize sedation during complex cases, and a skilled radiologist can help look for subtle radiographic clues that either makes an EMR contraindicated, or help identify complications in a timely manner.[25]

PREDICTORS OF SUCCESS – TOOLS AND TECHNIQUE
Before Patient's Arrival on the Unit

A successful EMR begins before the procedure itself. For instance, it is critical to educate the referring physicians that before referral, they should not attempt partial endoscopic resection, nor should they tattoo within 5 cm (or even underneath) the lesion, lest it results in massive submucosal fibrosis. This not only increases the technical complexity of the procedure (up to procedural failure) but also may increase the risk of complications including perforation. In fact, lesions that are obviously large and bulky, or are in an immediately recognizable landmark (eg, rectal vault, or cecal pit), do not need tattoo marking before referral for EMR. Similarly, referring gastroenterologists should avoid overly aggressive biopsies to reduce the risk of submucosal fibrosis.[26]

EMR Tools

Cap-assisted endoscopic mucosal resection

A cap attached to the distal end of the scope is a useful adjunctive method used to help with EMR, particularly among flat lesions. After submucosal injection or filling the lumen with water, suction or even gentle pressure can be applied so the tissue can fill into the cap for better tissue capture. Additionally, a cap can deflect folds allowing better visualization of the entire lesion.[27] Multiple caps exist (including purpose-designed cap EMR kits) which help facilitate the EMR procedure. Depending on the cap's snugness of fit onto the endoscope and the complexity of the EMR procedure, the use of waterproof anesthesia tape (Hy tape, Hy-Tape International, Patterson, NY) may help secure the cap onto the endoscope to reduce the likelihood of the cap from dislodging and unnecessarily distracting the endoscopist with a foreign body retrieval.[28]

Choice of snare
Multiple snares sizes and configurations exist; little data support the superiority of one snare choice over another. As reviewed in a recent European Society of Gastrointestinal Endoscopy (ESGE) clinical guideline, the most important determinant is an endoscopist's familiarity with the performance characteristics of a particular choice of snare. While monofilament snares may potentially allow faster tissue resection and therefore, reduced likelihood of colonic wall thermal injury (vs polyfilament snares may better grip the mucosa in flat polyps), this has not yet been systematically proven.[29]

Endoscopic Mucosal Resection Technique

Management of antithrombotic agents
The management of antithrombotic agents is discussed in detail in a separate chapter (Chapter 8).

Inspection
A high-quality inspection of the lesion is a necessity before performing EMR to determine if the lesion is appropriate for EMR. Lesions most suitable for EMR are either pedunculated or nonpedunculated laterally spreading lesions (LSL), which are nonpolypoid lesions larger than 10 mm in size.[30]

Inspection begins with viewing the lesion under high-definition white light and measuring the size of the lesion and location of the lesion. The next step is to determine if the lesion is granular or smooth. Nongranular LSL have a higher tendency to have submucosal invasion at 12% compared with 6% with granular LSL.[31] In a recent study, granular-mixed LSL has almost a 10% risk of having underlying submucosal invasive cancer, especially with lesions more than 4 cm or in the rectum.[32]

EMR should be limited to LSL that has superficial submucosal invasion or less than 1000 μm depth of invasion, which highlights the importance of accurate preprocedural inspection with endoscopic classifications such as the Kudo pit pattern or the Narrow Band Imaging International Colorectal Endoscopic (NICE)/Japan NBI Expert Team (JNET) classification (**Fig. 1**). Beyond this level of invasion, there is a high risk for incomplete resection with EMR, and other treatment modalities should be considered such as endoscopic submucosal dissection (ESD) or surgery. All 3 major endoscope manufacturers are equipped with optical imaging technology to emulate chromoendoscopy through various modalities, and are activated with a push of a button (narrowband imaging (NBI)—Olympus Corporation, Center Valley, PA; Fujinon Intelligent Chromoendoscopy (FICE) – FUJIFILM Corporation, Wayne, NJ; iSCAN – Pentax of America, Montvale, NJ), although a systematic review and meta-analysis of 17 randomized control trials failed to establish superiority of virtual chromoendoscopy over conventional dye chromoendoscopy for dysplasia detection in inflammatory bowel disease (IBD).[33] LSL that are brown to dark brown with disrupted or irregular vessels and irregular surface patterns are likely classified as NICE type 3 and has a

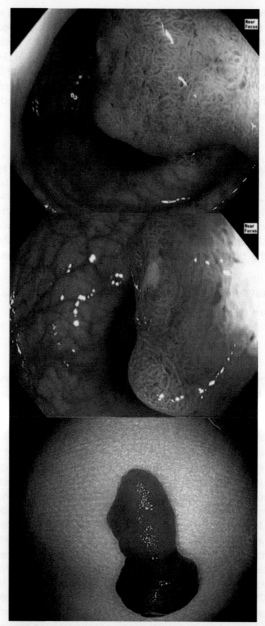

Fig. 1. Example of a JNET 2b pedunculated polyp. Based on the endoscopic appearance, the decision was made to perform EMR with contrast-enhanced submucosal injection. Pathology confirmed intramucosal cancer with wide negative margins (8 mm, Haggitt Level 0).

high probability of deep submucosal invasion.[34] The Paris Classification should also be used to help stratify which lesions are more likely to have advanced disease.[35] This highest risk configuration are LSL with a central depression; Paris 0-IIc lesions have an overall risk of 27%–36% for submucosal invasion with nearly all lesions greater than 20 mm having submucosal invasion.[36,37] After a thorough inspection of the lesion is performed and there is a low probability of deep submucosal invasion, preparation can be made for the EMR of the lesion.

Even if a lesion does not seem to have high-risk endoscopic features, a simplified scoring system may be invaluable in determining not only the EMR approach but also whether the lesion should even be resected by the endoscopist or instead be referred to a dedicated tertiary referral center. The "SMSA" score (with attendant components of Site, Morphology, Size, and Accessibility), first developed by Gupta and colleagues, is an easy-to-use, 4-Level scoring system which helps stratify an endoscopist's ability to undertake polypectomy of various polyp configurations, and more importantly may predict the likelihood of EMR technical failure. There was very high interobserver reliability for polyp scores (interclass correlation coefficient 0.93) and levels (K = 0.888). This was subsequently validated in a United Kingdom (UK)-based cohort of 114 patients; 20% of patients with a Level 4 polyp (8/41) experienced incomplete endoscopic resection, compared with no patients with a Level 2 polyp (0/9) (P < .001).[38,39]

Preparation for endoscopic mucosal resection

At the time of the procedure, before attempting EMR, it is imperative to be in an optimal endoscopic position for resection. This entails ensuring the scope is in a straight position without any looping. For lesions in the right colon, it may be necessary to retroflex to see the full extent of the lesion in the posterior aspect of an interhaustral valley. Similarly, the lesion should ideally be located at the 6 o'clock position whereby the biopsy channel is located to improve mechanical leverage of injection/snaring, which in turn increases the likelihood of technical success. Finally, the patient should be positioned so that any fluid will not settle in the resection site, as fluid (and potentially bleeding) can obscure the field of view and thereby increase the risk of complications or adenoma recurrence. Once an optimal position has been achieved, the next step involves lifting the polyp from the underlying submucosa to facilitate resection and minimize perforations and bleeding.

Injection-assisted endoscopic mucosal resection

Injection-assisted EMR involves injecting into the submucosa to lift the lesion from the muscularis propria to facilitate adequate resection and limit the risk of perforation. Numerous agents are available for submucosal injection. The ideal submucosal agent is one that provides a durable lift to reduce the need for frequent, repeated injections. Colloid plasma volume-expanding solutions such as sodium hyaluronate and hydroxyethyl starch have been shown to have a significant benefit over normal saline for sustained lift, increased rate of en bloc resection, and decreased risk for residual lesions.[40] However, at least one such FDA-approved lifting agent has been demonstrated, in a case series of 58 endoscopic resection specimens, to result in findings including severe submucosal fibrosis with multinucleated giant cells, and deposition of amorphous, pale blue-gray, finely granular material.[41] This has important clinical implications not only for the pathologist but also for the interventional endoscopists who may be referred cases of incomplete EMR resection from the community.

Staining dye such as methylene blue is also often added to the submucosal agent to facilitate the identification of the lateral margins of the LSL and also improve the recognition of inadvertent injury to the muscularis propria and perforation.[42] Additionally, dilute epinephrine (1:100,000–1:200,000) may also be added to the mixture to further enhance the submucosal cushion and decrease the risk of bleeding.[43]

The submucosal injection technique is important in obtaining an adequate lift. Dynamic injection should be performed rather than static injection. Dynamic submucosal injection involves injecting a small amount of solution to confirm entry into the submucosal space, followed by continued injection. As the solution is being injected, multiple maneuvers can be performed to enhance the lift including: the tip of the endoscope is deflected into the lumen, pulling back slightly of the needle catheter, and desufflating the lumen (**Fig. 2**).[44] It is important to note that there is a balance between not injecting enough and injecting too much—the goal of submucosal injection is to create a "sharp-peaked mountain" rather than a flat "rolling hill." Not only can the latter obscure the endoscopist's field of view but also it can produce excessive submucosal tension and reduce a snare's tissue grip, making EMR difficult.

After submucosal injection, it is important to assess for the adequate lift before proceeding to resection. If the lift is inadequate, either nonmalignant (submucosal fibrosis from an adjacent tattoo, prior attempts at resection or biopsies) or malignant (deep submucosal cancer invasion) causes may be responsible. Regardless of the cause, such lesions should be approached with caution, and if necessary, referred to an even higher level of care.[26]

Underwater-assisted endoscopic mucosal resection

An alternative to injection-assisted EMR to lift the lesion is underwater-assisted EMR. Instead of injecting into the submucosa to lift the agent, the entire lumen is filled with

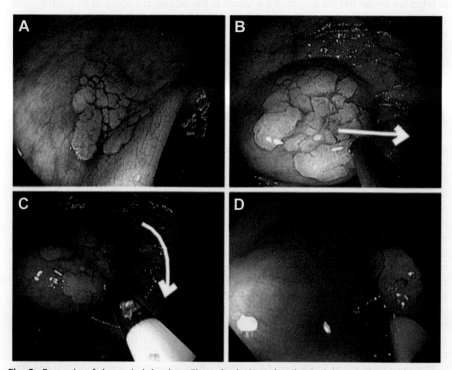

Fig. 2. Example of dynamic injection. First, the lesion's border is delineated with dilute indigo carmine (A). Next, during submucosal injection the endoscope is actively steered right (B), then clockwise (C). This promotes the desired direction of lift. Finally, the lesion is removed en-bloc via EMR (D). (From Soetikno R, Kaltenbach T. Dynamic submucosal injection technique. Gastrointest Endosc Clin N Am. 2010 Jul;20(3):497-502.)

water instead of gas, allowing for the mucosa and submucosa to involute and rise above the muscularis propria.[45] A meta-analysis of 7 studies with 1237 polyps revealed almost 2-fold increased rate of en-bloc resections using underwater EMR, especially for lesions ≥ 20 mm, which correlated with a 70% decreased risk for recurrence.[46]

Resection technique

Once adequate lesion lift has been achieved either through submucosal injection or underwater EMR technique, resecting the lesion can begin. In general, resection should begin at the area that is most difficult to access. The goal is to have en-bloc resection with a 2–3 mm margin of normal mucosa, which is possible for lesions 20 to 25 mm. A snare is used to capture the lesion; in situations of difficult-to-grasp lesions, enhanced measures may be necessary, including the use of specific snares such as crescent snares or braided snares, the use of a cap-fitted endoscope, wherein one suctions the lesion into the cap until "blue out" occurs, followed by immediate snare closure, or potentially even the use of hybrid ESD techniques. Once it is determined the grasped tissue is desired (ie, no obvious entrapment of muscularis propria), the snare is then lifted up into the lumen, and the lesion is resected.

Larger lesions resected with EMR require piecemeal resection. Piecemeal resection should be performed in an organized manner, using the edge of the previous mucosal defect as the next area for resection. This avoids leaving islands of adenoma. Efficient piecemeal resection includes repeating the following 3 steps: submucosal injection, 1 to 3 snare excisions, followed by cleaning and inspection of the mucosal defect. If the snare needs to be cleaned or exchanged, retrieving the resected pieces can typically be performed at the same time (**Fig. 3**).[25]

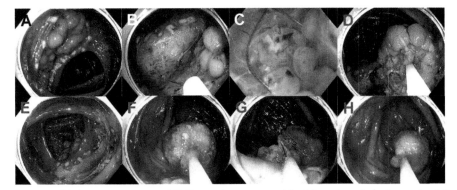

Fig. 3. Multiple core concepts of EMR are demonstrated in this series of photographs. (*A*) Using a cap-fitted colonoscope, the borders are marked using snare tip coagulation current prior to commencing. (*B*) The ileocecal valve is typically lipomatous; the fat seen is distinguished from a true perforation by the presence of blue-staining submucosa underneath the fat. (*B*) and (*C*) Flat components require various combinations of braided stiff snare, underwater EMR to promote mucosal floating, & lumen desufflation to promote a pseudopolyp formation (sometimes, to the point of "blue out"). (*D*) Wherever possible, dynamic injection should promote "sharp-peaked mountains." (*E*) In this example, polyp fragments are deposited in the cecal pit to promote efficient postprocedure fragment retrieval. (*F–H*) The retrieval basket (Roth Net, STERIS Corporation, Mentor, OH) with proper technique can be repeatedly closed, opened, & closed again, without losing prior fragments, to promote efficient fragment retrieval in a single pass.

Once the lesion has been completely removed, close inspection of the entire EMR field including the edges should be performed to evaluate for any adverse events including evaluating for any residual lesions, perforation, or bleeding.

Adverse Events

Residual lesion

For lesions larger than 25 mm, it is not typically possible for en-bloc resection with 2–3 mm of normal mucosal margin; instead, piecemeal resection is needed. Residual lesions can occur in up to 20% to 25% with piecemeal resections, especially in lesions greater than 40 mm in size, flat polyps, polyps in the right colon, and polyps in a difficult location such as the appendiceal orifice or ileocecal valve.[47] As discussed above, optimal technique for piecemeal resection is to resect in an organized manner at the edge of the previous resection. An adjunctive technique to decrease the risk of residual lesions includes ablating the edges of the EMR defect using argon plasma coagulation or snare tip coagulation. Using snare tip coagulation may be preferred because there is no additional cost of using the same snare for EMR as well as the snare tip for thermal ablation. This technique involves exposing 1 to 2 mm of the snare tip and gently moving along the margin of the EMR defect using soft coagulation to burn the edges. Margin thermal ablation can be very effective, with a multicenter randomized controlled trial revealing a 4-fold reduction in recurrence rates from 21% to 6%.[48]

In general, piecemeal resections should be followed with a surveillance colonoscopy in 6 months to assess for any residual lesions. Close inspection of the postmucosectomy scar with high-definition white light and NBI should be performed. A typical adenomatous pattern suggests residual lesions. Of note, if clips were placed previously, clip artifact can be present and should not be mistaken for residual lesions.[49] Clip artifact in general presents as a nodular elevation with normal pit pattern. Additionally, inflammatory nodules can be present, but these also should not be mistaken for residual lesions as they do not have the typical adenomatous pit pattern.

Perforation

Perforation is the most serious adverse event of EMR. A meta-analysis of 50 studies of EMR for lesions $\geq$ 20 mm revealed a perforation rate of 1.5%.[50] To decrease the risk of perforation, the first step is to ensure adequate lift of the submucosa. Another method to limit perforations is to ensure only the submucosa is captured in the snare. When one captures the desired tissue with the snare, before cutting, lift the tissue away from the wall to evaluate if it slightly mobile. If the muscularis propria is captured in the snare, the tissue will not move much, and the wall of the lumen may move instead. An additional sign that muscularis propria may be involved in the inability to transect the tissue within a reasonable amount of time (typically within 3–5 seconds of coagulation current pedal being depressed). In this instance, the snare should be relaxed and deflected upward to loosen the tissue.

The EMR defect should be inspected carefully for signs of deep mural injury or perforation. It is also important to evaluate the underside of the specimen and the EMR bed for the "target sign"/"reverse target sign," respectively. The target sign is composed of an inner white-gray circle, which is the muscularis propria, surrounded by the color of the dye in the submucosal agent used to lift, while the reverse target sign is an area of nonstaining on the EMR bed (**Fig. 4**).[51] Perforations can be often closed endoscopically with a reported success rate of 90%, highlighting the critical importance of prompt identification and if suitable, endoscopic management of the perforation.[52,53] Recently in a new classification system developed by Burgess and colleagues, multivariate analysis identified three risk factors associated with deep

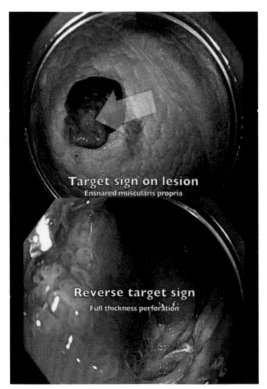

Fig. 4. Example of target sign (top) and reverse target sign (bottom) during EMR, indicating that perforation has occurred.

mural injury: transverse colon location (odds ratio (OR): 3.55, P = .028), en-bloc resection attempt (OR: 3.84, P = .005), and high-grade dysplasia or submucosal invasive cancer (OR: 2.97, P = .014).[54]

Bleeding
Bleeding is the most common post-EMR defect ranging from 2% to 11% in lesions greater than 20 mm.[55] Intraprocedural bleeding or bleeding recognized at the time of the procedure can usually be treated successfully without subsequent issues. However, delayed procedural bleeding can lead to increased morbidity for the patient given the need for possible admission, blood transfusions, and repeat colonoscopy. Risk factors for delayed bleeding include proximal colon location, polyp size, and intraprocedural bleeding.[55] Prophylaxis with clips or coagulation to prevent bleeding for all EMR sites has not been shown to be beneficial or cost-effective.[56] Moreover, clipping a wide-field EMR defect may not be possible. A 2019 multicenter randomized controlled trial did reveal certain patients may benefit from prophylactic clipping to prevent bleeding including lesions greater than 20 mm in the proximal colon.[57] Subsequently, a 2021 study investigating the cost-effectiveness of universal versus selective clipping in both Spanish and American economic contexts found that selective clipping was cost-effective only in a specific situation: those with a high risk of bleeding (based on a Spanish Endoscopy Society EMR group delayed bleed risk score (GSEED-RE2 score) > 6[58]), if the cost of the clip was below €394 or $154, respectively.[59]

Cold snare endoscopic mucosal resection

Traditionally, EMR has been performed using hot snare or with an electrosurgical current for possible increased efficacy of resection. However, hot snare EMR has been shown to have increased risk for delayed bleeding and perforation given the damage to deeper vessels and also deep mural injury, respectively.[60] Once a curiosity in

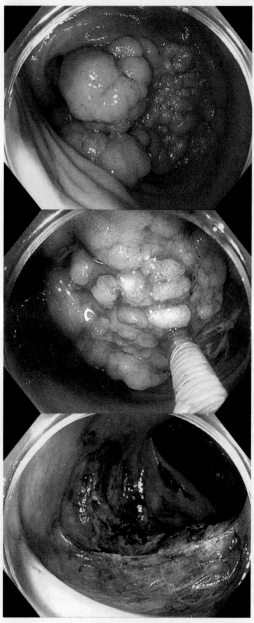

Fig. 5. Sequence of images showing cold snare EMR technique. Notice the lack of significant bleeding.

gastrointestinal literature,[61] in recent years cold snare polypectomy and EMR has become increasingly performed as an alternative to traditional hot snare EMR (**Fig. 5**. The benefit of cold snare EMR is the lack of any electrocautery-induced injury and therefore, a decreased risk in delayed bleeding and perforation. The possible concerns of cold snare EMR include possible difficulty in complete resection and subsequent decreased efficacy of complete removal of the lesion and risk of residual adenoma. One of the first applications of this technique was described in a 2015 series of 30 patients (15 duodenal polyps, 15 colon polyps). The median size of polyp was 20 mm in both locations, with the largest polyp being 60 mm and circumferential in the duodenum. All resections were successful, with only one patient in the duodenal cold snare EMR group requiring hospitalization for bleeding likely secondary to long-term anticoagulation requirements, and one patient in the colon cold snare EMR group requiring emergency room visit due to right lower quadrant pain 1 day after resecting a 20 mm polyp near the appendiceal orifice; after a negative workup, the patient was managed expectantly. There were no episodes of postpolypectomy syndrome or perforations.[62] Three years later, Tutticci and Hewett described cold snare EMR for 163 procedures across 99 patients. All procedures were successful. Only 2/163 lesions, or 1.2%, had positive margins which were again successfully treated with cold snare EMR. The side effect profile was similarly favorable—only 4 patients (4/99, or 4%) experienced any adverse events, with the only admission in the series most likely unrelated to the procedure itself.[63] Most recently, van Hattem and colleagues compared historical cohort of cold snare EMR (121 patients) to hot snare EMR (353 patients) in LSL $\geq$ 20 mm across 474 patients. The technical success rate for cold snare EMR was 100% and the residual adenoma rate was comparable between the 2 methods at 4% in 6 months. Furthermore, the study confirmed the superior safety profile of cold snare EMR, with no episodes of delayed bleeding nor deep mural injury, compared with hot snare EMR with 5.1% (18/353) having delayed bleeding and 3.4% (12/353) having deep mural injury.[64] However, this enthusiasm is somewhat tempered by a recent review by Suresh and colleagues of 310 polyps resected via cold snare EMR, among which a 34.8% recurrence rate (108/310) was noted. On multivariate analysis, risk factors included age ($P = .002$), polyp size ($P < .001$), and advanced polyp histology including tubulovillous adenoma or high grade dysplasia ($P = .023$).[65]

SUMMARY

With the most recent clinical guidelines recommending a start to CRC screening at age 45,[66] it is likely that the incidence of colonoscopic lesions requiring endoscopic resection will increase, thereby pushing the demand for EMR upward. In less than 70 years since Dr Rosenberg's first use of a saline wheal to protect against deep mural injury, using modern EMR techniques, the vast majority of lesions encountered today during colonoscopy are amenable to organ-preserving tissue resection techniques such as EMR, with excellent long-term clinical outcomes.

CLINICS CARE POINTS

- Proper bowel preparation (including split-dose preparation and simethicone tabs) is essential to a safe and effective procedure
- Referring physicians should be encouraged NOT to perform certain interventions which may cause submucosal fibrosis for subsequent EMR attempts. For instance, tattooing of the lesion should be performed 5 cm distal to the lesion, not underneath the lesion. A partial polypectomy attempt should similarly be avoided at all costs. Similarly, they should take care

with newer-generation, FDA-approved viscous lifting agents, as it is now reported to put the lesion at risk for significant submucosal fibrosis.

- The entire team plays a role in safe and efficient EMR. For instance, the nurses should be in the top 5% of the unit. High-performing nurses engage in closed-loop communication, are extremely familiar with various EMR devices, can troubleshoot problems, and have situational awareness to offer intelligent insight into the proper resection strategy for each lesion.

- Proper use of a distal attachment cap will facilitate EMR procedures by maintaining proper focal length between the colonoscope and the lesion. Caps also help splay open folds to improve visualization (eg, at colon turns and at interhaustral valleys).

- Wherever possible, keep the lesion above the waterline. Not only does this facilitate visualization but also it enhances safety in the event of bleeding or perforation

- Dynamic injection should be used to promote the proper shape to the submucosal injection—aim for a sharp-peaked valley, rather than a rolling hill

- After each resection, carefully inspect the underside of the specimen and EMR bed for signs of deep mural injury ("target sign"/"reverse target sign")

- In the event of perforation, keep the perforation above the waterline, and clip the defect closed in a timely manner.

ACKNOWLEDGMENT

The authors wish to acknowledge Gottumukkala S. Raju, MD, for his description of the four key requirements of success in EMR: the "Time, Team, Tools, Technique" concept.

DISCLOSURE

The authors have nothing to disclose.

REFERENCES

1. Rosenberg N. Submucosal saline wheal as safety factor in fulguration of rectal and sigmoidal polypi. AMA Arch Surg 1955;70(1):120–2.
2. Haber HP, Benda N, Fitzke G, et al. Colonic wall thickness measured by ultrasound: striking differences in patients with cystic fibrosis versus healthy controls. Gut 1997;40:406–11.
3. Wiesner W, Mortelé KJ, Ji H, et al. Normal colonic wall thickness at CT and its relation to colonic distension. J Comput Assist Tomogr 2002;26(1):102–6.
4. Deyhle P, Seuberth K, Jenny S, et al. Endoscopic polypectomy in the proximal colon. Endoscopy 1971;2:103–5.
5. Deyhle P, Largiader F, Jenny S, et al. A Method for Endoscopic Electroresection of Sessile Colon Polyps. Endoscopy 1973;5:38–40.
6. Inoue H, Takeshita K, Hori H, et al. Endoscopic mucosal resection with a cap-fitted panendoscope for esophagus, stomach, and colon mucosal lesions. Gastrointest Endosc 1993;39(1):58–62.
7. Tada M, Inoue H, Yabata E, et al. Colonic mucosal resection using a transparent cap-fitted endoscope. Gastrointest Endosc 1996;44(1):63–5.
8. Karita M, Tada M, Okida K, et al. Endoscopic therapy for early colon cancer: the strip biopsy resection technique. Gastrointest Endosc 1991;37:128–32.

9. Fukuzawa M, Gotoda T. History of endoscopic submucosal dissection and role for colorectal endoscopic submucosal dissection: A Japanese perspective. Gastrointest Interv 2012;1:30–5.

10. Takemoto T, Tada M, Yanai H, et al. Significance of strip biopsy, with particular reference to endoscopic "mucosectomy". Dig Endosc 1989;1(1):4–9.

11. Bond J. Polyp guideline: diagnosis, treatment, and surveillance for patients with colorectal polyps. Am J Gastroenterol 2000;95(11):3053–63.

12. Winawer SJ, Zauber AG, Ho MN, et al. Prevention of colorectal cancer by colonoscopic polypectomy. N Engl J Med 1993;329:1977–81.

13. Zauber AG, Winawer SJ, O'Brien MJ, et al. Colonoscopic polypectomy and long-term prevention of colorectal-cancer deaths. NEJM 2012;366:687–96.

14. Le Roy F, Manfredi S, Hamonic S, et al. Frequency of and risk factors for the surgical resection of nonmalignant colorectal polyps: a population-based study. Endoscopy 2016;48(3):263–70.

15. Raju GS, Lum PJ, Ross W, et al. Outcome of endoscopic mucosal resection as an alternative to surgery in patients with complex colon polyps. Gastrointest Endosc 2016;84(2):315–25.

16. Moss A, Bourke MJ, Williams SJ, et al. Endoscopic mucosal resection outcomes and prediction of submucosal cancer from advanced colonic mucosal neoplasia. Gastroenterology 2011;140:1909–18.

17. Ahmad NA, Kochman ML, Long WB, et al. Efficacy, safety, and clinical outcomes of endoscopic mucosal resection: a study of 101 cases. Gastrointest Endosc 2002;55:390–6.

18. Hwang JH, Vani Konda, Abu Dayyeh BK, et al. Endoscopic mucosal resection. Gastrointest Endosc 2015;82(2):215–26.

19. Jayanna M, Burgess NG, Singh R, et al. Cost analysis of endoscopic mucosal resection vs surgery for large laterally spreading colorectal lesions. Clin Gastroenterol Hepatol 2016;14(2):271–8.

20. Keswani R, Law R, Ciolino JD, et al. Adverse events after surgery for nonmalignant colon polyps are common and associated with increased length of stay and costs. Gastrointest Endosc 2016;84(2):296–303.

21. Law R, Das A, Gregory D, et al. Endoscopic resection is cost-effective compared with laparoscopic resection in the management of complex colon polyps: an economic analysis. Gastrointest Endosc 2016;83(6):1248–57.

22. Louis M, Johnston SA, Churilov L, et al. The hospital costs of complications following colonic resection surgery: A retrospective cohort study. Ann Med Surg (Lond) 2020;54(37–42):37.

23. Guo R, Wang Y, Liu M, et al. The effect of quality of segmental bowel preparation on adenoma detection rate. BMC Gastroenterol 2019;19:119.

24. Xirasagar S, Wu Y, Tsai MH, et al. Colorectal cancer prevention by CLEAR principles-based colonoscopy protocol: an observational study. Gastrointest Endosc 2020;91:905–16.

25. Klein A, Bourke MJ. How to perform high-quality endoscopic mucosal resection during colonoscopy. Gastroenterology 2017;152(3):466–71.

26. Kim HG, Thosani N, Banerjee S, et al. Effect of prior biopsy sampling, tattoo placement, and snare sampling on endoscopic resection of large nonpedunculated colorectal lesions. Gastrointest Endosc 2015;81(1):204–13.

27. Soetikno RM, Gotoda T, Nakanishi Y, et al. Endoscopic mucosal resection. Gastrointest Endosc 2003;57(4):567–79.

28. Sanchez-Yague A, Kaltenbach T, Yamamoto H, et al. The endoscopic cap that can (with videos). Gastrointest Endosc 2012;76:169–78.e2.

29. Ferlitsch M, Moss A, Hassan C, et al. Colorectal polypectomy and endoscopic mucosal resection (EMR): European Society of Gastrointestinal Endoscopy (ESGE) Clinical Guideline. Endoscopy 2017;49:270–97.

30. Kaltenbach T, Anderson JC, Burke CA, et al. Endoscopic removal of colorectal lesions - recommendations by the US Multi-Society Task Force on Colorectal Cancer. Gastroenterology 2020;158(4):1095–129.

31. Bogie RMM, Veldman MHJ, Snijders L, et al. Endoscopic subtypes of colorectal laterally spreading tumors (LSTs) and the risk of submucosal invasion: a meta-analysis. Endoscopy 2018;50(3):263–82.

32. D'Amico F, Amato A, Iannone A, et al. Risk of covert submucosal cancer in patients with granular mixed laterally spreading tumors. Clin Gastroenterol Hepatol 2021;19(7):1395–401.

33. Resende RH, Ribeiro IB, de Moura DTH, et al. Surveillance in inflammatory bowel disease: is chromoendoscopy the only way to go? A systematic review and meta-analysis of randomized clinical trials. Endosc Int Open 2020;8:E578–90.

34. Hayashi N, Tanaka S, Hewett DG, et al. Endoscopic prediction of deep submucosal invasive carcinoma: validation of the narrow-band imaging international colorectal endoscopic (NICE) classification. Gastrointest Endosc 2013;78(4):625–32.

35. The Paris endoscopic classification of superficial neoplastic lesions: esophagus, stomach, and colon: November 30 to December 1, 2002. Gastrointest Endosc 2003;58(6 Suppl):S3–43.

36. Soetikno RM, Kaltenbach T, Rouse RV, et al. Prevalence of nonpolypoid (flat and depressed) colorectal neoplasms in asymptomatic and symptomatic adults. JAMA 2008;299(9):1027–35.

37. Saitoh Y, Waxman I, West AB, et al. Prevalence and distinctive biologic features of flat colorectal adenomas in a North American population. Gastroenterology 2001; 120(7):1657–65.

38. Gupta S, Miskovic D, Bhandari P, et al. A novel method for determining the difficulty of colonoscopic polypectomy. Frontline Gastroenterol 2013;4:244–8.

39. Currie AC, Lucado AM, Gilani SNS, et al. Validation of the size morphology site access score in endoscopic mucosal resection of large polyps in a district general hospital. Ann R Coll Surg Engl 2019;101:558–62.

40. Yandrapu H, Desai M, Siddique S, et al. Normal saline solution versus other viscous solutions for submucosal injection during endoscopic mucosal resection: a systematic review and meta-analysis. Gastrointest Endosc 2017;85(4):693–9.

41. Olivas AD, Setia N, Weber CR, et al. Histologic changes caused by injection of a novel submucosal lifting agent for endoscopic resection in GI lesions. Gastrointest Endosc 2021;93:470–6.

42. Holt BA, Jayasekeran V, Sonson R, et al. Topical submucosal chromoendoscopy defines the level of resection in colonic EMR and may improve procedural safety (with video). Gastrointest Endosc 2013;77(6):949–53.

43. Hirao M, Hatakeyama H, Asanuma T, et al. [Endoscopic resection with local injection of hypertonic saline epinephrine for the treatment of early gastric cancer]. Gan To Kagaku Ryoho 1988;15(4):1466–72.

44. Soetikno R, Kaltenbach T. Dynamic submucosal injection technique. Gastrointest Endosc Clin N Am 2010;20(3):497–502.

45. Binmoeller KF, Weilert F, Shah J, et al. "Underwater" EMR without submucosal injection for large sessile colorectal polyps (with video). Gastrointest Endosc 2012; 75(5):1086–91.

46. Choi AY, Moosvi Z, Shah S, et al. Underwater versus conventional EMR for colorectal polyps: systematic review and meta-analysis. Gastrointest Endosc 2021; 93(2):378–89.
47. Sidhu M, Tate DJ, Desomer L, et al. The size, morphology, site, and access score predicts critical outcomes of endoscopic mucosal resection in the colon. Endoscopy 2018;50(7):684–92.
48. Klein A, Tate D, Jayasekeran V, et al. Thermal ablation of mucosal defect margins reduces adenoma recurrence after colonic endoscopic mucosal resection. Gastroenterology 2019;156(3):604–13.e3.
49. Pellise M, Desomer L, Burgess NG, et al. The influence of clips on scars after EMR: clip artifact. Gastrointest Endosc 2016;83(3):608–16.
50. Hassan C, Repici A, Sharma P, et al. Efficacy and safety of endoscopic resection of large colorectal polyps: a systematic review and meta-analysis. Gut 2016; 65(5):806–20.
51. Swan MP, Bourke MJ, Moss A, et al. The target sign: an endoscopic marker for the resection of the muscularis propria and potential perforation during colonic endoscopic mucosal resection. Gastrointest Endosc 2011;73(1):79–85.
52. Verlaan T, Voermans RP, van Berge Henegouwen MI, et al. Endoscopic closure of acute perforations of the GI tract: a systematic review of the literature. Gastrointest Endosc 2015;82(4):618–628 e5.
53. Baron TH, Wong Kee Song LM, Zielinski MD, et al. A comprehensive approach to the management of acute endoscopic perforations (with videos). Gastrointest Endosc 2012;76(4):838–59.
54. Burgess NG, Bassan MS, McLeod D, et al. Deep mural injury and perforation after colonic endoscopic mucosal resection: a new classification and analysis of risk factors. Gut 2017;66(10):1779–89.
55. Burgess NG, Metz AJ, Williams SJ, et al. Risk factors for intraprocedural and clinically significant delayed bleeding after wide-field endoscopic mucosal resection of large colonic lesions. Clin Gastroenterol Hepatol 2014;12(4):651–61.e1-3.
56. Boumitri C, Mir FA, Ashraf I, et al. Prophylactic clipping and post-polypectomy bleeding: a meta-analysis and systematic review. Ann Gastroenterol 2016; 29(4):502–8.
57. Pohl H, Grimm IS, Moyer MT, et al. Closure prevents bleeding after endoscopic resection of large colon polyps in a randomized trial. Gastroenterology 2019; 157(4):977–984 e3.
58. Albeniz E, Gimeno-García AZ, Fraile M, et al. Clinical validation of risk scoring systems to predict risk of delayed bleeding after EMR of large colorectal lesions. Gastrointest Endosc 2020;91(4):868–78.e3.
59. Albeniz E, Enguita-Germán M, Gimeno-Garcia AZ, et al. The Answer to "when to clip" after colorectal endoscopic mucosal resection based on a cost-effectiveness analysis. Am J Gastroenterol 2021;116(2):311–8.
60. Yamashina T, Fukuhara M, Maruo T, et al. Cold snare polypectomy reduced delayed postpolypectomy bleeding compared with conventional hot polypectomy: a propensity score-matching analysis. Endosc Int Open 2017;5(7):E587–94.
61. Waye JD. Polyps large and small (Editorial). Gastrointest Endosc 1992;38(3): 391–2.
62. Choksi N, Elmunzer BJ, Stidham RW, et al. Cold snare piecemeal resection of colonic and duodenal polyps ≥1 cm. Endosc Int Open 2015;3:E508–13.
63. Tuttici NJ, Hewett DG. Cold EMR of large sessile serrated polyps at colonoscopy (with video). Gastrointest Endosc 2018;87:837–42.

64. van Hattem WA, Shahidi N, Vosko S, et al. Piecemeal cold snare polypectomy versus conventional endoscopic mucosal resection for large sessile serrated lesions: a retrospective comparison across two successive periods. Gut 2021; 70(9):1691–7.

65. Suresh S, Zhang J, Ahmed A, et al. Risk factors associated with adenoma recurrence following cold snare endoscopic mucosal resection of polyps >= 20mm: a retrospective chart review. Endosc Int Open 2021;9:E867–73.

66. Shaukat A, Kahi CJ, Burke CA, et al. ACG Clinical Guidelines: Colorectal Cancer Screening 2021. Am J Gastroenterol 2021;116(3):458–79.

Colon Polypectomy with Endoscopic Submucosal Dissection and Endoscopic Full-Thickness Resection

Maham Hayat, MD[a], Nabeel Azeem, MD[b],
Mohammad Bilal, MD[b,c],*

KEYWORDS

- Polypectomy • Endoscopic resection • Endoscopic submucosal dissection
- Endoscopic full-thickness resection

KEY POINTS

- Endoscopic submucosal dissection (ESD) and endoscopic full-thickness resection (EFTR) are minimally invasive methods for the resection of advanced lesions in the colon.
- ESD in the colon is an effective method for treatment of large precancerous lesions, early colorectal cancer, and residual or recurrent colorectal adenomas.
- EFTR is more commonly used in lesions with suspected deeper submucosal invasion, lesions originating from muscularis propria, or those with advanced fibrosis.
- In the future, direction from leading GI societies will be crucial for the evaluation of competence and shaping training for EFTR and ESD.

INTRODUCTION

Endoscopic resection has become the gold standard for the management of most of the large colorectal polyps. Various endoscopic resection techniques include endoscopic mucosal resection (EMR), endoscopic submucosal dissection (ESD), and

Financial support: None.

Potential competing interests: None.

Copyrights: No images were used in this publication without prior permission from the original article's authors.

[a] Section of Digestive Diseases and Nutrition, University of Oklahoma Health Sciences Center, 800 Stanton L Young Boulevard, Oklahoma City, OK 73104, USA; [b] Division of Gastroenterology, Hepatology and Nutrition, University of Minnesota, Minneapolis, MN 55455, USA; [c] Advanced Endoscopy, Division of Gastroenterology & Hepatology, Minneapolis Veterans Affairs Medical Center, 1 Veterans Drive, Minneapolis, MN 55417, USA

* Corresponding author. Advanced Endoscopy, Division of Gastroenterology & Hepatology, Minneapolis Veterans Affairs Medical Center, 1 Veterans Drive, Minneapolis, MN 55417.

E-mail addresses: billa17@hotmail.com; mbilal@umn.edu

endoscopic full-thickness resection (EFTR). ESD is a minimally invasive method for resection of advanced lesions in the gastrointestinal (GI) tract to achieve en-bloc resection. It was first described in the 1990s by Ono and colleagues[1] and Oyama and colleagues[2] primarily for the resection of early gastric cancer. Over the past two decades, both the technique and utility of ESD have matured and it is currently being used in North America for a variety of indications throughout the GI tract including colorectal lesions. ESD is especially useful for lesions with limited submucosal invasion as a curative resection can be proven, and it allows for the accurate determination of lesion margin given the resection is en-bloc.

The utility of EMR and ESD can be limited in lesions that have evidence of invasion through the muscularis propria, such as nonlifting epithelial lesions, in areas of severe fibrosis and scarring, and lesions in difficult anatomic locations with higher chance of perforation and infection (peri-appendiceal, or within a diverticulum, etc.). Previously surgical resection was the predominant approach for the removal of these lesions. Now endoscopic full-thickness resection (EFTR) offers a less invasive treatment alternative, with the potential of complete avoidance of surgical intervention. In this review, we provide a brief overview of ESD and EFTR in the management of colon polyps.

ENDOSCOPIC SUBMUCOSAL DISSECTION
Indications

The ESD technique in the colon and rectum is an effective method for the resection of large lesions, usually > 2 cm that carry a risk of early colorectal cancer, which are often difficult to resect en-bloc via EMR. The American Gastroenterological Association (AGA) recommendations for colorectal ESD or advanced endoscopic resection are as follows:

- En bloc resection for lesions at risk for submucosally invasive cancer:
  - Type V Kudo pit pattern depressed component (Paris 0–IIc)
  - Complex morphology (0–Is or 0–IIa + Is)
  - Rectosigmoid location
  - Nongranular LST (adenomas), ≥20 mm in size
  - Granular LST (adenomas), ≥ 30 mm in size
- Residual or recurrent colorectal adenomas (**Fig. 1**)[3]

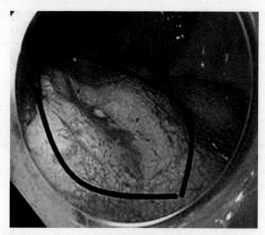

Fig. 1. Residual adenoma at the previous site of resection is outlined.

Related indications are summarized in **Table 1**.[4,5]

Lesion Assessment and Classifications

Appraisal of features of colonic polyps, especially to analyze if the polyp could have a component of invasive cancer is critical. This information helps determine which patients benefit from ESD over EMR vs surgery.

Several classifications have been introduced for the evaluation of colonic polyps.

(A) Paris Classification: Most recent guidelines by US Multi-Society Task Force on Colorectal Cancer, recommends the use of Paris classification for the surface morphology of colonic polyps.[6]

- Type 0-I indicates polypoid lesions:
  - 0-Ip Polypoid or pedunculated
  - 0-Is Sessile, broad-based
- Type 0-II indicates flat or superficial forms, namely
  - 0-IIa - Minimally elevated
  - 0-IIb - Completely flat
  - 0-IIc - Minimally depressed
- Type 0-III: Excavated/ulcerated

Type 0-IIc morphology suggests superficially invasive cancer that benefits from en bloc resection and type 0-III consistent with deeply invasive cancer that requires surgical resection.

Nonpolypoid lesions greater than 10 mm in diameter are referred to as laterally spreading tumors (LSTs), and are a subgroup of Type IIa lesions. Further subtypes are:

- LST - granular homogenous
- LST - granular nodular mixed (**Fig. 2**): nodular component carries risk for more advanced dysplasia
- LST - nongranular flat elevated
- LST - nongranular pseudodepressed (**Fig. 3**): much higher risk for advanced dysplasia including superficially invasive cancer

Table 1	
Indications of endoscopic submucosal dissection (ESD) in the colon	
1. Benefit from en-bloc Histologic Assessment	LST-NG, particularly LST-NG (PD) LST-G with nodular component(s) Depressed-type tumors (Paris 0-IIc) Lesions exhibiting a Kudo V-type pit pattern Cancers with predicted superficial submucosal invasion
2.	Mucosal lesions with submucosal fibrosis (prior resection attempt/aggressive biopsies/underlying tattoo)
3.	Lesions with underlying background of chronic inflammation (IBD)
4.	Local residual early cancers after endoscopic resection

Abbreviations: G, granular; LST, laterally spreading tumors; NG, Non-granular; PD, pseudodepressed.

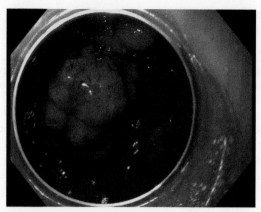

Fig. 2. A granular laterally spreading tumor, nodular subtype.

(B) The NICE classification is a widely adopted classification that incorporates narrow-band imaging (NBI) for the detailed assessment of colon polyps during colonoscopy for an optical diagnosis. NBI allows for the visualization of vessel and surface patterns. The classification of a lesion is based on color change compared with background, vascular patterns, and surface description of mucosa. Diagnosis based on NICE classification can be beneficial for predicting more advanced dysplasia within a polyp. NICE classification divides polyps into 3 categories: (i) Type 1 lesions are usually hyperplastic or serrated polyps, have a similar color to the surrounding mucosa, may have a lacy vascular pattern or lack any specific vascular pattern; (ii) Type 2 with adenomatous lesions, presenting with brown vessels surrounding white structures giving an overall browner appearance compared with the background mucosa; (iii) Type 3 with dark to brown background, disrupted or missing vessels and irregular

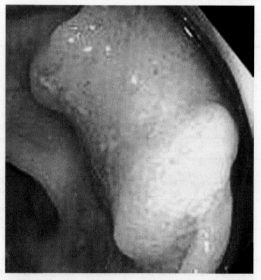

Fig. 3. A nongranular laterally spreading tumor, pseudodepressed subtype.

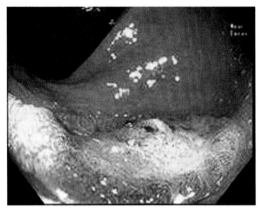

Fig. 4. NICE 3 lesion, brown background with disrupted vessels and irregular surface pattern.

surface pattern most likely to contain deeper submucosal invasion (**Fig. 4**). Using magnifying endoscopes available in some Asian countries, JNET classification can be used to further subdivide NICE type 2 classification into 2A and 2B with 2B having a more irregular vessel and surface pattern correlating to high-grade dysplasia or superficial cancer.

(C) Kudo Pit Pattern: Another classification system incorporating magnification endoscopy and chromoendoscopy was formulated by Kudo and colleagues[7] and describes "pit patterns" to predict histology. The Kudo classification classifies pit pattern as round/normal (Type I), asteroid (Type II), tubular or round pit smaller than normal pit (Type IIIS), tubular or round pit larger than normal pit (Type IIIL), gyrus/dendritic (IV), irregular arrangement (Vi), and loss of decrease of pits with amorphous structure (VN). Type I pattern is normal mucosa. Type II can be hyperplastic or a serrated lesion. Type IIIL an IV are just adenomas and endoscopic resection can be performed. Type IIIs represents polyps with high-grade dysplasia or superficial cancer and may benefit from en bloc resection. While those with type Vi and VN are suggestive of deeper invasive cancer requiring surgical resection with only select type Vi potentially being candidates for en bloc endoscopic resection.

Outcomes

Endoscopic treatment such as EMR and ESD for localized colorectal carcinoma and advanced polyps have comparable outcomes to surgical resection, while being remarkably safer and cost-effective. A population-based study looking at mid-term (2.5 years) and long-term (5 years) CRC-free survival rates showed no difference between endoscopic and surgical groups of early adenocarcinoma.[8] Another study of more than 13,000 patients with early colon cancer showed comparable outcomes for early cancer tumors located in the left colon, polypectomy yielded comparable 5-year early cancer-specific survival for all left-sided lesions, irrespective of size and all less than 20 mm right colon lesions as compared with surgery (94.5 vs 94.3%, *P* value = .94).[9] The economic implications of surgical resection of premalignant lesions are burdensome, increasing health care cost for patients and limiting surgical resources. Surgery for complex colonic polyps is three times more expensive than endoscopic resection ($18,717 vs $5,570 per patient), while adding less quality life adjusted years.[10] Endoscopic resection also has shown to shorten the duration of hospital stay by 2.81 nights, thus giving further priority to endoscopic resection as first-line therapy for advanced polyps.[11]

There is growing evidence in favor of complete resection and long-term efficacy of ESD. A multicenter, observational study of 1845 early colorectal neoplasms measuring ≥20 mm, looked at outcomes of treatment with EMR or ESD. En bloc resection rates and mean procedure times were 56.9% versus 94.5% and 18 ± 23 min versus 96 ± 69 min, respectively, for EMR and ESD.[12] Although ESD had longer procedure times, en bloc resection by EMR was not possible in more than 43% of cases, limiting histologic assessment in high-risk lesions. A large Australian study found that for colonic lesions greater than 20 mm, a type V Kudo pit pattern, depressed component (Paris 0–IIc), complex morphology (0–Is or 0–IIa + Is), rectosigmoid location, nongranular surface morphology were all associated with submucosal invasive cancer, and therefore, should undergo en bloc ESD as a first-line treatment as opposed to EMR.[13]

ESD is also associated with a lower risk of recurrence when compared with EMR, thus warranting less frequent surveillance. Multiple large studies and meta-analysis suggest that for benign LSTs, piecemeal EMR is curative in almost all cases, but it carries a higher short-term recurrence rate of 10% to 20% (compared with as low as 1%–2% for ESD).[14–16] A recent study analyzed 254 large colon polyps with high-grade dysplasia, either resected piecemeal fashion or en-bloc. After a median follow-up of 28.7 months for the entire cohort, 6 cases of local recurrence were all in the piecemeal cohort and none in the en-bloc resection (hazard ratio (HR): 11.4; 95% confidence interval (CI): 0.48–273).[17] Another large multi-center study in Japan also showed that en-bloc ESD resection has reduced local recurrence with only 1.4% recurrence rate for ESD as compared with 6.8% for EMR.[18] Relative risk of local resection was 0.9however, when comparing piecemeal ESD with piecemeal EMR thus highlighting that piecemeal resection, regardless of technique, is an important risk factor for recurrence.[18] ESD technique also enables the accurate measurement of submucosal and lymphovascular invasion ultimately determining if resection was curative and if surgical resection can be avoided.[19]

Equipment

For the successful execution of ESD, specialized equipment is needed which includes distal attachment clear cap, submucosal injection solution(s), electrocautery generator, coagulation devices, and dedicated ESD knives.

Distal attachments: Distal attachments are variable-sized transparent caps that can be attached to the end of a variety of endoscopes. They help maintain a suitable distance of 2 to 4 mm between the scope and targeted area of lumen, provide some degree of traction by separating the mucosa and muscularis propria layer while dissecting through the submucosa, pushing aside folds and stabilizing the tip of the endoscope.[20] They also have a side hole allowing the suction of fluid without interfering with the endoscopic view.

Submucosal Injectants: Submucosal injection is a key step for ESD. It helps lift the mucosa away from the muscularis to create a safe space for submucosal dissection. Normal saline is readily available and the cheapest options but dissipates much more readily than colloid-based injectants such as Hetastarch. Solutions are often mixed with a blue dye such as methylene blue or indigo carmine which high lights the submucosa and is not picked up by the muscularis aiding in the delineation of layers.

Endoscopic submucosal dissection knives

Broadly speaking, two types of ESD knives are used: needle-type knives (**Fig. 5**) and blunt-tip knives (**Fig. 6**) with variations between the two. The needle-type knives have

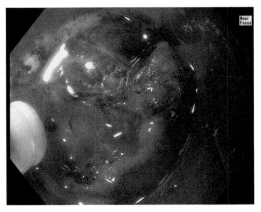

Fig. 5. Needle-type ESD knife.

a pointed tip allowing for precise control when dissecting in narrow spaces and providing high current density at the tip. The cutting motion of needle-type knives is often described as using a "fencing sword" whereby the knife thrusts away from the muscle layer. While using blunt-tip knives, the tip is often used to hook the tissue and dissection often occurs by dragging the knife laterally or pulling the knife toward the endoscope channel, which can often be conducted safely without a direct view of the dissection plane. These types of knives are often described as "slashing" type knives similar to a saber sword. One advantage of insulated tip knives is the lower risk of perforation.[21] The use of knives might vary in each case depending on anatomy and at the discretion and comfort level of the endoscopist.

Procedure

A guide to performing standard ESD includes important steps detailed later in discussion.[21,22]

A) *Accurate assessment of lesion margin and marking*

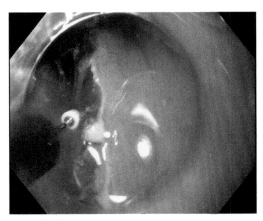

Fig. 6. Blunt tip-type ESD knife.

Resection with ESD is aimed at obtaining en bloc resection with negative margins. This step is critical when early carcinoma is suspected, as the patient can potentially avoid surgery if negative margins are documented. For colonic lesions, margins are usually easily identifiable under high-definition white-light endoscopy, NBI , and submucosal injection with a dye-based solution. In some circumstances, one may mark the lesion circumferentially at a 5 mm distance with either an ESD knife or with argon plasma coagulation (APC) to aid with the procedure.

B) *Incision*

Once the lesion is assessed or marked, submucosal injections to lift the perimeter of the lesion are performed. An initial mucosal incision (**Fig. 7**) is made with a needle knife roughly at the apex of the submucosal cushion to expose the submucosa and avoid injury to the muscularis propria. The incision can then be extended circumferentially (**Fig. 8**).

C) *Submucosal dissection*

Now that submucosa is exposed, this loose tissue can be taken down with the ESD knife and periodically injected with any lifting solution. Dissection continues generally at the mid-point between the mucosa and muscularis propria keeping the plane parallel to muscularis propria (**Fig. 9**), resulting in the safe removal of the lesion.

The two common modifications to the above ESD technique are the tunneling ESD and the pocket technique. A partial circumferential incision can be conducted before starting submucosal dissection, to limit fluid extravasation and resultant longer duration of lift, (pocket technique). Additionally, an incision on just the oral and anal side can be performed and submucosal dissection creating a tunnel beneath the lesion to connect the two openings can be conducted, also limiting fluid extravasation and improving traction (tunnel technique). Working within the pocket or tunnel helps stabilize the tip of the endoscope and at the same time providing good traction. This method has shown to have higher en bloc resection rate and R0 resection rates.[23,24]

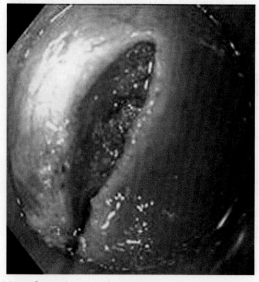

Fig. 7. Mucosal incision after submucosal injection.

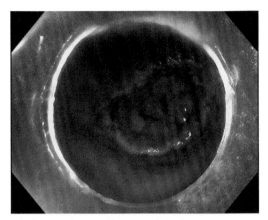

Fig. 8. Incision extended circumferentially around the lesion.

Traction devices
Lack of traction during dissection is one of the biggest challenges in ESD. Numerous traction methods and devices have been introduced to facilitate this.

"Clip and line" traction (**Fig. 10**) is an easy and simple way of maintaining tissue traction, described as tying a string, classically dental floss, to one of the jaws on an endoclip. With the string alongside/outside the endoscope, the clip is then deployed at the edge of the lesion. With gentle traction pressure applied to string from outside the patient, optimal stabilization and visualization of the lesion are obtained. Although cost-effective and simple, this method comes with the extra step of endoscope withdrawal, string attachment and reinsertion.[25] Several modifications have been described to this technique. One is that of an adapted clip-thread method.[26] Before the initiation of the procedure, a string is inserted through the therapeutic channel of endoscope, and pulled proximally outside from the channel, whereby the ends are tied. This end of the string is later tied to the endoclip, which is inserted through the scope, and ultimately saves the extra step of withdrawal and reinsertion.

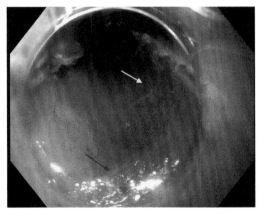

Fig. 9. Layers during ESD; Black arrow is pointing to mucosa; Yellow arrow is pointing to submucosa, also the plane of incision; Red arrow is pointing to plane of muscularis propria.

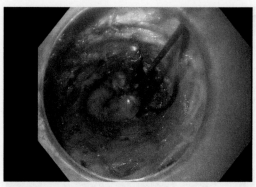

Fig. 10. Clip and line traction method demonstrated whereby a clip, tied to the end of a thread is deployed at one end of the lesion for maintained traction.

S-O clip is another traction device comprising of a 5 mm long spring attached to an endoclip on one end and a nylon loop on another end. With the clip first being applied to lesion margin, another clip's jaw is passed through the nylon loop and it's attached on the opposite bowel wall providing optimal traction. Use of this device in a randomized clinical trial (RCT) has shown to effectively shorten procedure times[27] . Other traction strategies described in literature include magnetic bead-assisted ESD,[28] thin endoscope-assisted ESD,[29] overtube type devices,[30] and double-balloon devices[31] to name a few.

Challenges

ESD is an advanced endoscopic procedure with a very steep learning curve. It should be performed by highly trained expert endoscopist. Although developed in Japan, it is currently being practiced at large tertiary referral centers across the United States. Despite the development and uptake of ESD being more prevalent in recent years, one study suggests that outcomes of ESD in the US are comparable to Asian countries whereby it is widely practiced.[32] In Asian countries, the practice of ESD is a step-wise approach starting from gastric lesions and onto colorectal lesions. Gastric ESD is typically safer and easier; however, early gastric cancer is far less common in the US limiting ideal cases for Western endoscopists to gain experience. European Society of Gastrointestinal Endoscopy ESGE recommends a dedicated curriculum, starting with smaller lesions and those in safer anatomic locations for at least the first 30 cases.[33] A clear pathway for training for ESD in the US is lacking, although recently a curriculum has been proposed by the ASGE training committee.[34] For physicians in the United States, lack of financial reimbursement of ESD is another discouraging factor. Essentially endoscopists will be incurring higher risk for lower financial reimbursement given the lack of billing codes for a procedure that can be very time-consuming.[35] Recent advocacy efforts by national gastroenterological organizations are underway to ensure appropriate reimbursement for ESD and other complex advanced endoscopic procedures.

Adverse Events

ESD of colorectal lesions is higher risk than that in other anatomic locations (eg, stomach). This is owed to thinner colonic walls especially in the cecum and ascending colon. It is also owed to the presence of lesions on tight flexures and challenging folds, alongside peristaltic movements of the colon.[36] A few common adverse events (AEs) of colonic ESD are:

a) Bleeding

Bleeding as an AE of ESD can either be immediate (intraprocedure/within 24 hours) or delayed (>48 hours), and is usually manageable endoscopically. Various studies of colorectal ESD have found the bleeding rate ranging from as low as 0.4% to 4.6%.[37-39] A meta-analysis by Fuccio and colleagues reported a pooled rate of 2.4%.[40] These findings interestingly are lower than large polyp EMR reported rates although direct-controlled comparisons have not been conducted. Antithrombotic use, antiplatelet use and larger size of resections are well-established risk factors for postprocedural bleeding.[41] Intraprocedural bleeding can be minimized by good choice of traction tools, adequate submucosal injection, step-wise dissection, allowing for the timely identification of the bleeding source and preventive coagulation of visible blood vessels during dissection.[42]

b) Perforation

Perforations are also classified as immediate (recognized mural defect with the visualization of peritoneum intraprocedurally) or delayed (diagnosed after the completion by the presence of free air on imaging). Fuccio and colleagues reported a pooled rate of 5.2% for perforation. [40] Risk factors such as tumor size, colonic location (cecum, right colon or sigmoid colon), submucosal fibrosis are well established to increase chances of ESD associated perforation.[43,44] A recent meta-analysis showed increased tissue fibrosis having an odds ratio (OR) for a perforation of 2.90.[45] Other identified risks such as proximal colonic location had an OR of 2.3 and increased size had an OR of 2.17. Expertise of the endoscopist showed, expectedly, proved to be a protective factor for perforation (OR: 0.96).[45]

c) Post-ESD coagulation syndrome

Post-ESD Coagulation syndrome, similar to postpolypectomy syndrome, is a result of electrocoagulation thermal injury to the bowel wall. The presentation is similar to that of a perforation, presenting as fever, pain, leukocytosis, and tenderness sometimes with rebound and guarding. A prospective multicenter observational trial showed the prevalence of CS of 14.2% after colorectal ESD.[46] It was more prevalent with female gender, cecal lesions, and associated with a longer procedural time.[46] Another study showed a rate of 4.8% of post-ESD CS, all improving with conservative management.[47]

Pathology

High-quality assessment of histopathology of resected lesions is the cornerstone of ESD, and therefore, all ESD specimens should be evaluated by an expert GI pathologist. To help maintain the original integrity and orientation of an en-bloc specimen, it is flattened and affixed to a cork or Styrofoam block with the aid of needles or pins before being put in formalin. This prevents the edges of the lesion from curling. In the pathologic analysis, the lesion is sectioned at 2-mm intervals in a plane perpendicular to the endoscopic resection plane. A thorough assessment of a specimen must comment on dimensions (depth of the lesion, involvement of both vertical and lateral margins), the histology (including the degree of pathologic differentiation), spread (absence or presence of lymphovascular involvement), and lastly the comment on tumor budding if present.[48] It is important to highlight that the colonic mucosa layer is the devoid of lymphatic drainage, and therefore, any dysplasia confined to only the mucosa carries no risk for lymph node metastasis.

Education

Despite robust evidence showing endoscopic resection to be more cost-saving and safer, recent data have shown an increasing rate of surgical removal of benign colonic polyps. A large national inpatient database study showed rates of surgery for nonmalignant colorectal polyps increased from 5.9 to 9.4 per 100,000 US adults from 2004 to 2014, despite colonoscopy volumes being stable.[49] Another study out of the Netherlands using prospective nationwide registry showed that surgical resection for large complex colorectal polyps is still performed very commonly.[50] This trend is alarming and highlights the need for continued physician education for better identification of lesions that could be removed endoscopically and appropriate referral for endoscopic resection or surgery. Importantly, adenocarcinoma in situ or intramucosal cancer should be considered equivalent to high-grade dysplasia in the colon, and essentially lesions that are endoscopically resectable are curable.[51] These lesions should be approached with EMR or ESD as the first-line treatment instead of surgery. Identifying lesions amenable to ESD is important along with timely referral to endoscopist with expertise in the area. The first attempt at resection carries the highest success rate.[52] Endoscopists who do not routinely perform advanced endoscopic resection, should therefore be educated to refrain from partial polypectomies or maneuvers potentially restricting endoscopic en bloc resection such as tattoo injection close to a lesion and extensive biopsies. These practices have been shown to increase the risk of tissue fibrosis and submucosal scarring, which ultimately has shown to be associated with higher risk of bleeding and perforation and lower rates of en-bloc resection.[53]

Future Advancements

Colorectal ESD is a time-consuming, technically challenging procedure that to date is not widely practiced in the US. However, in selected cases, it can prevent unnecessary surgery by proving curative endoscopic resections. The limitations enumerated previously should be addressed to allow for the global adoption of ESD by endoscopists. To ensure the procedure is being performed in a safe and effective manner, further research is needed to develop a curriculum for ESD. As proposed by the ASGE committee, the technical, nontechnical, and cognitive aspects of ESD training should be emphasized and instilled among trainees in ESD training programs.[34] Technology needs to continue to advance to better identify those lesions that benefit most from performing ESD, speed up the dissection process, make the technique less cumbersome and improve the safety margin of ESD. A separate billing code for ESD and reimbursement by third-party payors is also critical if the field is to gain widespread adoption in the US. The current enthusiasm among gastroenterologists as well as endoscopy devices companies is palpable and ESD practice is likely to increase in the future in the US.

ENDOSCOPIC FULL-THICKNESS RESECTION
Introduction

EFTR offers clinical advantages over other endoscopic techniques such as adequate tissue specimen for definitive diagnosis, absolute resection and potentially saving patients from multiple surveillance examinations. EFTR was first described in 2001 by Schurr and colleagues,[54] and the initial prototype constituted of a flexible shaft with the over-the-scope device with a multifunctional front-end which allowed the use of tissue graspers and a cutting mechanism. However, this device never gained widespread popularity due to its large dimensions and limited maneuverability in the GI tract. However, over the last two decades with advances in endoscopic technology, the technology has been refined, and now dedicated EFTR devices and other endoscopic techniques have allowed for growing use of EFTR in the resection of various GI tract lesions. EFTR differs from EMR and ESD in that both these techniques rely on the separation of the mucosa and submucosa from the muscle layer using submucosal injection. EFTR is, therefore, an effective technique for removal of lesions, especially in locations whereby EMR and ESD can be challenging.[55]

Indications

Indications for use of EFTR are evolving, but some indications are outlined in **Box 1** later in discussion.[56–58] Epithelial lesions with suspected deeper infiltration, especially involving or originating from the muscularis propria are not amenable to advanced endoscopic techniques such as EMR or ESD, but can be resected via EFTR. The same applies to neuroendocrine tumors, especially in the rectum given their higher malignant potential. Recurrent adenomas usually have a high degree of submucosal fibrosis owing to multiple resection attempts, thus inadequately lifting in response to submucosal injections and EFTR can be considered for the resection of these lesions. In lesions with no prior resection attempt, and still poor lift suspicion for infiltrative carcinomas should increase, and EFTR could be diagnostic and/or therapeutic in these circumstances. EFTR can also be used in the resection of incidentally found T1a carcinoma whereby a good assessment of negative margins was unable to be made on initial resection. Lastly, lesions in challenging location such as those involving appendiceal orifices or within diverticuli can be amenable to EFTR.[59,60]

Techniques and Devices

EFTR techniques are broadly divided into exposed EFTR and nonexposed EFTR.[61] The term "expose" refers to temporary exposure of the peritoneum before the closure of defect. So, in exposed EFTR, the resection precedes the closure of defect, thus creating a window for "exposure," albeit just temporarily. On the other hand, in nonexposed EFTR, the bowel wall on the serosal side is approximated before the resection of the isolated lesion thus hypothetically eliminating exposure of peritoneum to the GI cavity. This can be achieved by either dedicated EFTR devices or the clip assisted approach.

Nontunneled exposed endoscopic full-thickness resection
This approach is similar to ESD in many ways. It starts with submucosal injection to lift and demarcate lesion. This is followed by mucosal incision and dissection in

Box 1	
Indications for endoscopic full-thickness resection in the colon	
1.	Epithelial Tumors with Deeper Invasion
2.	Removal of subepithelial lesions
3.	Nonlifting lesions
4.	Recurrent adenomas with nonlifting signs.
5.	Lesions associated with significant fibrosis
6.	Lesions in difficult anatomic locations
7.	Sampling for accurate histologic analysis for neuromuscular gut disorders

submucosal space to expose deeper portion of the lesion. Then muscularis is dissected to ensure complete resection followed by extraction and eventual closure of defect. For closure of defect multiple tools have been used. A technique described by Ye and colleagues[62] describes the use of a nylon loop through a double-channel endoscope, in the augmentation of the clips for closure. The nylon loop is opened precisely over all clips to trap them and tighten them together in a ligature. Another approach is that the endoloop is opened over the defect and clips are applied over the loop at different points. The loop is then closed to approximate the edges of the defect.[56] Other tools used are large endoscopic clips such as over-the-scope clips (OTSC).[63] Endoscopic suturing has also been shown to be a safe and effective technique for closure of colonic defects.[64] However, the above approaches for defect closure can be cumbersome and also increasing risks for a perforation.

Tunneled exposed endoscopic full-thickness resection

This approach uses the same principle as peroral endoscopic myotomy (POEM), whereby a mucosal defect is made at a distance of approximately 5 cm from the margin of the lesion. A submucosal tunnel is then formed toward the lesion via dissection. The lesion is dissected and enucleated circumferentially and removed via tunnel. In this technique, only the mucosal defect at the initiation of the tunnel warrants closure, and full-thickness approximation is not needed.

Nonexposed endoscopic full-thickness resection

This "close then cut" technique involves the approximation and fixation of the serosal surface of both adjacent sides of the lesion, such that the lesion is retracted into the lumen allowing full-thickness resection. In this approach the defect is closed before resection, so technically peritoneum is never "exposed" to luminal contents. Devices used to achieve this goal are endoscopic sutures, over-the-scope clips and dedicated full-thickness resection device (FTRD), detailed later in discussion. The development of dedicated FTRDs has led to widespread use of this approach.

Nondedicated Clips for Clips-Assisted Endoscopic Full-Thickness Resection

The Padlock clip (STERIS Corporation Mentor, OH, USA) is a star-shaped, premounted clip available in Standard Padlock size (fits endoscope with 9.5–11 mm diameter), and Padlcok Pro-select (fits 11.5–14 mm). Its flat configuration facilitates snare positioning for the optimal resection of tissue above the clip. As opposed to the Over-The-Scope Clip OTSC (Ovesco Endoscopy GmbH, Tübingen, Germany) the wire for the deployment of Padlock clip is outside the endoscope freeing the working channel.[55]

The OTSC clip is also a premounted clip, using the working channel and a wheel for the deployment similar to standard banding. The OTSC clip comes in 3 sizes of 11 mm, 12 mm, and 14 mm and cap depths of both 3 mm and 6 mm. These clips also have different teeth configurations a (blunt teeth), type t (small spikes on teeth), and type gc (spikes on elongated teeth). For resections in colon, either the 12/6 or 14/6 type t can be used.[55]

These clips are used for nonexposed EFTRs with the close then cut strategy. The target lesion is retracted into the cap using grasping forceps or a retraction device, followed by clip deployment beneath that. The now protruding lesion can be resected with a snare.

One of the limitations to EFTR is lesion size. Studies have suggested adequate resection up to 25 to 30 mm[60,65] but this size is reduced further in cases with colonic scarring. The maximum volume of the lesion that can be incorporated into the device is about 3 cm³, limiting factor being the size of the cap. This is a critical factor in achieving true full-thickness resection. Tumor features and rigidity of the colonic wall are other factors that influence chances of successful resection.

Dedicated Devices

Full-thickness resection device (FTRD; Ovesco Endoscopy, Tübingen, Germany), is a dedicated device for EFTR which has been Food and Drug Administration (FDA) approved since 2017 in the US. The device integrates both an OTSC clip and electro-surgical snare, enabling one-step EFTR with deployment. It comprises a clear cap of a larger depth (23 mm or 21 mm vs 6 mm), preloaded with a modified 14-mm OTSC and a 13 mm monofilament snare integrated on the tip of the cap, with the snare catheter running alongside the shaft of endoscope, contained in a plastic sheath. For colonic lesions, the FTRD comes in 2 sizes, diagnostic (19.5 mm cap diameter and 23 mm cap depth) and colonic (21 mm cap diameter and 23 mm cap depth). The FTRD can be mounted on the standard colonoscope, pediatric colonoscope, or a modified single-channel therapeutic upper endoscope. After marking the margins of the target lesion with Argon Plasma Coagulation (APC) or a marking probe, the lesion is then s retracted into the cap with a grasping device, and the clip is deployed. The pre-loaded snare which is already mounted on the device is then closed and the lesion is resected using electrocautery.

Hybrid Endoscopic Mucosal Resection-Endoscopic Full-Thickness Resection

A hybrid technique incorporating EMR and EFTR is a relatively new and effective approach for the resection of lesions that are not amenable to EFTR alone. This is generally applicable to lesions that lift well, especially at the periphery. The edges of the lesion are injected and resected with cold snare in a piecemeal fashion. This step reduces the size of lesion circumferentially, allowing for the lesion to be amenable to EFTR. Fischer and colleagues were the first to describe this technique whereby the lesion in question was polypoid and exceeded the ideal size for EFTR. Cold snare resection of polyp followed by an EFTR of polyp base was performed.[66] Meier et al then analyzed this technique in 10 patients with 100% success rate and no major complications.[67] Most recently Bauermeister and colleagues published the largest case series of 17 patients with nonlifting colorectal lesions. They reported no major complications and histologic full-thickness resection in 94.1% of the cases and free lateral margins in 76.4% of the patients.[68] Follow-up endoscopy is critical in this subset of patient and ideally should be performed at 6 months after resection.[67,68] Site of resection should be examined carefully, and although most of the OTSC detach within this time frame, if it is still in-situ, there is now a commercially available device that can be used to remove the OTSC or FTRD clips called the remOVE System (Ovesco Endoscopy AG, Tübingen, Germany). This system has shown to be successful in greater than 97% of cases and very safe.[69]

Outcomes

A case series using OTSC targeting lesions in rectosigmoid colon and appendiceal orifice polyps, with mean size 8 mm ± 3 mm, showed 100% complete resection (R0), without any AEs.[70] Similarly, another case series used OTSC device primarily for the removal of colorectal lesions, showed a technical success of 94% and 100% R0 rate.[71] A prospective case series of colorectal EFTR using the padlock clip again showed 100% technical success rate with a 92% full-thickness resection rate.[72]

More robust evidence has been merging in support of the use of FTRD. A retrospective pilot study was published in 2015 suggesting for FTRD to be a safe and effective resection method.[60] To further validate the results, authors went on to conduct a prospective trial of 181 patients in 9 centers showing a technical technically success rate of 89.5%, and R0 resection rate of 76.9%.[73] The WALL RESECT trial is a prospective trial that was conducted across 9 centers in Germany, studying 181 patients who underwent adenoma resection with FTRD. 89.5% of cases were technically successful, with an RO resection rate of 76.9%. 9.9% of patients had some AEs with only 2.2% requiring surgery emergently.[73] Most recently published study augmenting data is an analysis of the German Colonic FTRD registry and is the largest study to date with results from 65 centers and 1178 EFTR procedures incorporated.[74] The study reported a technical success rate of 88.2% and 80% of cases with R0 resection . 58.0% of patient had endoscopic follow-up, with 13.5% showing residual/recurrent lesions warranting repeat endoscopic intervention in majority, with only 2% requiring surgical treatment. Multiple previously reported studies and case-series have yielded similar results.[65,75–77]

Two recent meta-analysis looking at EFTR both from FTRD and clip-assisted method in the whole GI tract showed R0 rate of 82% and 84.9%, full-thickness resection rate of 83% and 89.5%, and technical success rate of 95% and 94%, respectively.[78,79] Even in patient subset with severe neuromuscular disorders of the GI tract a case series showed FTRD for lesions with a mean diameter of 21 mm had a success rate of 100% and no complications.[80]

Adverse Events

The previously mentioned German study remarked EFTR as safe and effective for colorectal lesions.[74] Only 3.1% of 1178 enrolled patients had major AEs. These included 2.5% of the patients that had either immediate or delayed perforation and 0.6% of patients with obstructive or nonobstructive stenosis. About 9% had minor AEs, including 7.1% bleeding risk, 1.3% risk of inflammation or infection, 0.6% with the misplacement of FTRD clip or accidental clipping of grasping device.[74] EFTR near the appendiceal orifice comes with a high risk of appendicitis secondary to the closure of appendiceal orifice. In this study, 89 cases had adenomas at the appendiceal orifice and only 8% had appendicitis, and 3.4% required appendectomy.[74] WALL-RESECT trial showed a similar efficacy profile with 9.9% of patients having either major or minor AEs.[73] Only 3.3% (6/181) of patients had perforation, out of which only 2 patients required surgical closure while others were managed endoscopically. Bleeding was observed in 2.2% of the patients. Out of 34 cases with appendiceal adenoma resection, appendicitis was seen in only 3 patients (8.8%), with 1 patient requiring appendectomy.[73] A recently published meta-analysis showed a pooled estimate of bleeding risk to be 2.2% for bleeding and 0.19% for perforation. Postpolypectomy syndrome rate was estimated to be 2.3%.[79]

Challenges

Nonexposed EFTR remains of restricted utility still given only a small subset of lesions ideal for resection by these techniques. Anatomic location, size, and the chance of involvement of adjacent structures remain the biggest limitation in the safety and efficacy of the procedure. Any tumor with lymph node involvement is not eligible for resection via EFTR by default. For exposed EFTR, leakage of carbon dioxide (CO_2) hinders luminal distention and visibility. With any breach of the mucosal surface into deeper tissue and resultant translocation of GI contents comes the risk of higher infection and local inflammation.[81] In lesions with severe fibrosis the histologic assessment of the superficial mucosal layer may be difficult. This is due to mucosal tears that have inadvertently been made with the grasping forceps when pulling the lesion into the cap. Thus, superficial foci of hemorrhage may appear in the specimen and interfere with the pathologic evaluation.

Although proven to be reasonably effective for lesions ≤20 mm, increased size especially greater than 30 mm, tissue fibrosis and right-sided colonic lesions are at higher risk of incomplete resection.[73] FTRD use is hindered by restricted advancement along the colon owing to the plastic-wrapped endoscope. The increased cap depth, although beneficial for the volume of tissue capture, also restricts the field of view and maneuverability through sharp flexures, potentially increasing the chances of failure. An acute perforation owing to the malfunction of device such as snare dysfunction or failed clip deployment should always be a consideration.

Future Directions

One of the key issues in the further advancement of endoscopic full-thickness resection is the lack of head-to-head data comparing surgical resection to EFTR. It is well established that surgery enables precise resection with reliable closure of defects, and assessment of lymph nodes ideal for more advanced lesions.[82] EFTR is a minimally invasive and safe approach that is ideal for lesions with low risk of tumor seeding, small mesenchymal tumors, and early localized malignant lesions.[58] Although recent developments in technology have made EFTR more widely available with ease of use and acceptable safety profile, patient selection is key to improved outcomes. Additional prospective trials looking at safety, efficacy, degree of resection, and closure are needed. Areas of further research based on location, size, type of lesion, and risk of seeding will be crucial in determining subset lesions that EFTR is most efficacious in resecting.[56] Lastly as most advanced endoscopic resection procedures, a standardized protocol for EFTR training is lacking. In the future, direction from leading GI societies will be crucial for the evaluation of competence and shaping training for EFTR.[55]

CLINICS CARE POINTS

- When examining colonic lesions use NBI and surface features to help classify lesions according to NICE, Paris and Kudo classification to assess the risk of deep invasion.
- When considering referral for endoscopic resection, avoid excessive biopsy or tattooing of the lesion. Good assessment and photo documentation is critical.
- ESD has comparable outcomes to surgery for long-term efficacy.
- ESD has a much lower risk of lesion recurrence when compared with EMR.
- Multiple longitudinal studies have proven for EFTR to provide high R0 resection rates.
- Consider ESD/EFTR if lesion is amenable to either before surgical referral.

ACKNOWLEDGMENTS

None

DISCLOSURE

None.

REFERENCES

1. Ono H, Kondo H, Gotoda T, et al. Endoscopic mucosal resection for treatment of early gastric cancer. Gut 2001;48(2):225–9.
2. Oyama T. Esophageal ESD: technique and prevention of complications. Gastrointest Endosc Clin N Am 2014;24(2):201–12.
3. Draganov PV, Wang AY, Othman MO, et al. AGA Institute Clinical Practice Update: Endoscopic Submucosal Dissection in the United States. Clin Gastroenterol Hepatol 2019;17(1):16–25.e1.
4. Tanaka S, Kashida H, Saito Y, et al. JGES guidelines for colorectal endoscopic submucosal dissection/endoscopic mucosal resection. Dig Endosc 2015;27(4): 417–34.
5. Saito Y. Indication for colorectal ESD. In: Fukami N, editor. Endoscopic submucosal dissection: Principles and Practice. New York, (NY): Springer New York; 2015. p. 19–24.
6. Kaltenbach T, et al. Endoscopic Removal of Colorectal Lesions: Recommendations by the US Multi-Society Task Force on Colorectal Cancer. Am J Gastroenterol 2020;115(3):435–64.
7. Kudo S, et al. Diagnosis of colorectal tumorous lesions by magnifying endoscopy. Gastrointest Endosc 1996;44(1):8–14.
8. Mounzer R, et al. Endoscopic and surgical treatment of malignant colorectal polyps: a population-based comparative study. Gastrointest Endosc 2015; 81(3):733–40.e2.
9. Gangireddy VGR, et al. Polypectomy versus surgery in early colon cancer: size and location of colon cancer affect long-term survival. Int J Colorectal Dis 2018;33(10):1349–57.
10. Law R, et al. Endoscopic resection is cost-effective compared with laparoscopic resection in the management of complex colon polyps: an economic analysis. Gastrointest Endosc 2016;83(6):1248–57.
11. Jayanna M, et al. Cost Analysis of Endoscopic Mucosal Resection vs Surgery for Large Laterally Spreading Colorectal Lesions. Clin Gastroenterol Hepatol 2016; 14(2):271–8.e1-2.
12. Nakajima T, et al. Current status of endoscopic resection strategy for large, early colorectal neoplasia in Japan. Surg Endosc 2013;27(9):3262–70.
13. Burgess NG, et al. Risk Stratification for Covert Invasive Cancer Among Patients Referred for Colonic Endoscopic Mucosal Resection: A Large Multicenter Cohort. Gastroenterology 2017;153(3):732–42.e1.
14. Fujiya M, et al. Efficacy and adverse events of EMR and endoscopic submucosal dissection for the treatment of colon neoplasms: a meta-analysis of studies comparing EMR and endoscopic submucosal dissection. Gastrointest Endosc 2015;81(3):583–95.
15. De Ceglie A, et al. Endoscopic mucosal resection and endoscopic submucosal dissection for colorectal lesions: A systematic review. Crit Rev Oncol Hematol 2016;104:138–55.
16. Arezzo A, et al. Systematic review and meta-analysis of endoscopic submucosal dissection vs endoscopic mucosal resection for colorectal lesions. United European Gastroenterol J 2016;4(1):18–29.
17. Mehta N, et al. Recurrence with malignancy after endoscopic resection of large colon polyps with high-grade dysplasia: incidence and risk factors. Surg Endosc 2021;35(6):2500–8.

18. Oka S, et al. Local recurrence after endoscopic resection for large colorectal neoplasia: a multicenter prospective study in Japan. Am J Gastroenterol 2015; 110(5):697–707.
19. Saito Y, et al. How to Perform a High-Quality Endoscopic Submucosal Dissection. Gastroenterology 2021;161(2):405–10.
20. Sanchez-Yague A, et al. The endoscopic cap that can (with videos). Gastrointest Endosc 2012;76(1):169–78.e1-2.
21. Harlow C, et al. *Endoscopic submucosal dissection: an update on tools and accessories.* Therapeutic Advances in Gastrointestinal Endoscopy 2020;13. 2631774520957220.
22. Bhatt A, et al. Indications and Techniques for Endoscopic Submucosal Dissection. Am J Gastroenterol 2015;110(6):784–91.
23. Takezawa T, et al. The pocket-creation method facilitates colonic endoscopic submucosal dissection (with video). Gastrointest Endosc 2019;89(5):1045–53.
24. Yoshida N, Naito Y, Yasuda R, et al. The efficacy of the pocket-creation method for cases with severe fibrosis in colorectal endoscopic submucosal dissection. Endosc Int Open 2018;6(8):E975–83.
25. Oyama T. Counter traction makes endoscopic submucosal dissection easier. Clin Endosc 2012;45(4):375–8.
26. Yamasaki Y, Takeuchi Y, Hanaoka N, et al. A novel traction method using an endoclip attached to a nylon string during colonic endoscopic submucosal dissection. Endoscopy 2015;47. Suppl 1 UCTN: p. E238-9.
27. Ritsuno H, Sakamoto N, Osada T, et al. Prospective clinical trial of traction device-assisted endoscopic submucosal dissection of large superficial colorectal tumors using the S-O clip. Surg Endosc 2014;28(11):3143–9.
28. Ye L, Yuan X, Pang M, et al. Magnetic bead-assisted endoscopic submucosal dissection: a gravity-based traction method for treating large superficial colorectal tumors. Surg Endosc 2019;33(6):2034–41.
29. Uraoka T, et al. Advantages of using thin endoscope-assisted endoscopic submucosal dissection technique for large colorectal tumors. Dig Endosc 2010; 22(3):186–91.
30. Jawaid S, Yang D, Draganov PV. Tissue retractor system–assisted endoscopic submucosal dissection of a large rectal tumor with significant fibrosis from direct tattooing. VideoGIE 2019;4(2):84–6.
31. Sharma S, Momose K, Hara H, et al. Facilitating endoscopic submucosal dissection: double balloon endolumenal platform significantly improves dissection time compared with conventional technique (with video). Surg Endosc 2019;33(1): 315–21.
32. Draganov PV, Aihara H, Karasik MS, et al. Endoscopic Submucosal Dissection in North America: A Large Prospective Multicenter Study. Gastroenterology 2021; 160(7):2317–27.e2.
33. Pimentel-Nunes P, Pioche M, Albéniz E, et al. Curriculum for endoscopic submucosal dissection training in Europe: European Society of Gastrointestinal Endoscopy (ESGE) Position Statement. Endoscopy 2019;51(10):980–92.
34. Aihara H, Dacha S, Anand GS, et al. Core curriculum for endoscopic submucosal dissection (ESD). Gastrointest Endosc 2021;93(6):1215–21.
35. Rex DK, Hassan C, Dewitt JM. Colorectal endoscopic submucosal dissection in the United States: Why do we hear so much about it and do so little of it? Gastrointest Endosc 2017;85(3):554–8.
36. Saito Y, Otake Y, Sakamoto T, et al. Indications for and technical aspects of colorectal endoscopic submucosal dissection. Gut Liver 2013;7(3):263–9.

37. Toyonaga T, Nishino E, Man IM, et al. Principles of quality controlled endoscopic submucosal dissection with appropriate dissection level and high quality resected specimen. Clin Endosc 2012;45(4):362–74.

38. Lee EJ, Lee JB, Lee SH, et al. Endoscopic submucosal dissection for colorectal tumors–1,000 colorectal ESD cases: one specialized institute's experiences. Surg Endosc 2013;27(1):31–9.

39. Takeuchi Y, Ohta T, Matsui F, et al. Indication, strategy and outcomes of endoscopic submucosal dissection for colorectal neoplasm. Dig Endosc 2012;(24 Suppl 1):100–4.

40. Fuccio L, Hassan C, Ponchon T, et al. Clinical outcomes after endoscopic submucosal dissection for colorectal neoplasia: a systematic review and meta-analysis. Gastrointest Endosc 2017;86(1):74–86.e17.

41. Kataoka Y, Tsuji Y, Sakaguchi Y, et al. Bleeding after endoscopic submucosal dissection: Risk factors and preventive methods. World J Gastroenterol 2016; 22(26):5927–35.

42. Ahmed Y, Othman M. EMR/ESD: Techniques, Complications, and Evidence. Curr Gastroenterol Rep 2020;22(8):39.

43. Hong SN, Byeon JS, Lee B, et al. Prediction model and risk score for perforation in patients undergoing colorectal endoscopic submucosal dissection. Gastrointest Endosc 2016;84(1):98–108.

44. Kim ES, Cho KB, Park KS, et al. Factors predictive of perforation during endoscopic submucosal dissection for the treatment of colorectal tumors. Endoscopy 2011;43(7):573–8.

45. Santos JB, Nobre MRC, Oliveira CZ, et al. Risk factors for adverse events of colorectal endoscopic submucosal dissection: a systematic review and meta-analysis. Eur J Gastroenterol Hepatol 2020;34(3).

46. Arimoto J, Higurashi T, Kato S, et al. Risk factors for post-colorectal endoscopic submucosal dissection (ESD) coagulation syndrome: a multicenter, prospective, observational study. Endosc Int Open 2018;6(3):E342–9.

47. Ito S, Hotta K, Imai K, et al. Risk factors of post-endoscopic submucosal dissection electrocoagulation syndrome for colorectal neoplasm. J Gastroenterol Hepatol 2018;33(12):2001–6.

48. Pimentel-Nunes P, Dinis-Ribeiro M, Ponchon T, et al. Endoscopic submucosal dissection: European Society of Gastrointestinal Endoscopy (ESGE) Guideline. Endoscopy 2015;47(9):829–54.

49. Peery AF, Cools KS, Strassle PD, et al. Increasing Rates of Surgery for Patients With Nonmalignant Colorectal Polyps in the United States. Gastroenterology 2018;154(5):1352–60.e3.

50. Bronzwaer MES, Koens LB, Willem A, et al. Volume of surgery for benign colorectal polyps in the last 11 years. Gastrointest Endosc 2018;87(2):552–61.e1.

51. Bourke MJ, Neuhaus H, Bergman JJ. Endoscopic Submucosal Dissection: Indications and Application in Western Endoscopy Practice. Gastroenterology 2018; 154(7):1887–900.e5.

52. Moss A, Bourke MJ, Williams SJ, et al. Endoscopic mucosal resection outcomes and prediction of submucosal cancer from advanced colonic mucosal neoplasia. Gastroenterology 2011;140(7):1909–18.

53. Jeong JY, Oh YH, Yu YH, et al. Does submucosal fibrosis affect the results of endoscopic submucosal dissection of early gastric tumors? Gastrointest Endosc 2012;76(1):59–66.

54. Full thickness resection device (FTRD) for endoluminal removal of large bowel tumours: development of the instrument and related experimental studies. Minim Invasive Ther Allied Technol 2001;10(6):301–9.

55. Rajan E, Wong Kee LM. Song, Endoscopic Full Thickness Resection. Gastroenterology 2018;154(7):1925–37.e2.

56. Aslanian HR, Sethi A, Bhutani MS, et al. ASGE guideline for endoscopic full-thickness resection and submucosal tunnel endoscopic resection. VideoGIE 2019;4(8):343–50.

57. von Helden A, Hildenbrand R, Sido B, et al. Endoscopic full-thickness resection using an over-the-scope device for treatment of recurrent/residual colorectal neoplasia: a single-center case series. BMC Gastroenterol 2019;19(1):121.

58. Schmidt A, Meier B, Caca K. *Endoscopic full-thickness resection: Current status.* World J Gastroenterol 2015;21(31):9273–85.

59. Valli PV, Kaufmann M, Vrugt B, et al. Endoscopic resection of a diverticulum-arisen colonic adenoma using a full-thickness resection device. Gastroenterology 2014;147(5):969–71.

60. Schmidt A, Bauerfeind P, Gubler C, et al. Endoscopic full-thickness resection in the colorectum with a novel over-the-scope device: first experience. Endoscopy 2015;47(8):719–25.

61. Modayil R, Stavropoulos SN. A Western Perspective on "New NOTES" from POEM to Full-thickness Resection and Beyond. Gastrointest Endosc Clin N Am 2016; 26(2):413–32.

62. Ye L-P, Yu Z, Mao X, et al. Endoscopic full-thickness resection with defect closure using clips and an endoloop for gastric subepithelial tumors arising from the muscularis propria. Surg Endosc 2014;28(6):1978–83.

63. Guo J, Liu Z, Sun S, et al. Endoscopic full-thickness resection with defect closure using an over-the-scope clip for gastric subepithelial tumors originating from the muscularis propria. Surg Endosc 2015;29(11):3356–62.

64. Kantsevoy SV, Bitner M, Hajiyeva G, et al. Endoscopic management of colonic perforations: clips versus suturing closure (with videos). Gastrointest Endosc 2016;84(3):487–93.

65. Richter-Schrag HJ, Walker C, Thimme R, et al. [Full thickness resection device (FTRD). Experience and outcome for benign neoplasms of the rectum and colon]. Chirurg 2016;87(4):316–25.

66. Fischer A, Knoop RF, Walker C, et al. Resection of a large rectal polyp with the simultaneous combination of snare polypectomy and full-thickness resection device resection. Endoscopy 2015;47(Suppl 1):E607–8.

67. Meier B, Caca K, Schmidt A. Hybrid endoscopic mucosal resection and full-thickness resection: a new approach for resection of large non-lifting colorectal adenomas (with video). Surg Endosc 2017;31(10):4268–74.

68. Bauermeister M, Mende M, Hornoff S, et al. Hybrid resection of large colorectal adenomas combining EMR and FTRD. Scandinavian Journal of Gastroenterology 2021;56(8):978–83.

69. Caputo A, Schmidt A, Caca K, et al. Efficacy and safety of the remOVE System for OTSC(®) and FTRD(®) clip removal: data from a PMCF analysis. Minim Invasive Ther Allied Technol 2018;27(3):138–42.

70. Al-Bawardy B, Rajan E, Wong Kee LM. Song, Over-the-scope clip-assisted endoscopic full-thickness resection of epithelial and subepithelial GI lesions. Gastrointest Endosc 2017;85(5):1087–92.

71. Fähndrich M, Sandmann M. Endoscopic full-thickness resection for gastrointestinal lesions using the over-the-scope clip system: a case series. Endoscopy 2015;47(1):76–9.

72. Backes Y, Kappelle WFW, Berk L, et al. Colorectal endoscopic full-thickness resection using a novel, flat-base over-the-scope clip: a prospective study. Endoscopy 2017;49(11):1092–7.

73. Schmidt A, Beyna T, Schumacher B, et al. Colonoscopic full-thickness resection using an over-the-scope device: a prospective multicentre study in various indications. Gut 2018;67(7):1280–9.

74. Meier B, Stritzke B, Kuellmer A, et al. Efficacy and Safety of Endoscopic Full-Thickness Resection in the Colorectum: Results From the German Colonic FTRD Registry. Am J Gastroenterol 2020;115(12):1998–2006.

75. Aepli P, Criblez D, Baumeler S, et al. Endoscopic full thickness resection (EFTR) of colorectal neoplasms with the Full Thickness Resection Device (FTRD): Clinical experience from two tertiary referral centers in Switzerland. United European Gastroenterol J 2018;6(3):463–70.

76. Velegraki M, Trikola A, Vasiliadis K, et al. Endoscopic full-thickness resection of colorectal lesions with the full-thickness resection device: clinical experience from two referral centers in Greece. Ann Gastroenterol 2019;32(5):482–8.

77. Schmidt A, Damm M, Caca K. Endoscopic full-thickness resection using a novel over-the-scope device. Gastroenterology 2014;147(4):740–2.e2.

78. Brewer Gutierrez OI, Akshintala VS, Ichkhanian Y, et al. Endoscopic full-thickness resection using a clip non-exposed method for gastrointestinal tract lesions: a meta-analysis. Endosc Int Open 2020;8(3):E313–25.

79. Li P, Ma B, Gong S, et al. Efficacy and safety of endoscopic full-thickness resection in the colon and rectum using an over-the-scope device: a meta-analysis. Surg Endosc 2021;35(1):249–59.

80. Valli PV, Pohl D, Fried M, et al. Diagnostic use of endoscopic full-thickness wall resection (eFTR)-a novel minimally invasive technique for colonic tissue sampling in patients with severe gastrointestinal motility disorders. Neurogastroenterol Motil 2018;30(1).

81. Goto O, Takeuchi H, Kitagawa Y, et al. Endoscopic Submucosal Dissection (ESD) and Related Techniques as Precursors of "New Notes" Resection Methods for Gastric Neoplasms. Gastrointest Endosc Clin N Am 2016;26(2):313–22.

82. Meining A. Endoscopic full-thickness resection: the logical step toward more extended endoscopic oncologic resections? Endoscopy 2015;47(2):101–2.

Management of Antiplatelet and Anticoagulant Agents before and after Polypectomy

Jennifer J. Telford, MD, MPH, FRCPC, FACG, FCAG[a],*,
Neena S. Abraham, MD, MSc (Epi), FASGE, FACG, AGAF[b]

KEYWORDS

- Antithrombotic • Anticoagulant • Antiplatelet • Colonoscopy • Polypectomy
- Postpolypectomy bleeding • Cold snare polypectomy

KEY POINTS

- Antithrombotic use increases the risk of postpolypectomy bleeding.
- Careful consideration of thromboembolic risk versus postpolypectomy bleeding should be considered, as well as patient preferences.
- Cold snare polypectomy and prophylactic clipping of large polypectomy sites may help prevent postpolypectomy bleeding.

BACKGROUND

Several antithrombotic medications are available with different mechanisms of action, half-lives, and times to effect (**Table 1**). These are broadly divided into agents that affect platelet function and those that affect coagulation factors. Antiplatelet and anticoagulant agents are indicated to prevent thromboembolism in at-risk patients, as summarized later in discussion.

Antiplatelet agents

- Acute coronary syndrome
- Postcoronary stent
- Postperipheral artery stent
- Stroke/transient ischemic attack

Anticoagulant agents

- Atrial fibrillation

[a] Division of Gastroenterology, Department of Medicine, University of British Columbia, 770-1190 Hornby Street, Vancouver, British Columbia V6Z2K5, Canada; [b] Division of Gastroenterology and Hepatology, Department of Medicine, Mayo Clinic, 13400 E Shea Blvd, Scottsdale, AZ 85259, USA
* Corresponding author.
E-mail address: jtelford@telus.net

Gastrointest Endoscopy Clin N Am 32 (2022) 299–312
https://doi.org/10.1016/j.giec.2021.12.006
1052-5157/22/© 2021 Elsevier Inc. All rights reserved.

Table 1
Antithrombotic agents

	Mechanism of Action	When to Stop	When to Resume
Anticoagulant Agents			
Warfarin	Vitamin K antagonist	5 d	Same day
Direct-Acting Oral Anticoagulants			
Dabigatran	Thrombin inhibitor	1–2 d	Next day
Rivaroxaban	Factor Xa inhibitor	2 d	Next day
Apixaban	Factor Xa inhibitor	2 d	Next day
Edoxaban	Factor Xa inhibitor	2 d	Next day
Betrixaban	Factor Xa inhibitor	2 d	Next day
Antiplatelet Agents			
Acetylsalicylic Acid	Platelet cyclooxygenase-1 inhibitor	Do not stop	Do not stop
$P2Y_{12}$ Inhibitors			
Ticagrelor	Platelet $P2Y_{12}$ receptor antagonist	4 d	Optimal timing unknown; preferably within 24 h following the procedure
Clopidogrel	Platelet $P2Y_{12}$ receptor antagonist	7 d	Optimal timing unknown; preferably within 24 h following the procedure
Prasugrel	Platelet $P2Y_{12}$ receptor antagonist	7 d	Optimal timing unknown; preferably within 24 h following the procedure
Ticlopidine	Platelet $P2Y_{12}$ receptor antagonist	10–14 d	Optimal timing unknown; preferably within 24 h following the procedure

- Mechanical heart valve
- Venous thromboembolic disease
- Thrombophilia

It is now commonplace for a gastroenterologist to be asked for recommendations regarding antithrombotic management before and following colonoscopy. The risk of postpolypectomy bleeding without antithrombotic interruption is weighed against the risk of sustained thromboembolic complication due to antithrombotic interruption. Often, the patient's hematologist, cardiologist, or neurologist is involved in the peri-procedural antithrombotic management, particularly in the context of a patient at high risk of thromboembolism or a more advanced polyp resection.

There are very few randomized trials comparing different management strategies in patients on antithrombotic agents undergoing colonoscopy and polypectomy. Our best sources of evidence are derived from large, multicenter studies that include all surgeries and invasive procedures but do not report specific outcomes in the colonoscopy subgroup. Often, these trials exclude those patients at the highest risk of thromboembolism. Published cohort studies specific to colonoscopy are difficult to interpret due to confounding as patient and physician factors may influence peri-procedural antithrombotic management and decisions regarding the polypectomy approach. Also, there is an observed inconsistency between studies in outcomes definition and ascertainment, follow-up time, and polypectomy technique, including prophylactic measures to prevent postpolypectomy bleeding. Several guidelines address the management of antithrombotic medications before and following colonoscopy; however, these are based on low-quality evidence. As physicians incorporate these guidelines into their clinical practice, it is important to recognize that, in the absence of high-quality studies to inform decisions, patient preferences are essential to decisions regarding the interruption of antithrombotic drugs.

DISCUSSION
Patient Preferences and Shared Decision-Making

Perceptions and values regarding antithrombotic therapy vary among patients and between patients and their physicians.[1] Generally, patients will accept a higher gastrointestinal (GI) bleeding risk to prevent a stroke or an acute coronary event,[2–4] but these preferences are influenced by a patient's personal experience with bleeding or thromboembolism.[3]

Physicians may respond more strongly to the risk of postpolypectomy bleeding as it is an outcome they experience immediately and may treat following resumption of the antithrombotic agent.[1,5] Whereas a stroke may occur later, perhaps without the knowledge of the physician performing the colonoscopy. Physicians should be mindful of the potential for unconscious biases and ensure they identify the management strategy most in keeping with the patient's preferences.

A patient may elect to continue the antithrombotic agent for their procedure after a risk-benefit discussion with their gastroenterologist, cardiologist, hematologist, and/ or neurologist. During consent, gastroenterologists can specify that removing subcentimeter polyps by cold snare polypectomy is possible without the temporary interruption of antiplatelet or anticoagulant drugs; however, a repeat colonoscopy with medication discontinuation may be required to excise a larger polyp safely. Alternatively, an approach of universal temporary interruption can be adopted in the anticipation of performing small and large polypectomy at index colonoscopy after appropriate discussion with the patient. The latter approach may be favorable in the setting of open-access endoscopy.

Clinical Practice Guidelines Addressing Antithrombotics and Polypectomy

Several clinical practice guidelines address the management of antithrombotic medications in patients undergoing endoscopic procedures.[6–9] These recommendations distinguish between endoscopic procedures at low or high risk of postprocedure bleeding and categorize patients based on their risk of thromboembolism (**Table 2**).[10,11] All guidelines endorse the safety of colonoscopic biopsy without temporary interruption of antithrombotic drugs. In contrast, polypectomy has traditionally been considered a high-risk bleeding intervention for which antiplatelet agents, except for acetylsalicylic acid (ASA), and anticoagulants are temporarily interrupted. In addition to low and high-risk bleeding procedures, the Asian guidelines classified endoscopic submucosal dissection and endoscopic mucosal resection (EMR) of lesions greater than 2 cm as ultra-high-risk procedures and suggested withholding ASA.[8]

However, with increasing uptake of nonthermal polypectomy techniques, there is a growing acceptance to classify cold snare polypectomy of polyps (up to 1 cm) as a low-risk bleeding risk procedure. Such a low-risk procedure might be performed safely without temporary interruption of antiplatelet or anticoagulant drugs, which are appealing as most polyps discovered at colonoscopy will be less than 1 cm in size.[7,9] However, endorsement of this strategy is based on very limited data, as discussed later in this review.

Table 2
Risk of thromboembolism in patients prescribed an oral anticoagulant

Risk Category	Mechanical Heart Valve	Atrial Fibrillation	Venous Thromboembolism
High	• Mitral position (any) • Aortic position (older: caged-ball or tilting disc) • TIA/stroke within 3 mo	• CHADS$_2$ score 5 or 6 • CHA$_2$DS$_2$VASc score $\geq$ 7 • TIA/stroke within 3 mo • Rheumatic valvular heart disease	• VTE within 3 mo • Severe thrombophilia: ○ Protein C deficiency ○ Protein S deficiency ○ Antithrombin deficiency ○ Antiphospholipid antibodies • Multiple thrombophilias • Venocaval filter • Active cancer[a]
Moderate	• Bileaflet aortic valve prosthesis plus 1 of: ○ Atrial fibrillation ○ Prior TIA/stroke ○ Hypertension ○ Diabetes ○ Congestive heart failure ○ Age > 75 y	• CHADS$_2$ score 3 or 4 • CHA$_2$DS$_2$VASc score 5 or 6	• VTE within 3–12 mo • Recurrent VTE • Nonsevere thrombophilia • Cancer within 5 y
Low	• Bileaflet aortic valve prosthesis	CHADS$_2$ score $\leq$ 2	• Single VTE > 12 mo

[a] Consider pancreatic, gastric, brain, and myeloproliferative.
Data from Refs [10,11].

Colonic polyps greater than 1 cm pose a greater risk of immediate and delayed postpolypectomy bleeding,[12–16] and most require a short period of temporary interruption of the anticoagulant or non-ASA antiplatelet drug as outlined later in discussion.

Patients prescribed a non-ASA thienopyridine antiplatelet drug (clopidogrel, prasugrel) should be instructed to hold their antiplatelet agent for 7 days before the colonoscopy. Patients prescribed ticagrelor can discontinue their drugs for a shorter period of 4 days, as this nonthienopyridine is the only reversible platelet P2Y$_{12}$ receptor antagonist. Resumption is recommended once immediate hemostasis is achieved, ideally within 24 hours. However, as described later in discussion, gastroenterologists should avoid temporary interruption of these specific agents during periods when the patient is at the highest risk of thrombotic events and consider deferring the colonoscopy until the antiplatelet can be safely held.

For patients anticoagulated with warfarin, the accepted standard is to discontinue warfarin 5 days before the colonoscopy and polypectomy and resume the day of the procedure, provided endoscopic hemostasis was attained. Bridging during warfarin interruption is not required unless the patient has a high-risk thromboembolic condition (see **Table 2**), such as certain mechanical heart valves, atrial fibrillation plus mitral stenosis, or a high CHADS$_2$/CHA$_2$DS$_2$VASc score, or recent venous thromboembolism or cerebrovascular event. In this situation, bridge therapy, typically with low molecular weight heparin, is begun 3 days before the colonoscopy and polypectomy, held the day of the procedure, and then continued for 3 to 5 days following, until the patient's INR reaches the target range. Direct oral anticoagulants (DOAC) are discontinued 1 to 2 days before colonoscopy and polypectomy with resumption the day after the procedure if endoscopic hemostasis is achieved. Bridge anticoagulation is not required, as these agents achieve therapeutic levels within hours of resumption.[17]

Could Colonoscopy Be Deferred?

Among the patient group at the highest risk of thromboembolic events, there are several clinical scenarios in which antithrombotic medication should not be interrupted for a specified period.

Patients who have been diagnosed with one of the following in the previous 3 months:

- Transient ischemic attack,
- Stroke,
- Lower extremity deep vein thrombosis
- Pulmonary embolus, or
- Acute coronary syndrome event

Patients who have undergone coronary stent placement:

- Drug-eluting stent placement within the previous 6 months,
- Bare metal stent placement within the previous month,
- Acute coronary syndrome event *plus* drug-eluting stent placement within the previous 6 months, or
- Acute coronary syndrome event *plus* bare metal stent within the previous 2 months.

Whether colonoscopy can be safely deferred depends on the indication and the patient's risk of a thrombotic event (as highlighted above and in **Table 2**). Colonoscopy undertaken for average-risk screening, previous neoplastic polyps or colorectal cancer surveillance, or a family history of colorectal cancer could reasonably be deferred until the minimum period of antithrombotic therapy is complete. For patients with a positive fecal immunochemical test (FIT), a recent systematic review of 8 studies concluded that colonoscopy performed beyond 9 months of a positive FIT was associated with a higher incidence of colorectal cancer and advanced-stage colorectal cancer.[18] While most colon screening programs use 1 or 2 months as the benchmark time to complete colonoscopy following a positive FIT,[19,20] these data indicate it is reasonable to wait if aligned with the patient's wishes. Similarly, the urgency by which a luminal cause of iron deficiency anemia or abdominal symptoms is sought can be dictated by the patient's presentation, the risk for advanced luminal lesions, and their underlying thrombotic risk, which determines the safety of temporary interruption of the antithrombotic agent.

Through informed discussion, a shared decision is reached to either:

1) Defer colonoscopy in patients at higher risk of thromboembolism until the minimum period of necessary continuous antithrombotic therapy is complete, or
2) Undergo colonoscopy with the understanding that a repeat procedure may be necessary to remove larger polyps at higher risk of postpolypectomy bleeding.

Antithrombotic Agents and Polypectomy: What We Know to Date

Polypectomy and acetylsalicylic acid

ASA monotherapy is used for secondary cardioprevention in doses from 81 mg to 325 mg per day. In general, ASA does not need to be interrupted before colonoscopy and polypectomy. ASA interruption is associated with an increase in thromboembolic events, and the risk of postpolypectomy bleeding seems to be very low.[21,22] However, removal of large colonic polyps ($\geq$1 cm) will carry a higher bleeding risk, and this needs to be balanced against the patient's cardiovascular risk and their preferences regarding bleeding complications versus thromboembolic complications.

Polypectomy and P2Y$_{12}$ receptor inhibitors

P2Y$_{12}$ inhibitors, including the thienopyridine agents clopidogrel, prasugrel, and ticlopidine, and the nonthienopyridine agent ticagrelor, are used in the treatment of patients with coronary or peripheral artery stent placement, recent acute coronary syndrome event, and transient ischemic attack (TIA) or stroke.[23,24] The newer P2Y$_{12}$ agents have largely replaced ticlopidine due to a less favorable side effect profile. Dual antiplatelet therapy (DAPT) combines a P2Y$_{12}$ inhibitor with ASA and is recommended, often temporarily, for patients who have acute coronary syndrome with or without percutaneous coronary intervention.[25]

Whether P2Y$_{12}$ inhibitors should be interrupted before colonoscopy and polypectomy has been addressed in 2 randomized trials comparing continued clopidogrel to placebo, with or without ASA, in patients undergoing colonoscopy and polypectomy.[26,27] Chan and colleagues included various polypectomy techniques (42.8% cold biopsy or cold snare) and did not allow prophylaxis against postpolypectomy bleeding with clipping. There was no significant difference in the rate of immediate postpolypectomy bleeding, delayed postpolypectomy bleeding, or thromboembolic events between the clopidogrel and placebo groups. The delayed postpolypectomy bleeding rate was 3.8% and 3.6% in the clopidogrel and placebo arms, respectively. Won and colleagues included patients undergoing cold snare polypectomy of polyps $\leq$ 1 cm and reported similar delayed postpolypectomy bleeding rates between those randomized to continue DAPT (1/42%, 2.4%) versus ASA alone (0/45).[27] However, both trials had low numbers of postpolypectomy bleeding events and wide confidence intervals, raising concerns about whether the sample size was large enough to detect a true difference.[7]

Adding to our understanding of bleeding risk with uninterrupted thienopyridines is the prospective cohort study by Feagins and colleagues,[22] which reported 7.3% of patients on continuous P2Y$_{12}$ inhibitors experienced postpolypectomy bleeding (69.2% cold biopsy or cold snare). Immediate postpolypectomy bleeding was more common following cold forceps removal, while delayed bleeding was exclusively seen in patients who underwent hot snare polypectomy. A subsequent systematic review and meta-analysis including the Chan and Feagins studies reported a significant increase in the rate of delayed postpolypectomy bleeding in patients continued on clopidogrel.[28] This meta-analysis has methodologic concerns as it mislabels a cohort study as a randomized trial and pools randomized trials with observational studies.

Overall, these data suggest that hot-snare polypectomy without temporary interruption may be associated with an increased risk of delayed bleeding. An emerging body of literature suggests cold polypectomy techniques may be associated with less delayed postpolypectomy bleeding in patients who continue their P2Y$_{12}$ inhibitor, acknowledging the potential for increased intraprocedural bleeding.

Polypectomy and warfarin

Vitamin K antagonists (VKA), such as warfarin, were the only oral anticoagulants available until 2011, when the DOACs were approved to prevent stroke in patients with nonvalvular atrial fibrillation.[29] While most consensus guidelines recommend discontinuing warfarin before colonoscopic polypectomy, with heparin bridging depending on the underlying thromboembolic risk of the patient, the data to support this recommendation are lacking.[6–8]

Whether uninterrupted warfarin increases the risk of postpolypectomy bleeding, particularly in the context of nonthermal polypectomy techniques, has been addressed in a small trial randomizing patients with polyps up to 1 cm in size to continuous warfarin and cold snare polypectomy, versus interrupted warfarin with heparin bridging and hot snare polypectomy.[30] The former strategy was noninferior with no patients in the uninterrupted warfarin/cold snare group (0/30) and 12.0% (3/25) of patients in the interrupted warfarin/hot snare group sustaining major bleeding with a risk difference of 12.0% (95% CI: -0.7–24.7). This study failed to control for the polypectomy technique, evaluating 2 interventions simultaneously. Additional methodological issues include patient recruitment, which was not consecutive, that patients and physicians were not blinded to the patient's allocation, and the small sample size with few bleeding events. While this study is challenging to interpret, the results seem to support the evolving paradigm of cold snare excision of small polyps on uninterrupted warfarin.

Larger polyps, however, may require temporary interruption of warfarin with or without heparin bridging. The BRIDGE trial assessed the indication for heparin bridging. Patients with atrial fibrillation, who were not at high risk of embolism (see **Table 2**), undergoing an invasive procedure, including colonoscopy and polypectomy, were randomized to low molecular weight heparin bridging or placebo.[31] The control group was noninferior to the bridged group in the risk of arterial thromboembolism; however, the risk of postprocedural bleeding was lower in patients that were not bridged (Relative Risk 0.41, 95% CI: 0.02–0.78).

In summary, patients on warfarin may elect to continue anticoagulation with the removal of polyps up to 1 cm in size with cold snare polypectomy with the understanding that repeats colonoscopy with warfarin interruption may be indicated if a larger polyp is detected.

Polypectomy and direct oral anticoagulants

DOACs including, apixaban, dabigatran, edoxaban, and rivaroxaban, are used for secondary thromboembolic prevention, treatment of venous thromboembolism, and stroke prevention in patients with nonvalvular atrial fibrillation.[29] There is evolving data that GI bleeding risk varies among the DOACs, with apixaban associated with a more favorable GI bleeding and postpolypectomy bleeding profile.[32,33]

Direct oral anticoagulant agents offer several advantages over warfarin:

- Fixed dose,
- Rapid anticoagulation within 3 hours of the first dose,
- No monitoring, and
- No interaction with medications or foods

A limited number of studies are published assessing the approach to polypectomy in patients taking DOACs whereby there are 4 specific considerations: is temporary interruption beneficial, when should DOACs be resumed if a temporary interruption occurs, is bridge anticoagulation required, and the role of cold snare polypectomy in preventing postpolypectomy bleeding.

The PAUSE trial is the landmark study informing our understanding of patient outcomes associated with a standardized approach to peri-procedural interruption of DOACs. The PAUSE trial is a prospective cohort trial enrolling patients with nonvalvular atrial fibrillation on DOAC agents undergoing elective procedures, including colonoscopy and polypectomy.[17] A standardized protocol for DOAC interruption and resumption without heparin bridging was assessed. The DOAC was held the day before a low-risk bleeding procedure (the category that includes all GI procedures) and 2 days before a high-risk bleeding procedure. The DOAC was resumed 24 hours after low-risk bleeding procedures and 48 to 72 hours after high-risk bleeding procedures once hemostasis was attained. This standardized approach to DOAC interruption was shown to be safe. Of the 3007 patients enrolled, the rate of major bleeding at 30 days ranged from 0.90% to 1.85% and the rate of arterial thromboembolism ranged from 0.16% to 0.60%, depending on the DOAC used.

Our ability to apply the results of the PAUSE study to colonoscopy and polypectomy is supported by a retrospective analysis including 1590 patients on DOAC medications who underwent colonoscopy and polypectomy, including EMR, following a brief period of DOAC interruption.[34] Peri-procedural DOAC management was concordant with the ASGE guidelines[6]: held 1 to 3 days before the procedure and resumed within 48 hours. A small proportion, 1.6%, did receive heparin bridging. After adjusting for bridge anticoagulation, patient comorbidities, and procedure type, patients with DOAC did not have an increased risk of GI bleeding (0.63%, 95% CI: 0.3%–1.2%), stroke, myocardial infarction, or hospital admission following drug resumption compared with patients not on DOACs.

The recommendation to avoid heparin bridging in patients with nonvalvular atrial fibrillation who require a short peri-procedural interruption of their DOACs is aligned with the PAUSE trial, which did not use bridging anticoagulation in their population of patients with lower CHADS-VASC scores.[17] This no-bridge strategy is also supported by the results of the RE-LY trial, whereby an increased risk of procedural bleeding without a decrease in thromboembolic events was associated with heparin bridging.[35] Altogether, a short period of DOAC interruption without bridge anticoagulation seems to be safe as these agents achieve therapeutic levels within hours of resumption. If DOACs are continued for colonoscopy, cold snare polypectomy of sub-centimeter polyps may be preferable.

Strategies to Decrease Postpolypectomy Bleeding Risk

The risk of delayed postpolypectomy bleeding has been associated with larger polyp size,[12–16] proximal,[12,13,16,33] especially cecal,[36] location, and the use of antithrombotic medications.[12,15,34,37] In addition, a large, retrospective cohort of patients on oral anticoagulants reported the use of thermal techniques for polypectomy was independently associated with postpolypectomy bleeding.[33] Postpolypectomy bleeding definitions vary among studies but are often subgrouped into immediate (intraprocedural) bleeding or delayed bleeding (typically reported at 14- or 30-days following colonoscopy). In patients on antithrombotic agents, the risk of postpolypectomy bleeding is challenging to assess as this population of patients is often under-represented in clinical studies. Furthermore, patients prescribed antithrombotic agents tend to be at higher risk of bleeding due to increased age, comorbid medical conditions, and multiple medications, all contributing to altered metabolism and excretion of the antithrombotic drugs.[38]

The following summarizes 2 strategies that may decrease the risk of postpolypectomy bleeding: cold snare polypectomy and prophylactic clip placement at the polypectomy site.

Cold snare polypectomy

The American and European endoscopy societies recommend cold snare polypectomy for nonpedunculated polyps up to 1 cm in size.[39,40] Concerning postpolypectomy bleeding, a recent meta-analysis included 3 randomized controlled trials comparing cold snare polypectomy to hot snare polypectomy to remove polyps 4 to 10 mm in size.[41] The rate of delayed postpolypectomy bleeding was similar between the 2 groups, but the pooled sample size was unlikely to detect any difference. The meta-analysis did show an increase in adverse events in the cold snare polypectomy arm due to immediate bleeding. However, the previously mentioned studies excluded patients on antithrombotic medications, thus limiting our ability to extrapolate findings to this specific population.

In patients who are not on an antithrombotic agent, self-limited intraprocedural bleeding is common after cold-snare polypectomy.[42] Less is known about the severity of immediate bleeding following cold polypectomy techniques in patients who require prompt resumption of an antiplatelet or anticoagulant agent. Published studies vary in their definition of immediate bleeding. While some have described bleeding beyond 30 seconds as a significant adverse event, other studies have a less standardized protocol in which bleeding is considered a true complication when the endoscopist, at their discretion, applies hemostatic therapy. This behavior is subject to bias as an unblinded endoscopist may have a lower threshold for hemostatic therapy in a patient they know to be on an antithrombotic drug.

Takeuchi and colleagues clarified intraprocedural bleeding as poorly controlled bleeding at the time of colonoscopy requiring blood transfusion, surgery, or interventional radiology.[30] Recently, a greater effort has been made to define intraprocedural bleeding in a fashion that can be easily standardized and is consistent with expert consensus that suggested: "Immediate bleeding is not considered an adverse event unless it results in hospitalization, transfusion, or surgery."[43] This general statement did not apply specifically to patients on antithrombotics; and, the definition and importance of immediate postpolypectomy bleeding is an evolving area of controversy.

Two randomized trials have compared cold and hot snare polypectomy in patients on anticoagulant medications. Horiuchi and colleagues randomized 70 patients on continuous warfarin therapy with polyps less than 1 cm to cold or hot snare polypectomy.[44] Immediate bleeding, managed by clip placement, was observed in 5.7% of the cold snare group and 23% of the hot snare group. At 14-day follow-up, no patients in the cold snare arm experienced delayed bleeding versus 14% in the hot snare arm. This trial was at risk of bias due to a lack of blinding of the physician performing the colonoscopy and the outcome assessors. Furthermore, the lower risk of immediate postpolypectomy bleeding in the cold snare arm is incongruent with studies evaluating cold snare polypectomy in patients who are not on antithrombotics.[41] As discussed above, Takeuchi and colleagues demonstrated that cold snare polypectomy on continuous warfarin or DOAC was noninferior to hot snare polypectomy in patients with the anticoagulant interrupted and receiving heparin bridging.[30] However, in addition to the design flaws previously noted, the bridging strategy used in patients prescribed DOACs is not endorsed by national cardiology or hematology organizations in the United States.

Prophylactic clipping

Prophylactic clipping is attractive to many endoscopists following polypectomy of larger lesions in patients requiring antiplatelet or anticoagulant agents. Several prospective trials have studied the association between clipping and postpolypectomy bleeding.[12–14]

Feagin and colleagues did stratify randomization by antithrombotic use and presented different outcomes for different antithrombotic strategies.[12] Of the 1050 patients with polyps $\geq$ 1 cm, 5.7% were on $P2Y_{12}$ inhibitors (4% interrupted, 1.7% uninterrupted), 1.6% on uninterrupted DOACs, and 6.8% on interrupted warfarin therapy (2.6% bridged,

4.2% not bridged). Given the small numbers in each subgroup, it is not unexpected that a difference in postpolypectomy bleeding rate was not observed; however, the authors did find that bridging therapy and $P2Y_{12}$ inhibitor use—without discriminating between continuous and interrupted—were associated with postpolypectomy bleeding.

A recently published meta-analysis included the Feagin study and 8 additional randomized trials comparing postpolypectomy clip placement to a control group.[45] Overall, clipping did not significantly lower the rate of postpolypectomy bleeding (2.2% and 3.3%, respectively), yielding a pooled relative risk of 0.69 (95% CI 0.45%–1.08%). In subgroup analysis, there was a decrease in the bleeding rate for polyps ≥ 2 cm in size, particularly in the proximal colon. Despite pooling results of several studies, there was insufficient data to inform the question of prophylactic clipping of large postpolypectomy mucosal defects in patients that require prompt resumption of their antiplatelet or anticoagulant drugs.

In the absence of high-quality evidence, a recommendation cannot be made for or against routine clipping postpolypectomy at this time. Until data are available that demonstrates the benefit of mechanical hemostasis in this subgroup of patients, it makes intuitive sense to consider prophylactically clip closure of defects following excision of polyps greater than 1 cm in patients who require ongoing antithrombotic therapy.

SUMMARY

This review has highlighted several scenarios in which clinical decisions are made using low-quality data. Balancing the risk of postpolypectomy bleeding against the risk of a thrombotic event requires shared decision-making to ensure the patient understands the risks and benefits of antithrombotic drug management before and after colonoscopy with polypectomy. In all cases, this discussion should include the patient's preferences for preventing thromboembolism versus postpolypectomy bleeding risk. Consultation with the patient's cardiologist, hematologist, or neurologist is particularly important if the patient is at high risk of a thromboembolic event.

Polypectomy techniques may also dictate the risk of postpolypectomy bleeding. There is growing acceptance of cold snare polypectomy in subcentimeter polyps while on continuous antithrombotic medications, but further study is needed in patients requiring antithrombotic drugs. Does a patient need to temporarily interrupt an antithrombotic before colonoscopy and cold snare polypectomy? Currently, the data to answer this question are sparse. While clipping polyps larger than 2 cm seems to decrease postpolypectomy bleeding, the benefit of prophylactic clipping following polypectomy of polyps less than 2 cm in size in patients on antithrombotics has yet to be determined. Studies assessing patient preferences regarding antithrombotic interruption in the setting of colonoscopy planning would be a welcome addition to the current literature and help inform shared decision-making discussions.

CLINICS CARE POINTS

- A patient's underlying thrombotic risk and their personal preferences regarding postpolypectomy bleeding versus thrombotic events are essential to consider before undertaking any procedure whereby polypectomy is possible.

- The timing of colonoscopy, decisions concerning temporary interruption, and the endoscopist's choice of polypectomy technique should be dictated by the patient's underlying risk for thrombotic events and the size of the polyp removed.

- Colonoscopy should be deferred in patients during the period when the alteration of the antithrombotic regimen is associated with the greatest risk of adverse cardiac events.
- ASA can be continued for colonoscopy and polypectomy
- DOACs have a short half-life and rapid onset of action resulting in safe temporary interruption for colonoscopy and polypectomy 2 days before the procedure. Prompt resumption of the DOAC is recommended once endoscopic hemostasis is achieved, usually the day after the procedure. There is no need to bridge patients on DOACs with low molecular weight heparin.
- Polyps up to 1 cm in size removed by cold snare polypectomy may be treated as a low-risk bleeding procedure.
  ○ Consider continuing anticoagulant and antiplatelet therapy
- For polyps ≥ 1 cm, at higher risk of bleeding, consider temporary interruption of anticoagulant and antiplatelet therapy
- Reserve heparin bridging for patients on interrupted warfarin at high risk of thromboembolism
- Prophylactic clip placement of polyps ≥ 1 cm may help prevent postpolypectomy bleeding in patients requiring antithrombotic drugs.

DISCLOSURE

The authors have no disclosures

REFERENCES

1. Alonso-Coello P, Montori VM, Díaz MG, et al. Values and preferences for oral antithrombotic therapy in patients with atrial fibrillation: physician and patient perspectives. Health Expect 2015;18(6):2318–27.
2. Abraham NS, Naik AD, Street RL, et al. Complex antithrombotic therapy: determinants of patient preference and impact on medication adherence. Patient Prefer Adherence 2015;9:1657–68.
3. Lane D, Meyerhoff J, Rohner U, et al. Patients' perceptions of atrial fibrillation, stroke risk, and oral anticoagulation treatment: an international survey. TH Open 2018;02(03):e233–41.
4. Wilke T, Bauer S, Mueller S, et al. Patient preferences for oral anticoagulation therapy in atrial fibrillation: a systematic literature review. Patient - Patient-centered Outcomes Res 2017;10(1):17–37.
5. Doorey AJ, Weintraub WS, Schwartz JS. Should procedures or patients be safe? bias in recommendations for periprocedural discontinuation of anticoagulation. Mayo Clin Proc 2018;93(9):1173–6.
6. Acosta RD, Abraham NS, Chandrasekhara V, et al. The management of antithrombotic agents for patients undergoing GI endoscopy. Gastrointest Endosc 2016;83(1):3–16.
7. Veitch AM, Radaelli F, Alikhan R, et al. Endoscopy in patients on antiplatelet or anticoagulant therapy: British Society of Gastroenterology (BSG) and European Society of Gastrointestinal Endoscopy (ESGE) guideline update. Endoscopy 2021. https://doi.org/10.1055/a-1547-2282.
8. Chan FKL, Goh K-L, Reddy N, et al. Management of patients on antithrombotic agents undergoing emergency and elective endoscopy: joint Asian Pacific Association of Gastroenterology (APAGE) and Asian Pacific Society for Digestive Endoscopy (APSDE) practice guidelines. Gut 2018;67(3):405–17.

9. Abraham NS, Barkun AN, Douketis J, et al. American College of Gastroenterology-Canadian Association of Gastroenterology clinical practice guideline: peri-endoscopic management of anticoagulants and antiplatelets. Am J Gastroenterol, March 17, 2022. 10.14309/ajg.0000000000001627 doi: 10.14309/ajg.0000000000001627.

10. Douketis JD, Berger PB, Dunn AS, et al. The perioperative management of antithrombotic therapy. Chest 2008;133(6):299S–339S.

11. Spyropoulos AC, Brohi K, Caprini J, et al. Scientific and Standardization Committee Communication: guidance document on the periprocedural management of patients on chronic oral anticoagulant therapy: Recommendations for standardized reporting of procedural/surgical bleed risk and patient-specific thromboembolic risk. J Thromb Haemost 2019;17(11):1966–72.

12. Feagins LA, Smith AD, Kim D, et al. Efficacy of prophylactic hemoclips in prevention of delayed post-polypectomy bleeding in patients with large colonic polyps. Gastroenterology 2019;157(4):967–76.e1.

13. Pohl H, Grimm IS, Moyer MT, et al. Clip closure prevents bleeding after endoscopic resection of large colon polyps in a randomized trial. Gastroenterology 2019;157(4):977–84.e3.

14. Matsumoto M, Kato M, Oba K, et al. Multicenter randomized controlled study to assess the effect of prophylactic clipping on post-polypectomy delayed bleeding: Effect of prophylactic clipping. Dig Endosc 2016;28(5):570–6.

15. Repici A, Hassan C, Vitetta E, et al. Safety of cold polypectomy for < 10 mm polyps at colonoscopy: a prospective multicenter study. Endoscopy 2012;44(01):27–31.

16. Kothari ST, Huang RJ, Shaukat A, et al. ASGE review of adverse events in colonoscopy. Gastrointest Endosc 2019;90(6):863–76.e33.

17. Douketis JD, Spyropoulos AC, Duncan J, et al. Perioperative management of patients with atrial fibrillation receiving a direct oral anticoagulant. JAMA Intern Med 2019;179(11):1469.

18. Forbes N, Hilsden RJ, Martel M, et al. Association between time to colonoscopy after positive fecal testing and colorectal cancer outcomes: a systematic review. Clin Gastroenterol Hepatol 2021;19(7):1344–54.e8.

19. Segnan N, Patnick J, von Karsa L. European Commission, International Agency for Research on Cancer. In: European guidelines for quality assurance in colorectal cancer screening and diagnosis.Vol 1 Office for Official Publications of the European Communities; 2010.

20. Canadian Partnership Against Cancer. Colorectal Cancer Screening in Canada: Monitoring and Evaluation of Quality Indicators - Results Report, January 2011-December 2012. Published online 2014.

21. Yousfi M, Gostout CJ, Baron TH, et al. Postpolypectomy lower gastrointestinal bleeding: potential role of aspirin. Am J Gastroenterol 2004;99(9):1785–9.

22. Feagins LA, Iqbal R, Harford WV, et al. Low rate of postpolypectomy bleeding among patients who continue thienopyridine therapy during colonoscopy. Clin Gastroenterol Hepatol 2013;11(10):1325–32.

23. Kernan WN, Ovbiagele B, Black HR, et al. Guidelines for the prevention of stroke in patients with stroke and transient ischemic attack: a guideline for healthcare professionals from the American Heart Association/American Stroke Association. Stroke 2014;45(7):2160–236.

24. Gerhard-Herman MD, Gornik HL, Barrett C, et al. 2016 AHA/ACC guideline on the management of patients with Lower Extremity Peripheral Artery Disease: A Report of the American College of Cardiology/American Heart Association Task

Force on Clinical Practice Guidelines. Circulation 2017;135(12). https://doi.org/10.1161/CIR.0000000000000471.

25. Levine GN, Bates ER, Bittl JA, et al. 2016 ACC/AHA guideline focused update on duration of dual antiplatelet therapy in Patients With Coronary Artery Disease. J Am Coll Cardiol 2016;68(10):1082–115.

26. Chan FKL, Kyaw MH, Hsiang JC, et al. Risk of postpolypectomy bleeding with uninterrupted clopidogrel therapy in an industry-independent, double-blind, randomized trial. Gastroenterology 2019;156(4):918–25.e1.

27. Won D, Kim JS, Ji J-S, et al. Cold snare polypectomy in patients taking dual antiplatelet therapy: a randomized trial of discontinuation of thienopyridines. Clin Transl Gastroenterol 2019;10(10):e00091.

28. Li D, Chang X, Fang X, et al. Colonoscopic post-polypectomy bleeding in patients on uninterruptedclopidogrel therapy: a systematic review and meta-analysis. Exp Ther Med 2020;12. https://doi.org/10.3892/etm.2020.8597.

29. January CT, Wann LS, Calkins H, et al. 2019 AHA/ACC/HRS Focused Update of the 2014 AHA/ACC/HRS Guideline for the Management of Patients With Atrial Fibrillation: A Report of the American College of Cardiology/American Heart Association Task Force on Clinical Practice Guidelines and the Heart Rhythm Society in Collaboration With the Society of Thoracic Surgeons. Circulation 2019; 140(2). https://doi.org/10.1161/CIR.0000000000000665.

30. Takeuchi Y, Mabe K, Shimodate Y, et al. Continuous anticoagulation and cold snare polypectomy versus heparin bridging and hot snare polypectomy in patients on anticoagulants with subcentimeter polyps: a randomized controlled trial. Ann Intern Med 2019;171(4):229.

31. Douketis JD, Spyropoulos AC, Kaatz S, et al. Perioperative bridging anticoagulation in patients with atrial fibrillation. N Engl J Med 2015;373(9):823–33.

32. Abraham NS, Noseworthy PA, Yao X, et al. Gastrointestinal safety of direct oral anticoagulants: a Large Population-Based Study. Gastroenterology 2017; 152(5):1014–22.e1.

33. Lau LH, Guo CL, Yip TC, et al. Risks of post-colonoscopic polypectomy bleeding and thromboembolism with warfarin and direct oral anticoagulants: a population-based analysis. Gut 2021;22. gutjnl-2020-323600.

34. Yu JX, Oliver M, Lin J, et al. Patients prescribed direct-acting oral anticoagulants have low risk of postpolypectomy complications. Clin Gastroenterol Hepatol 2019;17(10):2000–7.e3.

35. Douketis JD, Healey JS, Brueckmann M, et al. Perioperative bridging anticoagulation during dabigatran or warfarin interruption among patients who had an elective surgery or procedure: Substudy of the RE-LY trial. Thromb Haemost 2015; 113(03):625–32.

36. Rutter M, Nickerson C, Rees C, et al. Risk factors for adverse events related to polypectomy in the english bowel cancer screening programme. Endoscopy 2014;46(02):90–7.

37. Aizawa M, Utano K, Nemoto D, et al. Risk of delayed bleeding after cold snare polypectomy in patients with antithrombotic therapy. Dig Dis Sci 2021;10.

38. Abraham NS. Antiplatelets, anticoagulants, and colonoscopic polypectomy. Gastrointest Endosc 2020;91(2):257–65.

39. Kaltenbach T, Anderson JC, Burke CA, et al. Endoscopic removal of colorectal lesions—recommendations by the US Multi-Society task force on colorectal cancer. Gastrointest Endosc 2020;91(3):486–519.

40. Ferlitsch M, Moss A, Hassan C, et al. Colorectal polypectomy and endoscopic mucosal resection (EMR): European Society of Gastrointestinal Endoscopy (ESGE) Clinical Guideline. Endoscopy 2017;49(03):270–97.
41. Jegadeesan R, Aziz M, Desai M, et al. Hot snare vs. cold snare polypectomy for endoscopic removal of 4 – 10 mm colorectal polyps during colonoscopy: a systematic review and meta-analysis of randomized controlled studies. Endosc Int Open 2019;07(05):E708–16.
42. Papastergiou V, Paspatis GA, Paraskeva KD. Immediate intraprocedural bleeding: true 'complication' of cold snare polypectomy? Endosc Int Open 2019;07(08):E1031–2.
43. Rex DK, Schoenfeld PS, Cohen J, et al. Quality indicators for colonoscopy. Gastrointest Endosc 2015;81(1):31–53.
44. Horiuchi A, Nakayama Y, Kajiyama M, et al. Removal of small colorectal polyps in anticoagulated patients: a prospective randomized comparison of cold snare and conventional polypectomy. Gastrointest Endosc 2014;79(3):417–23.
45. Spadaccini M, Albéniz E, Pohl H, et al. Prophylactic clipping after colorectal endoscopic resection prevents bleeding of large, proximal polyps: meta-analysis of randomized trials. Gastroenterology 2020;159(1):148–58.e1.

Clinical, Pathologic, and Molecular-Genetic Aspects of Colorectal Polyps

Quinn Miller, MD, Omer Saeed, MD, Hector Mesa, MD*

KEYWORDS

- Colonic polyps • Colorectal neoplasms • Pathology • Surgical • Molecular genetics
- Review

KEY POINTS

- Polyps are the most common colorectal neoplasms and are precursors of cancer.
- Polyps can be clinically divided into sporadic and syndromic and can be associated with inflammatory bowel disease.
- Pathologically polyps fall in one of the following categories: adenomatous, serrated, juvenile/retention, and Peutz-Jeghers.
- The combination of clinical, pathologic, and molecular-genetic abnormalities allows separating these lesions into discrete groups with predictable risk of progression to colorectal cancer.

In this article, the authors review the histologic classification of polyps, the different clinical scenarios in which polyps may be encountered, and the molecular genetic advances that allow segregating polyps into specific clinical-pathologic-molecular-genetic groups with inherent risks to progression to colorectal cancer (CRC).

The term polyp is often loosely applied to any discrete lesion of the colonic mucosa (raised, flat, depressed, pediculated, sessile). Histologically, however, only epithelial mucosal lesions are considered true polyps. Four histologic categories of epithelial polyps are recognized: (1) Adenomatous, (2) serrated, (3) juvenile/retention, and (4) Peutz-Jeghers. Clinically, they occur in 3 main scenarios: (1) Sporadic, (2) syndromic, and (3) associated with inflammatory bowel disease (IBD). The combination of the specific histologic category with the clinical scenario gives rise to many different clinicopathologic diagnostic categories, each with a different risk of progression to CRC.[1]

Most polyps (∼90%) are sporadic, occur in individuals older than 50 years of age, and are more common in men. Less than 10% of polyps occur in the context of

Department of Pathology and Laboratory Medicine, Indiana University School of Medicine, IU Health Pathology Laboratory, 350 West 11th Street, Indianapolis, IN 46202, USA
* Corresponding author.
E-mail address: hmesa@iu.edu

Gastrointest Endoscopy Clin N Am 32 (2022) 313–328
https://doi.org/10.1016/j.giec.2021.12.007
giendo.theclinics.com

inherited or acquired genetic mutations, affect children or young individuals, are associated with markedly increased risk of developing CRC, and/or occur in large numbers. Less than 1% of CRC arises from polyps in the context of IBD.[1]

Whether sporadic, syndromic, or IBD associated, it is accepted that most CRC arises from polyps with adenomatous change/dysplasia through a years-long multistep process designated the "adenoma-carcinoma sequence." This model provides a rationale for implementing screening, surveillance, and eradication strategies tailored for specific clinicopathologic scenarios developed by public health organizations and/or professional gastroenterological or multidisciplinary societies.[2,3]

In syndromic polyps, the lifetime risk for progression is inherent to the underlying genetic abnormality, being almost universal for familial adenomatous (FAP) and mutY DNA glycosylase (MUTYH)-associated polyposis (MAP), moderate (40%–70%) for Lynch (LS), juvenile polyposis (JPS), and Peutz-Jeghers (PJS) syndromes, and much lower (<15%) for Cowden syndrome.[1]

In IBD-associated polyps/lesions, the risk of progression is directly proportional to the extent, duration, and severity of the disease. In general, lesions that are endoscopically characteristic of sporadic polyps are treated as such, whereas unusual-appearing mass-forming lesions are frequently associated with CRC and are usually treated by endoscopic mucosal resection or more extensive surgery.[1–3]

In the much more common sporadic polyps, the risk of dysplasia and progression is much lower (<5%) and influenced by age, gender, ethnicity, environmental factors, size, location, and number of polyps.[2]

Environmental Factors

Obesity, smoking, and meat and alcohol consumption have been proven to induce a direct mutational effect on the DNA or nonmutational (epigenetic) modifications of the genome.[4,5] Protective factors, such as dietary fiber, consumption of fruits and vegetables, and chemoprevention using calcium and nonsteroidal anti-inflammatory drugs among others, have also been established.[6]

Location

Although any type of polyp can occur at any location, in aggregate, specific morphologies and/or molecular-genetic signatures are much more common on the right or the left colon; for example, sessile serrated lesions and microsatellite (MS) unstable lesions are more likely to occur and to progress on the right colon, whereas adenomatous, MS stable lesions without epigenetic abnormalities are more common and more likely to occur and progress in the rectosigmoid. Different patterns of epigenetic modifications have also been documented for right- and left-sided adenomas.[7] These regional differences in the molecular profile of neoplasms of the right and left colon most likely reflect embryologically determined regional molecular heterogeneity of the stem cells at these sites that lead to site-specific genetic and epigenetic susceptibilities.[8] For this reason, it is relevant to submit lesions resected at different sites in different containers to the pathology laboratory.

Size

Diminutive polyps (<5 mm) have been shown to have no risk of malignant transformation. Small polyps (<1 cm) may harbor areas of high-grade dysplasia in less than 1% of cases but almost never invasive carcinoma.[9] Essentially all carcinomas arise in lesions greater than 1 cm, and the risk increases with increasing polyp size and is overall estimated to be less than 5%. Polyps ≥2 cm have also been shown to be a risk factor for metachronous CRC.[10] For lesions resected piecemeal, pathologists rely on the endoscopic measure; for lesions resected in toto, pathologists rely on the gross description.

Number of Polyps

Provided an optimal examination is performed, the number of polyps identified at a screening colonoscopy is an indirect measure of the deleterious environmental effects on the genome of colonic stem cells of a particular individual. Statistically significant differences in the risk for metachronous malignancy have been shown in patients with 1 to 5, 6 to 9, and ≥10 polyps at screening colonoscopy.[3] When endoscopists submit many polyps in the same container, including polyps that have been resected piecemeal and others that were not, pathologists may only be able to confirm the presence or absence of adenomatous change, high-grade dysplasia, or different types of polyps.

ADENOMATOUS POLYPS
Epidemiology

Adenomatous polyps are the most common type, comprising ~70% of epithelial polyps. Their frequency increases with age, and in the United States, there is an overall prevalence of ~35% (male: 40%; female: 29%) at age 60 in autopsy studies and is associated with an ~4% lifetime risk of CRC.[10,11]

Pathology

Microscopically, there are 3 variants: tubular (TA), tubulovillous (TVA), and villous adenomas (VA). All show evidence of markedly increased proliferative activity manifested by increased density of glands, increased number of cells within glands, and increased mitotic and apoptotic activity, a phenomenon described as "adenomatous change" and equivalent to low-grade dysplasia (**Fig. 1**). When proliferation markers, such as Ki-67, are applied, there is a displacement and expansion of the proliferative compartment from its normal location at the base of the gland, to the neck and surface areas. With increasing polyp size, the proliferative compartment may expand further to comprise the entire gland.[12]

TAs are the most common type; most are less than 1 cm and have a smooth surface. As the lesions increase in size greater than 1 cm, fingerlike projections become apparent or predominant, and the lesions are classified as TVA if the villous component is greater than 25% or VA if greater than 75%.[1] In larger lesions, foci of increased cytologic atypia characterized by increased nuclear to cytoplasmic ratios, rounded nuclei with prominent nucleoli and loss of polarity, and architectural complexity characterized by cribriform architecture may begin to appear and are considered evidence of progression to "high-grade dysplasia." If glands with high-grade dysplasia invade through the muscularis mucosa, the lesion is classified as invasive adenocarcinoma. **Fig. 2** shows a flow chart with criteria used for the histologic classification of adenomatous polyps. Advanced adenomas are adenomatous polyps associated with increased risk of local recurrence and progression when resected piecemeal or incompletely excised and are defined as any polyp greater than 1 cm, and/or with a villous component, and/or with high-grade dysplasia. These polyps are also considered markers of increased risk of metachronous CRC or familial CRC.[3,13]

Molecular Genetic Aspects of Sporadic Adenomatous Polyps

The underlying cause of polyps is spontaneous sporadic mutations in colonic stem cells. The rate of mutation is affected by age, gender, the biome, and exposure to

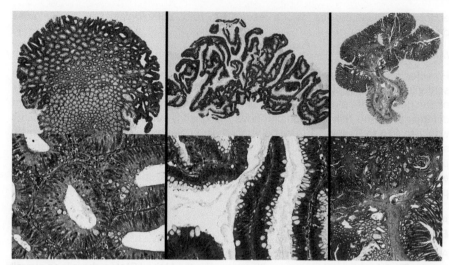

Fig. 1. Adenomatous polyps. The left panel shows a TA. At low magnification (*top*, hematoxylin-eosin [H&E], ×20), the surface appears smooth and dark, because of displacement of the proliferative compartment from the bottom of the crypts to the surface of the polyp. At high magnification (*bottom*, H&E, ×600), the nuclear pseudostratification, high nuclear density, and increased mitotic/apoptotic activity characteristic of adenomatous change are apparent. The middle panel shows a VA. The low power (*top*, H&E, ×20) shows thin tentacular projections that contrast with the appearance of the TA on the left. At high magnification (*bottom*, H&E, ×400), thin fibrovascular cores lined by adenomatous epithelium are seen. The right panel shows a malignant polyp. At very low magnification captured with a digital slide scanner (*top*, H&E, ×0.25), a large pediculated TA has a subset of glands invading the upper third of the stalk (*circle*). The base of the polyp is widely free of lesion. At low magnification (*bottom*, H&E, ×20), the invading glands show cribriform architecture and are surrounded by desmoplastic stroma (*circle*).

endogenous and exogenous carcinogens and protective agents in the feces and/or the blood. Epigenetic modifications of colonic stem cells are affected by the individual's environment and habits. The mutational effect of all these factors is time-dependent, and therefore, prevalence of polyps increases with age. Most small (<1 cm) sporadic adenomas are diploid and do not show chromosomal instability (CIN) or any molecular feature associated with progression. Molecular abnormalities in small TA are rare (≤5%) and include low-level CpG island methylator phenotype (CIMP), APC, and KRAS mutations.[14,15]

Advanced adenomas, by contrast, share the molecular abnormalities identified in CRC, which can be divided into 3 groups: (1) CIN pathway, (2) MS instability pathway, (3) CIMP.

Chromosomal instability pathway

These lesions show a progressive accumulation of mutations that induce a "mutator phenotype" and result in complex numerical and structural cytogenetic abnormalities that manifest morphologically as worsening dysplasia. A common early event is inactivating mutation of APC followed by activating mutations of KRAS or BRAF and additional mutations or losses of SMAD4, PIK3CA, TP53, and numerous other genes, of which less than 15 are considered critical for progression to invasive

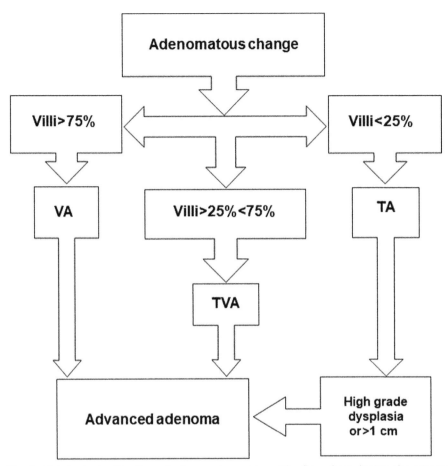

Fig. 2. Histologic classification of adenomatous polyps. The flow chart depicts the criteria used for the classification of adenomatous polyps based on the percentage of villous component. Advanced adenoma includes polyps with significant villous components or size >1 cm, or presence of high-grade dysplasia.

adenocarcinoma.[16] Although testing for many of the targetable recurrent mutations of the CIN pathway is currently standard for CRC, it is not usually done for adenomatous lesions.

Microsatellite instability pathway
These lesions result owing to acquired mutations in the DNA mismatch repair (MMR) system. The MMR proteins (MLH1, MSH2, MSH6, and PMS2) are needed to correct replication errors that occur in error-prone repetitive sequences of the DNA called microsatellites (MS). In the absence of MMR, these errors accumulate producing a microsatellite instability-high (MSI-H) phenotype. Sporadic MSI-H is detected in approximately 3% to 20% of all CRCs,[17,18] and it is usually due to silencing of the MLH1 gene through methylation of its promoter in the context of environmentally driven global hypermethylation.[18] In contrast to the CIN pathway, most sporadic MSI-H lesions are diploid, but given the tumorigenesis mechanism, they contain a high mutational

burden, a fact that has gained much relevance because metastatic lesions arising from these tumors can be targeted with immune checkpoint inhibitors.

CpG island methylator phenotype

The promoter regions of many genes contain cytosine-guanine (CG) dinucleotide-rich areas, defined as greater than 50% CG content per 200 base-pairs, which are susceptible to epigenomic silencing through methylation. Silencing of genes through methylation is much more common than through mutations. CIMP+ is responsible for most sporadic MSI-H lesions, but greater than 50% of CIMP+ lesions are MS stable. In those cases, CIMP+ is involved in silencing multiple tumor-suppressor genes and microRNAs. This abnormal methylation seems to occur due to an abnormal activation of an established epigenetic system that normally has a role in marking embryonic genes for repression and is mediated by H3 trimethylated on Lys27 (H3K27me3) and the Enhancer of zeste homolog 2 (EZH2)-containing polycomb complex.[19] Activation of this system can be indirectly induced by BRAF or KRAS mutations.[20,21]

Molecular Genetic Aspects of Syndromic Adenomatous Polyps

Adenomatous polyps are characteristic lesions of syndromes, including FAP, attenuated FAP (AFAP), FAP variants: Gardner and Turcot$_{subset}$, LS, LS variants: Muir-Torre and Turcot$_{subset}$, MAP, and polymerase proofreading-associated polyposis (PPAP).

All these syndromes are autosomal dominant, except for MAP, which is recessive.[1]

FAP and variants (AFAP, Gardner, Turcot) are characterized by germline mutations of the APC tumor-suppressor gene. The mutated protein loses its microtubule-binding sites, which are needed for its function as a regulator of cytoskeletal proteins that participate in contact inhibition of proliferation, and for interaction with proteins of the mitotic spindle. Loss of these functions leads to expansion of the mutant clone and CIN, respectively.[22,23]

MAP clinically resembles AFAP. Rarely, it may present as serrated polyposis syndrome (SPS) or with mixed adenomatous and serrated polyps. The underlying abnormality is biallelic germline mutations in the MUTYH gene, which codifies an enzyme involved in the repair of DNA damage induced by oxidative stress. Loss of function leads to the accumulation of mutations in several genes and high mutational burden, like the MMR pathway, making these lesions susceptible to be targeted with immune checkpoint inhibitors.[24] APC and KRAS are particularly susceptible to oxidative damage[25]; for this reason, MAP-associated polyps and CRC may show features of either the CIN pathway, the MSI pathway, or both.

LS and variants (Muir-Torre, Turcot$_{subset}$) are characterized by a germline mutation in one of the 4 MMR genes encoding the proteins that form the heterodimers MSH2/MSH6 and MLH1/PMS2. The loss of expression of these proteins is usually demonstrated by immunohistochemistry (IHC). Loss of 1 protein of the heterodimer usually leads to loss of expression of its partner. Rarely, MSH2 is silenced through methylation owing to a deletion of EPCAM/TACSTD1.[26] The MSH6 gene contains a MS and its expression can be lost because of a MSI-H phenotype induced by MLH1 or PMS2 mutation, resulting in an MLH1/PMS2/MSH6 triple loss of expression by IHC. Very rarely, germline mutations in the 4 MMR genes occur and result in a cancer predisposition syndrome called "constitutional MMR deficiency syndrome (CMMRD)." It is associated with a high risk of developing different types of malignancies that include lymphomas, gliomas, and CRC and that usually manifest before age 18 years. Patients with CMMRD show clinical features of neurofibromatosis type I associated with a polyposis syndrome.[27] The MSI status is determined through conventional polymerase chain reaction amplification/gel electrophoresis of 5 standardized MS loci known as the Bethesda panel.[28] MSI-H is defined as alteration in ≥ 2 of the 5 loci or greater than 40% of loci in larger panels. Common additional mutations in LS include mutations in the β-catenin or APC genes, but in contrast to sporadic MSI-H lesions, it is not associated with BRAF mutations.

PPAP is a relatively new addition to the list of polyposis syndromes and is characterized by germline mutations in the proofreading domains of POLE or POLD1, two DNA polymerases. Defects in DNA polymerase proofreading can lead to propagation of mistakes or mutations to daughter cells during cellular replication resulting in a mutator phenotype. Unlike LS, PPAP is MS stable with progression to CRC occurring via the CIN pathway.[29] The lifetime risk of progression of PPAP is high, at 36%.[30]

SERRATED POLYPS
Epidemiology

Serrated polyps are the second most common type comprising ~30% of epithelial polyps.[31] Although initially regarded as benign, it is now clear that these lesions also have a potential for progressing to carcinoma, albeit with lesser frequency than adenomatous polyps.

Pathology

Microscopically there are 3 variants: hyperplastic (HP), sessile serrated polyp/lesion (SSL), and traditional serrated adenoma (TSA). Although HP and SSL are very common, TSA is rare. **Fig. 3** shows a flow chart with the criteria for the histologic classification of serrated polyps. Serrated polyps are almost always sessile, and the superficial portion shows a characteristic saw-toothed architecture when the glands are sectioned longitudinally or appear star-shaped when sectioned transversally (**Fig. 4**). All serrated polyps have an aberrant immunophenotype with expression of the gastric-type mucin MUC5AC. In HP and SSL, the proliferative compartment remains at the base, and there is no adenomatous change/dysplasia. Their abnormal growth is due to inhibition of apoptosis, which causes an abnormal migration/maturation pattern of epithelial cells along the crypt.[32] Two types of HP are recognized, microvesicular and goblet cell rich. The former is more common and characterized by preponderance of variably vacuolated non–goblet cells and only scattered goblet cells; the latter shows preponderance of goblet cells and less prominent serrations and may be underrecognized.[33] Although the proliferative compartment in HP is well defined, in SSL it may be asymmetric and may expand beyond the base. HP are usually ≤ 5 mm, whereas SSL are typically larger than 5 mm and are more common on the right colon. Histologically, SSL differ from HP because the crypts appear dilated and complex at the base adjacent to the muscularis mucosa. In cases with ambiguous morphology between HP and SSL, most pathologists use site and size as additional parameters for classification: ambiguous right-sided lesions greater than 5 mm are usually defaulted to SSL; lesions less than 5 mm are usually defaulted to HP; and for the remaining lesions, variability in their classification is to be expected. Large SSL may show foci of conventional dysplasia and are classified as SSL with dysplasia. Right-sided SSL larger than 1 cm or with foci of dysplasia have an increased risk of progressing to CRC if incompletely excised and have been shown to be a risk factor for metachronous CRC; for these reasons, they are considered equivalent to "advanced adenoma" for surveillance purposes.[33] Carcinomas arising from SSL are designated "serrated pathway carcinomas."

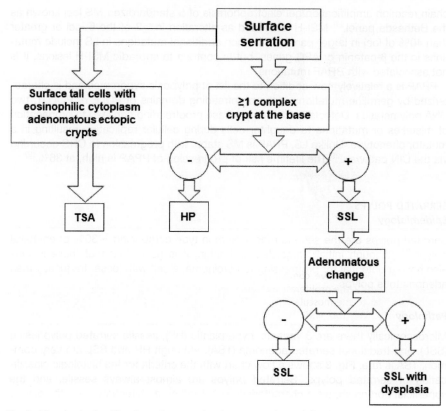

Fig. 3. Histologic classification of serrated polyps. HP and SSL differ by the complexity of the crypt bases, which reflect differences in the regulation of their proliferative compartments located at the base of the crypts. In HP, crypt bases are narrow and simple; in SSL, at least one, but usually many crypt-bases show branching and/or cystic dilatation indicative of greater dysregulation. TSA show superficial serrations like HP and SSL, but their surface cells are distinctively tall and pink, and the proliferative compartment is located in ectopic crypts along the villi and away from the muscularis mucosa.

In contrast to HP and SSL, TSA always shows adenomatous change. It occurs more frequently on the left colon of elderly individuals.[34] The superficial portion resembles small intestinal villi with slitlike serrations, scattered goblet cells, and surface epithelium with abundant eosinophilic cytoplasm. Ectopic crypt formation defined as the presence of crypt bases along the villous projections and away from the muscularis mucosa is characteristic. Ki-67 immunostain facilitates the recognition of the ectopic crypts and shows that the proliferative compartment is limited to these.[35] A subset of TSA arises from HP or SSL, and a residual precursor can often be recognized at the periphery of the polyp.[36] For surveillance purposes, they are considered equivalent to other adenomatous polyps; criteria for classifying them as advanced adenomas include size greater than 1 cm and/or presence of high-grade dysplasia.

Molecular Genetic Aspects of Sporadic Serrated Polyps

All serrated polyps have 3 molecular alterations in common: (1) Activation of mitogen-activated protein kinase-extracellular signal-regulated kinases (MAPK/ERK pathway),

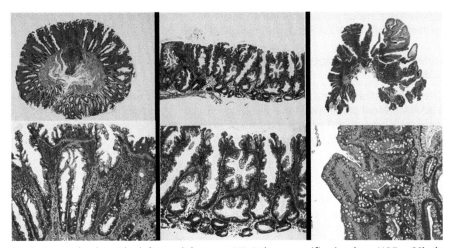

Fig. 4. Serrated polyps. The left panel shows an HP. At low magnification (*top*, H&E, ×20), the upper two-thirds of the gland appear lighter and display serrations. The deep portion of the crypts with the proliferative compartment appears darker. At intermediate magnification (*bottom*, H&E, ×200), the proliferative compartment lacks complex branching, and the glands are perpendicular to the muscularis mucosa (MM). The middle panel shows a sessile serrated lesion. At low power (*top*, H&E, ×20) the serrations are more prominent than the HP on the left. At intermediate magnification (*bottom*, H&E, ×200), the deep portions of the crypts appear complex and assume an orientation parallel to the MM. The right panel shows a TSA. At very low magnification captured with a digital slide scanner (*top*, H&E, ×0.5), a characteristic filiform architecture is apparent. At intermediate magnification (*bottom*, H&E, ×200), the surface epithelium consists of tall cells with abundant pink cytoplasm next to variably complex adenomatous ectopic crypts that hallmark the displacement of the proliferative compartment within the villi and away from its normal location next to the MM.

(2) inhibition of apoptosis, (3) epigenomic silencing of many tumor-suppressor genes through methylation.[37] Most HP, SSL, and TSA show mutually exclusive mutations of *BRAF* or *KRAS*, associated with a CIMP+ phenotype. *BRAF* mutations are more common on the right side and usually lead to CIMP+ and *MLH1* methylation, whereas *KRAS* mutations are more common on the left and have an overall low risk of progression to CRC. In general, *MLH1* methylation is responsible for the increased frequency of right-sided MSI-H CRC in tumors arising through the serrated pathway. TSA are more common in the left colon and therefore usually show *KRAS* mutations, associated with methylation of *the DNA repair gene O-6-methylguanine-DNA methyltransferase.*[37]

Molecular Genetic Aspects of Syndromic Serrated Polyps (SPS)

SPS is clinically defined as : (1) ≥5 serrated polyps proximal to the sigmoid with ≥2 of these being ≥1 cm, (2) any number of SSL proximal to the sigmoid in an individual with a first-degree relative with SPS, (3) greater than 20 SSL throughout the colon.[1] Two clinical variants are recognized: type 1: includes few proximal SSLs and has an increased risk of CRC; and type 2: includes only HPs and is not associated with CRC. Most affected patients are adults with a median age of 66 years. Genetic testing of reported cases have shown heterogenous results with most patients being negative for germline mutations,[38] except for rare familial cases in which germline mutations in *RING-type E3 ubiquitin ligase* (*RNF43*), an inhibitor of the *Wnt* pathway, have been found.[39] A subset of patients with MAP meets the criteria for SPS, but they should be considered MAP, and not an overlap syndrome.[40] CRC arising in the context of SPS usually show the typical molecular signature of serrated pathway: BRAF+/CIMP+/MSI-H. Whether sporadic or syndromic, the lifetime risk of CRC in SPS type 1 is high, at 29%.[41]

JUVENILE/RETENTION POLYPS
Epidemiology

Juvenile/retention polyps are the most common polyps in children, but one-third occur in adults.[42] Most present as rectal bleeding in patients younger than 10 years. In 50% of children, more than 1 polyp is present on colonoscopy; however, concern for a polyposis syndrome is not warranted if there is no family history and fewer than 5 polyps are present.[42]

Pathology

These polyps are usually pedunculated and less than 3 cm. Upon sectioning, mucus-filled cystic spaces are grossly apparent, and for this reason, they are also called "retention" polyps. Microscopically, they consist of cystically dilated glands with reactive changes, separated by edematous, variably inflamed stroma (**Fig. 5**). Ulceration and granulation tissue formation are common on the surface. Polyps with a single stalk but multiple heads may occur in syndromic cases.[1]

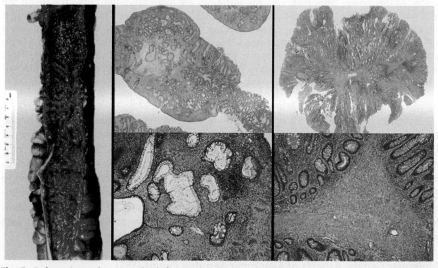

Fig. 5. Polyposis syndromes. The left panel shows a prophylactic colectomy specimen from a patient with FAP polyposis with innumerable small polyps. Histologically, these polyps would be adenomatous. The middle panel shows a juvenile/retention polyp from a young patient with JPS. At very low magnification captured with a digital slide scanner (*top*, H&E, ×0.5), the polyp appears pediculated, shows abundant edematous fibrous stroma and variably dilated hypermucinous glands. At intermediate magnification (*bottom*, H&E, ×200), cystic glands with distended goblet cells alternate with glands with regenerative changes and decreased mucin. The fibrous stroma contains increased inflammatory cells and lymphoid aggregates. The right panel shows a colonic Peutz-Jeghers polyp. At very low magnification captured with a digital slide scanner (*top*, H&E, ×0.25), the characteristic arborizing bundles of smooth muscle can be observed. At intermediate magnification (*bottom*, H&E, ×200), thick bundles of skeletal muscle compartmentalize the mucosa that shows mild hyperplastic changes and rectified gland contours characteristic of mucosal prolapse.

Table 1
Clinical-pathologic-molecular-genetic classification of polyps and their risk of progression to colorectal cancer

Clinical Presentation	Type of Polyp	Molecular Genetics	Risk of CRC	Extracolonic Neoplasms
Sporadic	Adenomatous	CIN pathway MSI pathway CIMP-high	Minimal if <1 cm; annual risk of progression if >1 cm or high-grade dysplasia: <5%	None
Familial adenomatous polyposis AFAP Gardner syndrome Turcot syndrome		Germline APC mutation, dominant	Lifetime risk: 70%–100%	Desmoid, osteomas, epidermoid cysts, fibromas, lipomas, gliomas
Lynch syndrome Muir-Torre syndrome Turcot syndrome		Germline mutation of MMR genes, dominant	Lifetime risk: 40%–70%	Endometrium, ovary, breast, prostate
Polymerase proofreading-associated polyposis MUTYH-associated polyposis		Germline mutation of POLE or POLD1, dominant Germline mutation MUTYH, recessive	Lifetime risk: 36% Lifetime risk: 40%–70%	Endometrial, ovarian, brain, upper gastrointestinal tract Gastrointestinal tract, thyroid
Sporadic	Serrated	MAPK/ERK pathway, BRAF or KRAS mutations leading to CIMP-high and MLH1 methylation	Hyperplastic polyp: none SSL/TSA: minimal if <1 cm; annual risk of progression if >1 cm or with dysplasia: <5%	None
Serrated polyposis syndrome		BRAF mutation, CIMP-high, MSI-high. Not inherited in most cases, rare familial cases associated with RNF43 mutations	Lifetime risk: 29%	None
Sporadic Juvenile polyposis syndrome	Juvenile	KRAS mutation Germline mutations of SMAD4 or BMPR1A, dominant	None Lifetime risk: 21%–68%	None SMAD4: stomach
Cowden syndrome Bannayan-Riley-Ruvalcaba syndrome		Germline mutation PTEN, dominant	Lifetime risk: <15%	Breast, thyroid, renal, uterine
Sporadic Peutz-Jeghers syndrome	Peutz-Jeghers	Somatic mutation STK11 Germline mutation STK11, dominant	None Lifetime risk: 39%	None Breast

Molecular Genetic Aspects of Sporadic Juvenile Polyps

KRAS mutations and absence of APC mutations have been found in sporadic juvenile polyps.[43]

Molecular Genetic Aspects of Syndromic Juvenile Polyps

Juvenile polyps are associated with JPS, Cowden (CS), and its variant Bannayan-Riley-Ruvalcaba (BRRS) syndromes.[1]

The molecular features underlying JPS include germline abnormalities in the SMAD4 and BMPR1A genes in ~60% of the cases and various genes in the remaining cases. The genes involved in JPS are part of the transforming growth factor-beta pathway, which regulates the transcription of genes involved in cell growth and division. Mutations of SMAD4 are also associated with hereditary hemorrhagic telangiectasia (HHT) syndrome, and these patients present with JPS/HHT overlap syndrome.[44] Both genes predispose patients to CRC, and SMAD4 also predisposes to gastric cancer.

The underlying abnormality in CS and BRRS is germline mutations of the PTEN tumor-suppressor gene. Given the broad spectrum of clinical manifestations of patients with PTEN mutations, the term PTEN hamartoma tumor syndrome (PHTS) has been gaining traction to encompass any clinical syndrome with proven PTEN abnormalities. PTEN is the most important negative regulator of the PI3K signaling pathway, which exerts its actions through the AKT/mTOR axis. It has a plethora of effects that include negative regulatory effect of growth factor–mediated cell proliferation and survival, ERK1/cyclin D1–mediated transcription, translation and chromosomal stability, angiogenesis, stem cell self-renewal, and maintenance of tumor microenvironment.[45] Somatic mutations of PTEN also occur in ~6% of sporadic CRC and is more common in tumors arising through the serrated pathway.[46] PTEN-mutated neoplasms are potentially targetable with EGFR and MAPK-inhibitor therapies.

Characteristic extraintestinal manifestations of PHTS include glycogenic acanthosis of the esophagus, trichilemmomas, and mucocutaneous papillomas. Germline mutations of PTEN are more commonly associated with breast, thyroid, renal, and endometrial carcinomas than CRC.

PEUTZ-JEGHERS POLYPS
Epidemiology

Peutz-Jeghers polyps are more common in the small bowel than in the colon, and 40% to 72% are associated with a polyposis syndrome.[47]

Pathology

The most conspicuous finding in these polyps is the presence of ramifying bundles of smooth muscle fibers emanating from the muscularis mucosa. The glandular component is less distinctive and shows features of mucosal prolapse with mucous hypersecretion, regenerative changes, and angulated/rectified gland borders (see **Fig. 5**). Although PJS is associated with an increased risk of CRC, dysplasia is exceedingly rare in PJ polyps. The risk of extraintestinal neoplasms is high, especially breast cancer in female patients.[1]

Molecular Genetic Aspects of Peutz-Jeghers Polyps

The underlying molecular abnormalities are mutations in the LKB1/STK11 gene, somatic mutations in sporadic cases, and germline mutations in syndromic cases. STK11 is a tumor suppressor that exerts negative regulation over the mTOR pathway; inactivating mutations lead to overactivation of this pathway involved in cell metabolism, growth, and proliferation. The use of mTOR inhibitors for chemoprevention of polyps/tumors in PJS has been limited by drug toxicities.[48]

SUMMARY

For a long time, it has been known that all disease processes are affected in varying proportions by genetic and environmental factors. The increasing use of molecular-genetic technologies in clinical studies is finally allowing us to decipher the intricate interplay of these factors in sporadic and syndromic polyps, and to predict more accurately their risk of progressing to CRC. As these sophisticated technologies become progressively integrated in the routine workup of pathology specimens, a clinical-pathologic-molecular-genetic classification of polyps is emerging (**Table 1**), which is being used to refine existing surveillance and eradication strategies for patients and their relatives, getting us closer to the long-held dream of personalized medicine.

CLINICS CARE POINTS

- Most polyps (~90%) are sporadic, occur in individuals greater than 50 years of age, are more common in men, and have a low risk (<5%) of progressing to colorectal cancer.

- Polyps in children or young adults are uncommon, may be associated with inherited or acquired genetic mutations, and are associated with markedly increased risk of developing colorectal cancer. Pertinent genetic testing should be considered.

- Diminutive polyps (<5 mm) have no risk of malignant transformation. Small polyps (<1 cm) may harbor areas of high-grade dysplasia in less than 1% of cases but almost never invasive carcinoma. Essentially all carcinomas arise in lesions greater than 1 cm, and the risk increases with increasing polyp size.

- The number of polyps identified at a screening colonoscopy is an indirect measure of the mutation rate of colonic stem cells. Statistically significant differences in the risk of synchronous or metachronous malignancy have been shown in patients with 1 to 5, 6 to 9, and ≥10 polyps.

- Advanced adenomas are defined as any polyp greater than 1 cm, and/or with a villous component, and/or with high-grade dysplasia. These polyps are associated with increased risk of local recurrence and progression when resected piecemeal or incompletely excised, and with metachronous or familial colorectal cancer.

- Right-sided sessile serrated lesions larger than 1 cm or with foci of dysplasia are considered equivalent to "advanced adenoma" for surveillance purposes.

- In 50% of children, greater than 1 juvenile polyp is present on colonoscopy; concern for a polyposis syndrome is not warranted if there is no family history and fewer than 5 polyps are present.

- Peutz-Jeghers polyps are associated with a polyposis syndrome in up to 72% of the cases. The risk of breast cancer in female patients with Peutz-Jeghers syndrome is much higher than the risk of colorectal cancer.

CONFLICT OF INTEREST DISCLOSURE

The authors do not have conflict of interest to declare.

REFERENCES

1. Bosman FT, Carneiro F, Hruban RH, et al, editors. WHO classification of tumours of the digestive system. Lyon: IARC; 2010. p. 139–73.

2. Rex DK, Boland CR, Dominitz JA, et al. Colorectal cancer screening: recommendations for physicians and patients from the U.S. Multi-Society Task Force on Colorectal Cancer. GIE 2017;86(1):18–33.

3. Rutter MD, East J, Rees CJ, et al. British Society of Gastroenterology/Association of Coloproctology of Great Britain and Ireland/Public Health England post-polypectomy and post-colorectal cancer resection surveillance guidelines. Gut 2020;69(2):201–23.

4. Otani T, Iwasaki M, Yamamoto S, et al. Japan Public Health Center-based Prospective Study Group. Alcohol consumption, smoking, and subsequent risk of colorectal cancer in middle-aged and elderly Japanese men and women: Japan Public Health Center-based prospective study. Cancer Epidemiol Biomarkers Prev 2003;12(12):1492–500.

5. Giovannucci E. An updated review of the epidemiological evidence that cigarette smoking increases risk of colorectal cancer. Cancer Epidemiol Biomarkers Prev 2001;10(7):725–31.

6. Sawicki T, Ruszkowska M, Danielewicz A, et al. A review of colorectal cancer in terms of epidemiology, risk factors, development, symptoms and diagnosis. Cancers (Basel) 2021;13(9):2025.

7. Koestler D, Li J, Baron J, et al. Distinct patterns of DNA methylation in conventional adenomas involving the right and left colon. Mod Pathol 2014;27:145–55.

8. Mesa H, Manivel JC, Larson WS, et al. Immunophenotypic comparison of neoplasms of the appendix, right colon, and left colon in search of a site-specific phenotypic signature. Int J Surg Pathol 2020;28(1):20–30.

9. Ponugoti PL, Cummings OW, Rex DK. Risk of cancer in small and diminutive colorectal polyps. Dig Liver Dis 2017;49(1):34–7.

10. Wieszczy P, Kaminski MF, Franczyk R, et al. Colorectal cancer incidence and mortality after removal of adenomas during screening colonoscopies. Gastroenterology 2020;158(4):875–83.

11. Rutter CM, Yu O, Miglioretti DL. A hierarchical non-homogenous Poisson model for meta-analysis of adenoma counts. Stat Med 2007;26(1):98–109.

12. Sheikh RA, Min BH, Yasmeen S, et al. Correlation of Ki-67, p53, and Adnab-9 immunohistochemical staining and ploidy with clinical and histopathologic features of severely dysplastic colorectal adenomas. Dig Dis Sci 2003;48(1):223–9.

13. Corley DA, Jensen CD, Marks AR, et al. Adenoma detection rate and risk of colorectal cancer and death. N Engl J Med 2014;370:1298–306.

14. Miyaki M, Konishi M, Kikuchi-Yanoshita R, et al. Characteristic of somatic mutation of the adenomatous polyposis coli gene in colorectal tumors. Cancer Res 1994;54:3011–20.

15. Nando Y, Watari J, Ito C, et al. Genetic instability, CpG island methylator phenotype, and proliferative activity are distinct differences between diminutive and small tubular adenoma of the colorectum. Hum Pathol 2017;60:37–45.

16. Wood LD, Parsons DW, Jones S, et al. The genomic landscapes of human breast and colorectal cancers. Science 2007;318:1108–13.

17. De Palma FDE, D'Argenio V, Pol J, et al. The molecular hallmarks of the serrated pathway in colorectal cancer. Cancers (Basel) 2019;11(7):1017.

18. Druliner BR, Ruan X, Sicotte H, et al. Early genetic aberrations in patients with sporadic colorectal cancer. Mol Carcinog 2018;57(1):114–24.

19. Schlesinger Y, Straussman R, Keshet I, et al. Polycomb-mediated methylation on Lys27 of histone H3 pre-marks genes for de novo methylation in cancer. Nat Genet 2007;39:232–6.

20. Fang M, Ou J, Hutchinson L, et al. The BRAF oncoprotein functions through the transcriptional repressor MAFG to mediate the CpG Island Methylator phenotype. Mol Cell 2014;55:904–15.

21. Serra RW, Fang M, Park SM, et al. A KRAS-directed transcriptional silencing pathway that mediates the CpG island methylator phenotype. eLife 2014;3: e02313.

22. Fodde R, Kuipers J, Rosenberg C, et al. Mutations in the APC tumour suppressor gene cause chromosomal instability. Nat Cell Biol 2001;3(4):433–8.

23. Sieber OM, Heinimann K, Gorman P, et al. Analysis of chromosomal instability in human colorectal adenomas with two mutational hits at APC. Proc Natl Acad Sci USA 2002;99(26):16910–5.

24. Nielsen M, de Miranda NF, van Puijenbroek M, et al. Colorectal carcinomas in MUTYH-associated polyposis display histopathological similarities to microsatellite unstable carcinomas. BMC Cancer 2009;15(9):184.

25. Yamaguchi S, Ogata H, Katsumata D, et al. MUTYH-associated colorectal cancer and adenomatous polyposis. Surg Today 2014;44(4):593–600.

26. Rumilla K, Schowalter KV, Lindor NM, et al. Frequency of deletions of EPCAM (TACSTD1) in MSH2-associated lynch syndrome cases. J Mol Diagn 2011; 13(1):93–9.

27. Bakry D, Aronson M, Durno C, et al. Genetic and clinical determinants of constitutional mismatch repair deficiency syndrome: report from the Constitutional Mismatch Repair Deficiency Consortium. Eur J Cancer 2014;50(5):987–96.

28. Boland CR, Thibodeau SN, Hamilton SR, et al. National Cancer Institute Workshop on Microsatellite Instability for Cancer Detection and Familial Predisposition: development of international criteria for the determination of microsatellite instability in colorectal cancer. Cancer Res 1998;58:5248–57.

29. Church JM. Polymerase proofreading-associated polyposis: a new, dominantly inherited syndrome of hereditary colorectal cancer predisposition. Dis Colon Rectum 2014;57(3):396–7.

30. Buchanan DD, Stewart JR, Clendenning M, et al. Risk of colorectal cancer for carriers of a germ-line mutation in POLE or POLD1. Genet Med 2018;20:890–5.

31. Crockett SD, Nagtegaal ID. Terminology, molecular features, epidemiology, and management of serrated colorectal neoplasia. Gastroenterology 2019;157: 949–66.

32. Higuchi T, Jass JR. My approach to serrated polyps of the colorectum. J Clin Pathol 2004;57(7):682–6.

33. Choi EY, Appelman HD. A historical perspective and exposé on serrated polyps of the colorectum. Arch Pathol Lab Med 2016;140(10):1079–84.

34. Bettington ML, Chetty R. Traditional serrated adenoma: an update. Hum Pathol 2015;46(7):933–8.

35. Torlakovic EE, Gomez JD, Driman DK, et al. Sessile serrated adenoma (SSA) vs. traditional serrated adenoma (TSA). Am J Surg Pathol 2008;32(1):21–9.

36. Chetty R, Hafezi-Bakhtiari S, Serra S, et al. Traditional serrated adenomas (TSAs) admixed with other serrated (so-called precursor) polyps and conventional adenomas: a frequent occurrence. J Clin Pathol 2015;68:270–3.

37. Kim KM, Lee EJ, Ha S, et al. Molecular features of colorectal hyperplastic polyps and sessile serrated adenoma/polyps from Korea. Am J Surg Pathol 2011;35(9): 1274–86.

38. Cauley CE, Hassab TH, Feinberg A, et al. Sessile serrated polyposis: not an inherited syndrome? Dis Colon Rectum 2020;63(2):183–9.

39. Quintana I, Mejias-Luque R, Terradas M, et al. Evidence suggests that germline RNF43 mutations are a rare cause of serrated polyposis. Gut 2018;67(12): 2230–2.

40. Boparai KS, Dekker E, Van Eeden S, et al. Hyperplastic polyps and sessile serrated adenomas as a phenotypic expression of MYH associated polyposis. Gastroenterology 2008;135:2014–8.

41. IJspeert JEG, Rana SAQ, Atkinson NSS, et al. Clinical risk factors of colorectal cancer in patients with serrated polyposis syndrome: a multicentre cohort analysis. Gut 2017;66:278–84.

42. Durno CA. Colonic polyps in children and adolescents. Can J Gastroenterol 2007;21(4):233–9.

43. Wu TT, Rezai B, Rashid A, et al. Genetic alterations and epithelial dysplasia in juvenile polyposis syndrome and sporadic juvenile polyps. Am J Pathol 1997; 150(3):939–47.

44. Blatter R, Tschupp B, Aretz S, et al. Disease expression in juvenile polyposis syndrome: a retrospective survey on a cohort of 221 European patients and comparison with a literature-derived cohort of 473 SMAD4/BMPR1A pathogenic variant carriers. Genet Med 2020;22(9):1524–32.

45. Milella M, Falcone I, Conciatori F, et al. PTEN: multiple functions in human malignant tumors. Front Oncol 2015;5:24.

46. Day FL, Jorissen RN, Lipton L, et al. PIK3CA and PTEN gene and exon mutation-specific clinicopathologic and molecular associations in colorectal cancer. Clin Cancer Res 2013;19(12):3285–96.

47. Stanich PP, Pearlman R, Hinton A, et al. Prevalence of germline mutations in polyposis and colorectal cancer-associated genes in patients with multiple colorectal polyps. Clin Gastroenterol Hepatol 2019;17(10):2008–15.

48. De Brabander J, Eskens FALM, Korsse SE, et al. Chemoprevention in patients with Peutz-Jeghers syndrome: lessons learned. Oncologist 2018;23(4):399, e33.

Quality Indicators for the Detection and Removal of Colorectal Polyps and Interventions to Improve Them

Angela Y. Lam, MD[a], Anna M. Duloy, MD[b],
Rajesh N. Keswani, MD, MS[c],*

KEYWORDS

- Colonoscopy • Quality • Detection • Polypectomy • Improvement

KEY POINTS

- The quality of polyp detection and removal during colonoscopy is operator-dependent. Suboptimal quality of lesion detection and removal may increase the risk of postcolonoscopy colorectal cancer.
- While numerous quality metrics for polyp detection, such as adenoma detection rate, have been developed and implemented into practice, quality metrics for polypectomy have been less studied. Measures currently include skills assessment tools and complete resection rates, though applicability outside of research studies remains a challenge.
- Multi-component interventions may be effective in improving the quality of neoplastic lesion detection and removal during colonoscopy, and are summarized in this review.

INTRODUCTION

While colorectal cancer (CRC) incidence has been decreasing over the last several decades, CRC remains the third leading cause of cancer-related deaths in the United States.[1] The beneficial effect of screening colonoscopy on reducing CRC incidence and mortality are largely derived from early detection and removal of neoplastic lesions.[2–4] However, the magnitude of this benefit varies based on examination quality—primarily, the ability of colonoscopists to detect and completely resect

Conflict of interest statement: R. Keswani is a consultant for Boston Scientific and Neptune Medical. All other authors disclosed no financial relationships.
[a] Department of Gastroenterology, Kaiser Permanente San Francisco Medical Center, 2350 Geary Boulevard, San Francisco, CA 94115, USA; [b] Division of Gastroenterology and Hepatology, University of Colorado Anschutz Medical Center, 1635 Aurora Court, Aurora, CO 80045, USA; [c] Division of Gastroenterology and Hepatology, Northwestern University Feinberg School of Medicine, 676 North Street, Clair, Suite 1400, Chicago, IL 60611, USA
* Corresponding author.
E-mail address: Raj-keswani@northwestern.edu

Gastrointest Endoscopy Clin N Am 32 (2022) 329–349
https://doi.org/10.1016/j.giec.2021.12.010

Abbreviations	
AAMR	advanced adenoma miss rate
ACE	assessment of competency in endoscopy
ADR	adenoma detection rate
AMR	adenoma miss rate
APC	adenomas per colonoscopy
BBPS	Boston bowel preparation scale
CADe	computer-aided detection
CIR	cecal intubation rate
CRC	colorectal cancer
CSPAT	cold snare polypectomy assessment tool
DOPyS	Direct Observation of Polypectomy Skills
HD-WLE	high-definition white light endoscopy
IRR	incomplete resection rate
PCCRC	post-colonoscopy colorectal cancer
SDR	sessile lesion detection rate
USMSTF	United States Multi-Society Task Force
WT	withdrawal time

precancerous polyps. While the ideal gold standard is that each colonoscopy "negative" for cancer has truly excluded CRC, postcolonoscopy colorectal cancers (PC-CRC) still occur. PC-CRC is defined as cancer appearing after a colonoscopy in which no cancer is diagnosed, encompassing interval cancers and noninterval cancers.[5] Etiologies include missed lesions, incomplete polypectomy, rapidly growing tumors[5,6] and iatrogenic tumor seeding.[7,8] The development of PC-CRC is the direct clinical outcome by which the effectiveness of colonoscopy in detecting and preventing CRC would ideally be measured, and root-cause analysis of each PC-CRC should be undertaken to understand etiology and contribution from potentially modifiable factors. However, the rarity of PC-CRC precludes feasible measurement as a quality metric.

To systematically optimize the quality of screening colonoscopy for the detection and prevention of neoplastic colorectal lesions, evidence-based quality metrics and interventions to guide improvement are crucial. This article aims to provide an overview of quality indicators for the detection and removal of colorectal polyps and review the evidence for interventions designed to improve them (summarized in **Fig. 1**).

ASSESSING THE QUALITY OF COLORECTAL POLYP DETECTION
Adenoma Detection Rate

The adenoma detection rate (ADR) measures the proportion of screening colonoscopies in which at least one adenoma is detected, and an inverse association with PC-CRC rate has been well-established in large studies performed in community-based populations.[9,10] When modeled as a continuous variable, each 1% increase in ADR predicted a 3% decrease in risk of PC-CRC.[10] Improvements in ADR over time have also been associated with subsequently reduced risk of PC-CRC.[11,12] Currently, the US Multi-Society Task Force (USMSTF) recommends ADR benchmarks of $\geq$30% for men, $\geq$20% for women, and $\geq$25% combined,[13] though data suggest there may be an additional benefit on the prevention of PC-CRC and related mortality with higher ADRs up to 33.5%.[10] Thus, recent guidance suggests that an optimal ADR may be greater than 35%.[14] In screening programs using fecal immunochemical tests (FITs), benchmark ADRs for subsequent colonoscopies performed for FIT-positive indication are $\geq$45% in men and $\geq$35% in women.[15]

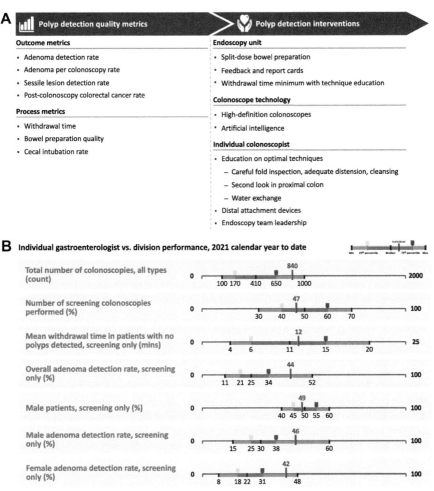

Fig. 1. (*A*) Overview of polyp detection quality metrics and interventions. (*B*) Sample adenoma detection report card.

While the current definition of ADR is restricted to screening colonoscopies, recent data from a sample of Veterans Affairs patients have suggested that a simplified overall ADR calculated from all colonoscopies does not significantly differ from conventional ADR.[16] These findings need to be validated in larger, more diverse patient populations before adoption into clinical practice.

Adenoma Per Colonoscopy Rate

While ADR has been extensively validated by a clear inverse association with PC-CRC rate and mortality,[9,10] there are limitations to consider. One concern is the "One and Done" theory,[17,18] referring to the potential practice of performing lower quality examination after the detection of one adenoma, as ADR does not credit the colonoscopist's ability to detect additional adenomas. The metric of adenomas per colonoscopy (APC) overcomes this theoretical concern. In a systematic review and meta-analysis to assess adenoma miss rates (AMR) and advanced adenoma miss rates (AAMR) on tandem colonoscopies, APC was more effective in monitoring AMR compared with ADR.[19] Importantly, APC (measured in positive index colonoscopies) was the only quality metric associated with AAMR. While APC generally correlates with ADR, APC has also been shown to be a greater differentiating metric between endoscopists compared with ADR alone.[20] Current barriers to adopting APC measurement in practice include increased pathology costs of bottling each adenoma separately, challenging methods of computation,[19] and lack of studies demonstrating an independent association with PC-CRC.

Sessile Serrated Lesion Detection Rate

Sessile serrated polyps are not currently factored into the calculation of ADR. This is chiefly related to significant interobserver variation between reading pathologists when discerning sessile serrated lesions from hyperplastic polyps, as well as the fact that serrated lesion detection rate (SDR) correlates significantly with ADR. However, PC-CRCs are more likely than screening-detected CRCs to develop from the sessile serrated pathway (CIMP-high, MSI-high), particularly in the proximal colon[17,21,22] highlighting the difficulty in detecting these lesions. Dedicated calculation of SDR addresses this gap, and SDR is calculated similarly to ADR as the proportion of screening colonoscopies with one or more sessile serrated lesion detected. SDR benchmarks of 7% to 11% have been suggested based on data from the New Hampshire Colonoscopy Registry.[23]

However, varying definitions of SDR and interobserver variation among pathologists distinguishing between sessile serrated polyps and hyperplastic polyps remain challenges to clinical implementation. The computation of SDR has varied across studies, some dependent on experienced pathologists.[24] In one study evaluating colonoscopies performed across 4 clinical sites with polyp specimens read by 48 pathologists, SDR was estimated to range from 0.5% to 12.0% depending on the reading pathologist.[25] As SDR correlates well with ADR, and uptake of ADR measurement is already suboptimal with only 61.5% of VA sites nationwide reporting ADR data,[26] it may be reasonable to focus on maximizing ADR uptake in clinical practice in settings with limited resources.

Withdrawal Time

Colonoscopy withdrawal time (WT) is a process measure defined as the time elapsed from when the colonoscope reaches the cecum to when it is withdrawn from the anus, excluding time taken for additional maneuvers such as polypectomy.[27] The rationale for implementing a minimum WT as a colonoscopy quality metric is that meticulous, high-quality mucosal examination requires time. Supporting this practice, an inverse correlation between WT of at least 6 minutes and PC-CRC rates was initially reported in the literature.[28] More recently, data have supported WT of at least 9 minutes to maximize the detection of neoplasia.[29] Of note, in practice, the WT is calculated on those colonoscopies whereby no polyps are biopsied or removed to increase the feasibility of this metric. However, one confounding factor to consider is that the withdrawal technique is the likely causal mechanism underlying the correlation between WT and PC-CRC rates. Measuring WT alone without a concomitant focus on withdrawal technique may miss the key causal element in the association with PC-CRC, though is much simpler to calculate. Consistent with this, mandating longer WT alone has not been shown to improve colorectal polyp detection.[30] Using WT as a quality metric may be most meaningful in evaluating the root cause of substandard ADRs, to identify avenues for improvement.

Withdrawal Technique

Ideal colonoscopy withdrawal technique focuses on 3 methods of improving neoplastic lesion detection: careful fold examination, adequate distension, and cleansing to obtain unobstructed views of the underlying colorectal mucosa. The first study to evaluate components of optimal withdrawal technique compared 2 colonoscopists in a tandem colonoscopy study, and found that the colonoscopist with lower AMR accrued higher scores for techniques focused on distension, cleansing, and time spent viewing and examining the proximal aspects of folds compared with the colonoscopist with higher AMR.[31] A follow-up study found that withdrawal technique scores were nearly 2-fold higher in colonoscopists with higher ADRs compared with those with lower ADRs; notably, there was no significant difference in WT.[32] Additionally, a study measuring colonoscopy inspection quality found that the scores correlated with ADR and SDR.[33] Measurement of withdrawal technique scores directly emphasizes the quality of colonic examination versus time spent in the procedure, though is labor-intensive to measure with limited feasibility outside of research studies at this time.

Bowel Preparation Quality

Adequate bowel preparation has been associated with colorectal lesion detection and ADR, primarily from improved detection of smaller lesions.[34–36] Inadequate bowel preparation has similarly been associated with a higher AMR in a systematic review and meta-analysis.[19] The validated Boston Bowel Preparation Scale (BBPS) is favored for the measurement of bowel preparation quality due to its high reliability.[37] Furthermore, BBPS scores have been shown to predict polyp detection rates[37] and the risk of missed neoplasia.[38] Currently, the benchmark for endoscopy units advises that 90% or above of screening colonoscopies should be scored adequate or better (overall BBPS score of ≥ 6, with each segment score of ≥ 2) in endoscopy units.[14]

Cecal Intubation Rate

Achieving cecal intubation is expected in all colonoscopies for the complete evaluation of the colorectum, and the performance target for screening examinations is $\geq 95\%$ based on the American Society for Gastrointestinal Endoscopy (ASGE)/American College of Gastroenterology (ACG) Task Force on Quality in Endoscopy.[14,17] Cecal intubation is defined as passing the colonoscope tip proximal to the ileocecal valve to visualize the entire cecal caput and should be documented through written reports and photographs of the appendiceal orifice and ileocecal valve. High cecal intubation rates are associated with lower risk of PC-CRC, particularly in the proximal colon.[39]

INTERVENTIONS TO IMPROVE THE DETECTION OF COLORECTAL POLYPS
High-Definition Colonoscopes

Observational studies initially detected that transitioning from standard-definition to high-definition colonoscopes was associated with higher ADR.[40] These findings have been validated in a recent systematic review and meta-analysis of 6 randomized controlled trials comparing high-definition white-light endoscopy (HD-WLE) to standard-definition colonoscopy, whereby ADR was significantly higher in the pooled HD-WLE arm compared with standard colonoscopy (40% vs 35%, risk ratio (RR): 1.13, 95% confidence interval (CI): 1.05–1.22).[41] Upgrading older, standard-definition colonoscopes to high-definition colonoscopes is an effective and sustainable intervention to improve ADR for entire endoscopy units and health care organizations.

Split-Dose Bowel Preparation

Administering bowel preparation in a split dose between the evening before and the morning of a colonoscopy has been shown to improve bowel preparation quality. Morning administration of bowel preparation was originally investigated as a strategy to address higher rates of inadequate bowel preparation in afternoon procedures,[42] and in an early prospective study was associated with improved bowel preparation quality as well as patient tolerability compared with traditional day-before preparation. In a subsequent meta-analysis of 47 trials, split-dose preparations were found to provide significantly better colon cleansing compared with day-before preparation (odds ratio (OR): 2.51; 95% CI: 1.86–3.39).[43] Furthermore, a higher proportion of patients were willing to repeat split-dose preparation (OR: 4.95; 95% CI: 1.05–3.46). Finally, in a multicenter endoscopist-blinded randomized trial of 690 patients, a split-dose bowel regimen was associated with a higher ADR compared with day-before preparation (53% compared with 30.9%, RR: 1.22, 95% CI: 1.03–1.46).[44] Notably, detection rates for advanced adenomas were also significantly higher in the split-dose preparation group (26.4% compared with 20.0% in day-before preparation arm, RR: 1.35, 95% CI: 1.06–1.73). Thus, transitioning from day-before bowel preparation to split-dose bowel preparation is an effective, patient-centered intervention that improves colorectal polyp detection through superior colon cleansing.

Simplifying Bowel Preparation Instructions

To optimize the quality of bowel preparation, instructions given to patients should be straightforward and easy to follow. Maximizing the ease and accessibility of bowel preparation instructions for all patients requires the consideration of socioeconomic disparities that inform health care disparities. Importantly in the United States, colorectal screening participation remains suboptimal in underserved populations including uninsured patients, recent immigrants, and racial/ethnic minorities.[45] Compounding this issue, in a study of 764 patients receiving care in primary care clinics and federally qualified health centers, comprehension of bowel preparation instructions was generally low and significantly worse among patients with low health literacy.[46] Simplification and standardization of instructions has rapidly improved preparation quality in real-time quality improvement initiatives.[47] Furthermore, simplified instructions provided at a 6th grade reading level was associated with improved bowel preparation and reduced procedural cancellation rates in a safety-net health care system.[48] Additional interventions that show promise in improving comprehension and accessibility of bowel preparation instructions include patient navigation programs,[49] educational videos,[50] and smartphone technologies.[51]

Continuous Audit with Endoscopist Feedback and Report Cards

Monitoring colonoscopy quality metrics and providing feedback to individual colonoscopists has been associated with improved ADR in a meta-analysis of 12 predominantly observational studies (RR: 1.21, 95% CI: 1.18–2.23).[52] Notably, colonoscopists with lower baseline ADRs derived greater benefit from this intervention compared with colonoscopists with higher baseline ADRs (RR: 1.62, 95% CI: 1.18–2.23 compared with RR: 1.06, CI: 0.99–1.13, respectively). While one single-center study also showed improvement in cecal intubation rates from 95.6% to 98.1% with quarterly report cards,[53] there was no significant improvement in cecal intubation rate nor WT in a larger meta-analysis.[52] Establishing minimum standards of practice alongside report card feedback may also augment ADR improvement.[54] A more recent longitudinal study from New Zealand demonstrated that continuous audit at a single institution demonstrated that the bulk of ADR and polyp detection rate improvement (from 25.8% to 28.3%) occurred in the first 2 years of auditing, and was primarily driven by increased detection of smaller adenomas and sessile serrated polyps.[55] Collectively, these studies highlight the value of continual assessment as a critical lever for improvement.

Where possible, coupling quality metric reporting with feedback and education on technique (particularly for low performers) is ideal. In a single-center randomized trial, an educational intervention for colonoscopists focused on best-practice techniques (careful fold examination, washing, recognition of subtle flat lesions, and classification of polyps) improved ADR from 36% to 47%, whereas the control group remained stagnant at 35% (OR: 1.73, 95% CI: 1.24–2.41).[56] Improvement was durable in a follow-up study,[57] though extension to multiple centers showed less differentiation between control and intervention sites.[58] In a separate study pairing colonoscopy inspection quality report cards (assessing fold examination, cleansing, and distension) with instructional videos, ADR and SDR modestly improved among colonoscopists with lower baseline ADR.[59] In a Polish study of 40 colonoscopy centers with inadequate ADR randomized to a leadership training program (skills assessment, hands-on training, and posttraining feedback for each center's leader) or audit and feedback only, the training arm demonstrated a larger improvement in ADR (3.9% absolute difference in mean ADR improvement, OR: 1.25, 95% CI: 1.04–1.50).[60] While programmatic training may be resource-intensive, the simpler alternative of educational support to facilitate improvement for low-performing colonoscopists should be available at all endoscopy units.

Optimizing Endoscopic Technique

The protective effect of colonoscopy against CRC is attenuated in the proximal colon, where a disproportionate fraction of PC-CRCs arise.[61–64] Proposed techniques to improve neoplasia detection in the proximal colon include right colon retroflexion as well as a second forward-viewing examination. In one observational single-center study, right-sided colon retroflexion identified a per-adenoma miss rate of 9.8% and per-patient AMR of 4.4% in the proximal colon, associated with increasing age, male sex, and the presence of polyps on forward view.[65] In a larger, multi-center prospective study, right-sided retroflexion resulted in a statistically significant but small increase in ADR (24.64% to 26.4%, 95% CI: 1.00–2.55).[66] A meta-analysis of 8 studies evaluating the effect of right colon retroflexion on adenoma detection found that the per-adenoma miss rate in the right colon was 16.9% (95% CI: 12.5%–22.5%).[67] However, right colon retroflexion may be technically challenging in some patients due to colonoscope looping, with an overall success rate of 91.9%.[67] Furthermore, cecal retroflexion is infrequently performed in practice and is often of inadequate quality.[68] Reexamination of the right colon in forward view yielded similar incremental ADR improvement compared with right colon retroflexion in a randomized controlled trial (ADR 46% compared with 47%, $P = .75$).[69] The number of adenomas per patient was also similar between groups (0.9 in second forward-viewing examination and 1.1 in retroflexion view, $P = .075$). High-quality reexamination of the proximal colon with either retroflexion or a second forward view examination are both effective in optimizing neoplasia detection.

Water exchange colonoscopy is another technique that may increase the detection of colorectal lesions via improved bowel cleansing. In a network meta-analysis of 17 randomized controlled trials comparing water exchange, gas insufflation, and water immersion colonoscopy, water exchange was associated with the highest overall ADR (OR: 1.40, 95% CI: 1.22–1.62 when compared with air insufflation, and OR:

1.31, 95% CI: 1.12–1.55 when compared with water immersion).[70] This effect was primarily linked to superior bowel preparation quality, as BBPS scores were highest in patients undergoing water exchange colonoscopy. An added benefit of water-aided colonoscopy (both exchange and immersion) was decreased insertion pain. It remains unclear whether water exchange provides any additional ADR benefit in patients who already have high BBPS scores.

Mandating Withdrawal Time Minimum

Mandating minimum WT have led to mixed results in observational studies. Two of the largest studies were published in 2008. Barclay and colleagues mandated an 8-minute WT among a group of 12 colonoscopists, and observed significantly greater rates of overall and advanced neoplasia detection during screening colonoscopy (34.7% vs 23.5% and 0.08 vs 0.055, respectively).[71] Notably, the intervention also included inspection technique education (insufflation, flexure and fold examination, suctioning, repetitive examination, and adequate time) at the beginning of the study period for all included colonoscopists, and segmented the 8-minute minimum into 2-minute minimums in each of 4 colonic sections using a timer. In contrast, Sawhney and colleagues implemented a 7-minute minimum WT policy across 42 colonoscopists and did not observe an effect on polyp detection.[30] While all colonoscopists were informed of the mandate, there was no further intervention regarding inspection technique or how to subdivide the 7 minutes. Both studies highlight the importance of technique, and limitation of WT as a process measure—while proper technique and meticulous examination require time, more time does not necessarily translate into better technique or examination.

Distal Attachment Devices

Distal attachment devices are mechanically designed to help colonoscopists better evaluate mucosa between haustral folds. An early meta-analysis of 4 studies demonstrated that cap-assisted colonoscopy demonstrated statistically significant improvement in proximal colon ADR (23% compared with 17%, respectively; OR: 1.49, 95% CI: 1.08–2.05).[72] Accordingly, there are now multiple devices better designed to expose and flatten haustral folds. In a multi-center randomized trial comparing high-definition colonoscopy alone compared with colonoscopy assisted by Endocuff, EndoRings, and full-spectrum endoscopy, the APC for Endocuff-assisted colonoscopy was highest at 1.82 (compared with 1.55 for EndoRings, 1.53 for standard high-definition colonoscopy, and 1.30 for full-spectrum endoscopy).[73] Multiple follow-up studies have demonstrated higher ADR, APC, and sessile lesion detection rates with Endocuff Vision-assisted colonoscopy compared with cap-assisted and standard colonoscopy.[74,75] AMRs were also lower while using Endocuff Vision.[74] Finally, a recent meta-analysis of 8 randomized controlled trials comparing Endocuff Vision to standard colonoscopy confirmed that the device was associated with significant ADR improvement (49.8% compared with 45.6, RR: 1.12, $P = .02$).[76] Notably, this difference was especially pronounced in colonoscopists with lower baseline ADR (<30%) with a subgroup ADR improvement of 9.4% ($P = .03$). The cuff device was also associated with shorter WT (by 0.93 minutes, $P<.01$), suggesting that the device facilitates efficient examination. While studies on non-Endocuff devices are scarcer, the AmplifEYE device was demonstrated to be noninferior to Endocuff Vision for adenoma detection.[77] The G-EYE device, a reusable balloon designed to flatten haustral folds and prevent slippage, was also found to significantly improve the detection of adenomas and sessile serrated polyps compared with standard colonoscopy.[78] Distal attachment devices mechanically reduce the workload of careful fold inspection, thereby improving detection in colonoscopists with lower ADR and offer the added benefit of increasing efficiency for high detectors.

Artificial Intelligence

Artificial intelligence is emerging as a novel technology that effectively improves ADR. A meta-analysis of 5 randomized controlled trials studying computer-aided detection (CADe) compared with standard colonoscopy control found that pooled ADR was significantly higher in the CADe group (36.6% compared with 25.2%, respectively, RR: 1.44, 95% CI: 1.27–1.62).[79] APC was also higher in the CADe group compared with control (RR: 1.70, 95% CI: 1.53–1.89). Notably, the low control group ADR generated concerns regarding generalizability to practice settings with higher baseline ADRs.[80] However, one trial demonstrated a significantly improved ADR of 54.8% in the CADe group compared with 40.4% in the control group, without a significant difference in WT.[81] Another recent prospective study evaluating colonoscopy aided by a CADe device (Skout) found that Skout-aided colonoscopy was associated with significantly higher screening ADR compared with historical controls (53.6% and 30.8%, respectively, $P = .024$).[82] Participating colonoscopists had an average ADR of 32.6% before the study period, supporting the effectiveness of artificial intelligence-aided polyp detection in settings with higher baseline ADRs.

Chromoendoscopy

Direct, dye-spray chromoendoscopy increased screening ADR in large randomized trials,[83,84] albeit marginally in settings with higher baseline ADR. While chromoendoscopy is used for screening in select high-risk patient populations,[85] the dye-spray process is considered too time and labor-intensive for routine screening colonoscopies. In a promising randomized controlled trial, delivery of methylene blue dye through a multi-matrix capsule improved ADR by 8.5% compared with placebo (OR: 1.46; 95% CI: 1.09–1.96), primarily through improved detection of diminutive adenomas and serrated polyps.[86] However, the drug was denied by the FDA until additional data from a confirmatory phase 3 trial are available. Electronic chromoendoscopy may also be effective in improving ADR, particularly through improved detection of diminutive flat adenomas in the proximal colon, though data are mixed.[85,87–90] The role of chromoendoscopy in routine colonoscopy remains an area of ongoing study.

Multiple Observers

The style of endoscopy team leadership may contribute to variation in detection rates. In a focus group study, endoscopy nurses identified physician leadership style as a factor affecting polyp detection—in particular, whether physicians set a collaborative team approach to the procedure in which all members are engaged in detecting lesions on the screen.[91] A small meta-analysis showing significantly higher ADR with nurse participation in polyp detection supports this hypothesis,[92] as did a broader meta-analysis of 23 studies comparing detection rates in colonoscopy performed by a single observer (colonoscopists alone) to those with dual observers (involving a nurse, trainee, and/or technician).[93] Framing neoplastic lesion detection as a team task in which all present staff members should engage is a simple practice that may improve ADR.

ASSESSING THE QUALITY OF POLYPECTOMY
Direct Polypectomy Outcomes

Optimizing polypectomy quality involves maximizing the effectiveness, safety, and efficiency of polypectomy technique.[94] The most direct measure of polypectomy effectiveness is to evaluate rates of complete resection, as the primary objective of polypectomy is complete lesion removal. Furthermore, incomplete polyp resection is a risk factor for PC-CRC. Polypectomy completeness is best assessed by biopsies of the postpolypectomy site, and in some cases, by close examination of the lateral and deep margins of snared polyp specimens.[95,96] In a prospective study wherein the resection margin was biopsied after "complete" polypectomy, 10.1% of polyps were found to be incompletely resected with rates increasing with polyp size (17.3% for polyps 10–20 mm, and 6.8% for polyps 5–9 mm) and with incomplete polypectomy rates varying between providers.[97] In a recent systematic review and meta-analysis evaluating incomplete resection rates (IRRs) of colon polyps up to 20 mm, overall IRR for snare removal was 13.8% and similarly increased with the size of the polyp (15.9% for polyps 1–10 mm and 20.8% for polyps 10–20 mm).[98] These data demonstrate alarming variability in resection quality, bringing attention to another dimension of colonoscopy quality that is less well-studied compared with polyp detection.

Unfortunately, the feasibility of measuring polypectomy completeness through resection margin biopsies and/or histologic examination of en bloc resection specimens is limited outside of research studies due to the additional time, labor, and costs required. Structured competency skills assessment tools, therefore, serve as theoretical proxy measures by scoring elements of resection best practices and are summarized in **Fig. 2**. However, research evaluating correlations between these tools and direct polypectomy outcomes (such as IRR) is lacking. As best practice guidelines for polypectomy emerge, adherence to recommendations will likely also become a focus of polypectomy quality assessment.

Direct Observation of Polypectomy Skills Tool

The direct observation of polypectomy skills (DOPyS) tool is the first validated method to measure polypectomy competence[99] and was designed to address the gap in methods to assess technical skills in polypectomy.[100] Polypectomy tasks were deconstructed to develop DOPyS, which includes a structured checklist of 34 individual components and a global assessment scale to assess overall polypectomy competence (**Fig. 2**B). The tool is applicable to live and videotaped polypectomy (though optimized for live assessment), and components (scored on a scale of 1–4)

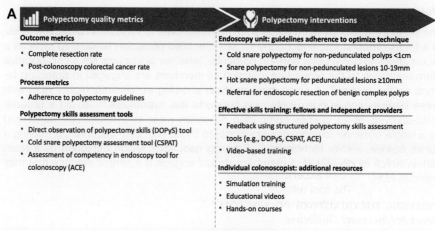

Fig. 2. (A) Overview of polypectomy quality metrics and interventions. (B) Direct observation of polypectomy skills (DOPyS). (C) Cold snare polypectomy assessment tool (CSPAT).

B DOPyS: Polypectomy Assessment Score Sheet

Date:_____

Assessor:_____

Endoscopist:_____

Case ID:_____

A separate sheet should be used for each case. Up to five polyps from one patient may be documents on the same DOPyS score sheet.

Scale and Criteria Key

4	Highly skilled performance
3	Competent and safe throughout procedure, no uncorrected errors
2	Some standards not yet met, aspects to be improved, some errors uncorrected
1	Accepted standards not yet met, frequent errors uncorrected
N/A	Not applicable/Not assessable

Generic	Polyp 1	Polyp 2	Polyp 3	Polyp 4	Polyp 5
Optimising view of / access to the polyp:					
1. Attempts to achieve optimal polyp position					
2. Optimises view by aspiration/insufflation/wash					
3. Determines full extent of lesion (+/- use of adjunctive techniques e.g. bubble breaker, NBI, dye spray etc) if appropriate					
4. Uses appropriate polypectomy technique (e.g. taking into account site in colon)					
5. Adjusts/stabilises scope position					
6. Checks all polypectomy equipment (forceps,snare,clips,loops) available					
7. Checks (or asks assistant to) snare closure prior to introduction into the scope					
8. Clear instructions to and utilisation of endoscopy staff					
9. Checks diathermy settings are appropriate					
10. Photo-documents pre and post polypectomy					
Stalked polyps: Generic, then					
11. Applies prophylactic haemostatic measures if deemed appropriate					
12. Selects appropriate snare size					
13. Directs snare accurately over polyp head					
14. Correctly selects en-bloc or piecemeal removal depending on size					
15. Advances snare sheath towards stalk as snare closed					
16. Places snare at appropriate position on the stalk					
17. Mobilises polyp to ensure appropriate amount of tissue is trapped within snare					
18. Applies appropriate degree of diathermy					
Sessile lesions / Endoscopic mucosal resection: Generic, then					
19. Adequate sub mucosal injection using appropriate injection technique, maintaining views					
20. Only proceeds if the lesion lifts adequately					
21. Selects appropriate snare size					
22. Directs snare accurately over the lesion					
23. Correctly selects en-bloc or piecemeal removal depending on size					
24. Appropriate positioning of snare over lesion as snare closed					
25. Ensures appropriate amount of tissue is trapped within snare					
26. Tents lesion gently away from the mucosa					
27. Uses cold snare technique or applies appropriate diathermy, as applicable					
28. Ensures adequate haemostasis prior to further resection					
Post polypectomy					
29. Examines remnant stalk/polyp base					
30. Identifies and appropriately treats residual polyp					
31. Identifies bleeding and performs adequate endoscopic haemostasis if appropriate					
32. Retrieves, or attempts retrieval of polyp					
33. Checks for retrieval of polyp					
34. Places tattoo competently, where appropriate					
Polyp size	mm	mm	mm	mm	mm
Polyp site: C/AC/TC/DC/SC/Rectum					
Overall Competency at Polypectomy: 4/3/2/1					
Comments:					

Fig. 2. continued.

include preprocedural or generic skills, specific skills depending on polyp size and morphology, and postpolypectomy skills. Scores of 1 and 2 indicate unacceptable and suboptimal competence, and scores of 3 and 4 indicate adequate and highly skilled competence, respectively. Validity was established in a study of 32 video-recorded polypectomies collected from colonoscopists of varying skill levels, assessed blindly by 4 experienced colonoscopists, 2 of whom were previously trained to use DOPyS. The tool reliably differentiated between polypectomies performed by colonoscopists of different experience levels when used by the previously trained assessors. However, DOPyS did not reliably differentiate the polypectomies graded by the 2 assessors who were unfamiliar with the tool beforehand. Thus, familiarity in skills assessment using DOPyS is a prerequisite to its use in clinical practice.

C

	4: Highly Skilled (perfect)	3: Competent and safe, no uncorrected errors (adequate)	2: Some standards not yet met, aspects to be improved, some errors uncorrected (sub-optimal)	1: Accepted standards not met, frequent errors uncorrected (unacceptable)
Achieves optimal polyp position	Ensures good polyp position (5-6 o'clock) with no errors during entire polypectomy.	Maintains polyp at 5-6 o'clock position during most of polypectomy with attempts at position correction	Does not maintain polyp at 5-6 o'clock position. Few attempts made at position correction	Does not maintain polyp in the optimal position at any time during the procedure
Optimizes view by aspiration/insufflation/wash	Maintains clear polyp views throughout the procedure	Attempts to obtain clear polyp views through aspiration, insufflation, and lens wash	Clear polyp views not maintained	Poor polyp views throughout the procedure with no attempts at correction
Adjusts/stabilizes scope position	Maintains stable colonoscope position Throughout polypectomy	Adjusts and stabilizes colonoscope position before polypectomy	Colonoscope not stabilized adequately. Little or no attempts made to reposition scope	Unstable colonoscope position throughout procedure with no attempts made at correction
Directs snare accurately over the lesion	Steers snare accurately over the lesion head with no errors	Steers snare accurately over the lesion head with minimal difficulty	Clumsy steering of snare over the lesion head	Clumsy steering of snare causing mucosal injury
Anchors sheath of snare several mm distal (downstream) to polyp	Efficiently and accurately positions and anchors snare several mm distal to polyp	Achieves adequate positioning of snare several mm distal to polyp, though with some inefficiency	Does not anchor sheath distal to polyp. Polypectomy may be adequate, but without border of normal tissue	Does not anchor sheath distal to polyp resulting in residual polyp tissue
Keeps tools close to scope	Keeps tool close to scope at all times	Keeps tool close to scope most of the time and in a way that does not preclude adequate polypectomy	Does not keep tool close to scope, but achieves adequate polypectomy	Does not keep tool close to scope resulting in inadequate polypectomy
Appropriate positioning of snare over lesion as snare closed	Accurately positions snare over lesion as snare closed gradually	Advances snare sheath in a controlled fashion toward stalk as snare is closed	Closes snare too rapidly or in an uncontrolled fashion	Closes snare too rapidly, cutting or shearing through the polyp tissue
Ensures appropriate amount of tissue is trapped within snare	Always ensures no additional tissue is trapped within snare	Ensures no additional tissue is trapped within snare	Does not ensure that additional tissue is not trapped within snare.	Does not check for additional tissue trapped within snare before resecting polyp.
Ensures rim of normal tissue is resected around polyp	Rim of normal tissue around entire polyp	Rim of normal tissue around most of polyp, but some areas resected at polyp border, adequate polypectomy	Most of polyp border without normal rim of tissue	No normal tissue around polyp resulting in residual polyp
Examines post-polypectomy site	Full visualization of post-polypectomy site using water jet to clear debris/blood	Visualization of post-polypectomy site, but some residual debris/blood	Sub-optimal visualization of post-polypectomy site where observer cannot tell whether resection was complete	No visualization of post polypectomy site
Identifies and appropriately treats residual polyp	Identifies and resects any residual tissue accurately	Identifies and resects any residual tissue	Does not adequately identify or treat visible residual polyp tissue	Leaves residual polyp tissue behind
Retrieves, or attempts, retrieval of polyp	Retrieves polyp by using method appropriate to polyp/size	Retrieves or attempts retrieval of polyp. May not use method appropriate to polyp/size	Inadequate attempt at retrieval of polyp	No attempts made at polyp retrieval
RATE THE OVERALL POLYPECTOMY Polypectomy time: _____ Polyp size: _____ Polyp morphology: ☐ Sessile ☐ Flat ☐ Pedunculated				

Fig. 2. continued.

Cold Snare Polypectomy Assessment Tool

The cold snare polypectomy assessment tool (CSPAT) was adapted from the DOPyS to assess the recommended technique to remove polyps <1 cm, which constitutes the majority of polyps detected during colonoscopy.[94,101] CSPAT includes 12 individual metrics and a global competence score designed for video-based assessment (see **Fig. 2**C). The individual metrics focus on evaluating skill in polyp inspection, positioning relative to the working channel, appropriate snare capture to include a rim of normal tissue, specimen retrieval, and postpolypectomy site inspection. Similar to the DOPyS, each component of the tool is scored from 1 (unacceptable) to 4 (highly skilled). The tool was validated through expert review of 55 colonoscopy videos, with a moderate degree of agreement in 10 metrics and a substantial degree of agreement in 2, suggesting adequate interrater reliability.[101] Average CSPAT scores also demonstrated moderate correlation to average DOPyS scores, indicating external validity. Compared with the DOPyS, the CSPAT is abbreviated and thus more efficient to use while also incorporating the assessment of skills specific to cold snare polypectomy. However, the CSPAT does not assess the ability to choose the correct polypectomy technique nor the quality of resection techniques outside of cold snare polypectomy.

Assessment of Competency in Endoscopy Tool for Colonoscopy

The assessment of competency in endoscopy (ACE) tool was adapted from the prior Mayo colonoscopy skills assessment tool by the ASGE Training Committee to evaluate cognitive and motor skills in colonoscopy. Skills assessed extend beyond polypectomy (such as loop reduction techniques, depth of independent scope advancement, management of patient discomfort, and lumen identification), though include the general assessment of knowledge and ability to apply therapeutic tools. In a large prospective multicenter trial of 93 gastroenterology fellows, the average fellow achieved all cognitive and motor skill endpoints after 250 procedures.[102] ACE is a broad colonoscopy skills assessment tool used in training that may approximate polypectomy competence, but is not designed to assess specific polypectomy technique.

Adherence to Recommended Polypectomy Practices

In 2020, the USMSTF published clinical practice guidelines outlining best practice recommendations for endoscopic removal of colorectal lesions.[94] These recommendations reflect a growing evidence base supporting the use of cold snare polypectomy to remove polyps <1 cm, aligning with previously published European Society of Gastrointestinal Endoscope (ESGE) guidelines.[103] Multiple studies have demonstrated higher complete resection rates with cold snare compared with cold forceps polypectomy in resecting polyps up to 10 mm in size.[104,105] One exception may be jumbo forceps polypectomy, which was noninferior to cold snare polypectomy for the resection of diminutive polyps up to 5 mm in a recent randomized controlled trial.[106] Cold resection techniques have also been favored where possible over electrocautery due to an enhanced safety and efficiency profile.[103,107–110] The 2020 USMSTF guidelines additionally suggest snare polypectomy (cold or hot) for nonpedunculated lesions between 10 and 19 mm, hot snare polypectomy for pedunculated lesions ≥10 mm, and endoscopic mucosal resection for nonpedunculated lesions ≥20 mm.[94] Establishing standardized and specific polypectomy guidelines in the United States provides an important foundation from which potential quality metrics may be developed and studied in the future.

Polypectomy Guidelines for Best Practice

With formal USMSTF guidelines recently published to guide polypectomy practice in the United States,[94] adherence to recommendations will be an area of interest. Implementation of polypectomy guidelines by the ESGE in 2010 had mixed results on selection of resection method in one European cohort study of screening colonoscopies.[111,112] Of polyps ≥5 mm in size, 46% were resected using forceps despite guidelines encouraging snare polypectomy. Following the implementation of guidelines, forceps polypectomy of lesions ≥5 mm decreased significantly in hospitals, but there was no improvement in forceps use in private practices—notably, forceps use for polyps greater than 10 mm in private practices even increased. In a recent single-center study in the United States, completed before USMSTF guideline implementation, 90% of diminutive polyps (1–3 mm), and 46.2% of small polyps (4–9 mm) were removed with cold forceps despite subjective survey results indicating that the study colonoscopists preferred cold snare polypectomy.[113–125] These results stress the need for additional studies evaluating resection techniques based on polyp size to gauge appropriateness, particularly after guideline implementation in the United States.

SUMMARY

Ensuring optimal quality of colorectal polyp detection and removal is fundamental to maximizing the protective effect of colonoscopy against CRC. By measuring the current state of practice, validated quality indicators provide an important starting point toward the goal of improving colonoscopy quality. Quality metrics for colorectal lesion detection are well-developed and integrated into clinical practice, with ADR in particular providing a reliable proxy measurement for the rate of post-colonoscopy CRCs. While quality metrics for polypectomy competence are scarce in comparison, current methods include the measurement of complete polypectomy rates, complication rates, and skills assessment tools, such as the DOPyS and CSPAT. While these resource-intensive methods are infrequently used in clinical practice, implementation of structured skills assessment in UK training programs has been successful. Continuous audit of quality metrics paired with multi-component interventions may improve the quality of polyp detection and removal, and reduce variation based on operator technique, colonoscope technology, and endoscopy unit practices.

CLINICS CARE POINTS

- When practicing colonoscopy withdrawal, focus attention on careful fold inspection, perform a second look in the proximal colon, involve the entire endoscopy team, and consider the use of a distal attachment device to improve polyp detection.

- When performing polypectomy for nonpedunculated polyps <1 cm, use cold snare technique to improve complete resection rates. Careful examination of the polypectomy base should be performed after all polypectomies to confirm complete resection.

- When teaching polypectomy to trainees, consider using a structured skills assessment tool, such as Direct Observation of Polypectomy Skills (DOPyS) or cold snare polypectomy assessment tool (CSPAT), to standardize and organize feedback.

REFERENCES

1. Siegel RL, Miller KD, Fuchs HE, et al. Cancer statistics, 2021. CA. Cancer J Clin 2021;71:7–33.

2. Winawer SJ, Zauber AG, Ho MN, et al. Prevention of colorectal cancer by colonoscopic polypectomy. N Engl J Med 1993;329:1977–81.

3. Zauber A, Winawer S, O'Brien M, et al. Colonoscopic polypectomy and long-term prevention of colorectal-cancer deaths. N Engl J Med 2012;366:687–96.

4. Tinmouth J, Vella ET, Baxter NN, et al. Colorectal cancer screening in average risk populations: evidence summary. Can J Gastroenterol Hepatol 2016; 2016:1–18.

5. Rutter MD, Beintaris I, Valori R, et al. World endoscopy organization consensus statements on post-colonoscopy and post-imaging colorectal cancer. Gastroenterology 2018;155:909–25.e3.

6. Anderson R, Burr NE, Valori R. Causes of post-colonoscopy colorectal cancers based on world endoscopy organization system of analysis. Gastroenterology 2020;158:1287–99.e2.

7. Backes Y, Seerden TCJ, Gestel RSFE, et al. Tumor seeding during colonoscopy as a possible cause for metachronous colorectal cancer. Gastroenterology 2019;157:1222–32.e4.

8. East JE. Can colonoscopy sow the seeds of colorectal cancer? Gastroenterology 2019;157:1192–5.

9. Kaminski MF, Regula J, Kraszewska E, et al. Quality indicators for colonoscopy and the risk of interval cancer. N Engl J Med 2010;362:1795–803.

10. Corley DA, Jensen CD, Marks AR, et al. Adenoma detection rate and risk of colorectal cancer and death. N Engl J Med 2014;370:1298–306.

11. Kaminski MF, Wieszczy P, Rupinski M, et al. Increased rate of adenoma detection associates with reduced risk of colorectal cancer and death. Gastroenterology 2017;153:98–105.

12. Lam A, Li Y, Gregory D, et al. Association between improved adenoma detection rates and interval colorectal cancer rates after a quality improvement program. Gastrointest Endosc 2020;92:355–64.e5.

13. Rex DK, Boland CR, Dominitz JA, et al. Colorectal cancer screening: recommendations for physicians and patients from the U.S. multi-society task force on colorectal cancer. Gastroenterology 2017;153:307–23.

14. Keswani RN, Crockett SD, Calderwood AH. AGA clinical practice update on strategies to improve quality of screening and surveillance colonoscopy: expert review. Gastroenterology 2021;161:701–11.

15. Robertson DJ, Lee JK, Boland CR, et al. Recommendations on fecal immunochemical testing to screen for colorectal neoplasia: a consensus statement by the US multi-society task force on colorectal cancer. Gastroenterology 2017; 152:1217–37.e3.

16. Kaltenbach T, Gawron A, Meyer CS, et al. Adenoma detection rate (ADR) irrespective of indication is comparable to screening ADR: implications for quality monitoring. Clin Gastroenterol Hepatol 2021;19:1883–9.e1.

17. Rex DK, Schoenfeld PS, Cohen J, et al. Quality indicators for colonoscopy. Gastrointest Endosc 2015;81:31–53.

18. Kaminski M, Robertson D, Senore C, et al. Optimizing the quality of colorectal cancer screening worldwide. Gastroenterology 2020;158:404–17.

19. Zhao S, Wang S, Pan P, et al. Magnitude, risk factors, and factors associated with adenoma miss rate of tandem colonoscopy: a systematic review and meta-analysis. Gastroenterology 2019;156:1661–74.e11.

20. Wang HS, Pisegna J, Modi R, et al. Adenoma detection rate is necessary but insufficient for distinguishing high versus low endoscopist performance. Gastrointest Endosc 2013;77:71–8.

21. Hoffmeister M, Bläker H, Jansen L, et al. Colonoscopy and reduction of colorectal cancer risk by molecular tumor subtypes: a population-based case-control study. Am J Gastroenterol 2020;115:2007–16.

22. Sawhney MS, Farrar WD, Gudiseva S, et al. Microsatellite instability in interval colon cancers. Gastroenterology 2006;131:1700–5.

23. Anderson JC, Butterly LF, Weiss JE, et al. Providing data for serrated polyp detection rate benchmarks: an analysis of the New Hampshire Colonoscopy Registry. Gastrointest Endosc 2017;85:1188–94.

24. Abdeljawad K, Vemulapalli KC, Kahi CJ, et al. Sessile serrated polyp prevalence determined by a colonoscopist with a high lesion detection rate and an experienced pathologist. Gastrointest Endosc 2015;81:517–24.

25. Gourevitch RA, Rose S, Crockett SD, et al. Variation in pathologist classification of colorectal adenomas and serrated polyps. Am J Gastroenterol 2018;113:431.

26. Gawron AJ, Lawrence P, Millar MM, et al. A nationwide survey and needs assessment of colonoscopy quality assurance programs in the VA. Fed Pract 2018;35:26–32.

27. May FP, Shaukat A. State of the science on quality indicators for colonoscopy and how to achieve them. Am J Gastroenterol 2020;115:1183–90.

28. Barclay RL, Vicari JJ, Doughty AS, et al. Colonoscopic withdrawal times and adenoma detection during screening colonoscopy. N Engl J Med 2006;355:2533–41.

29. Butterly L, Robinson CM, Anderson J, et al. Serrated and adenomatous polyp detection increases with longer withdrawal time: results from the new hampshire colonoscopy registry NIH public access. Am J Gastroenterol 2014;109:417–26.

30. Sawhney MS, Cury MS, Neeman N, et al. Effect of institution-wide policy of colonoscopy withdrawal time ≥ 7 minutes on polyp detection. Gastroenterology 2008;135:1892–8.

31. Rex DK. Colonoscopic withdrawal technique is associated with adenoma miss rates. Gastrointest Endosc 2000;51:33–6.

32. Lee RH, Tang RS, Muthusamy VR, et al. Quality of colonoscopy withdrawal technique and variability in adenoma detection rates (with videos). Gastrointest Endosc 2011;74:128–34.

33. Duloy A, Yadlapati RH, Benson M, et al. Video-based assessments of colonoscopy inspection quality correlate with quality metrics and highlight areas for improvement. Clin Gastroenterol Hepatol 2019;17:691–700.

34. Harewood GC, Sharma VK, Garmo P. Impact of colonoscopy preparation quality on detection of suspected colonic neoplasia. Gastrointest Endosc 2003;58:76–9.

35. Adler A, Wegscheider K, Lieberman D, et al. Factors determining the quality of screening colonoscopy: a prospective study on adenoma detection rates, from12 134 examinations (Berlin colonoscopy project 3, BECOP-3). Gut 2013;62:236–41.

36. Shaukat A, Oancea C, Bond JH, et al. Variation in detection of adenomas and polyps by colonoscopy and change over time with a performance improvement program. Clin Gastroenterol Hepatol 2009;7:1335–40.

37. Lai EJ, Calderwood AH, Doros G, et al. The Boston Bowel Preparation Scale: a valid and reliable instrument for colonoscopy-oriented research. Gastrointest Endosc 2009;69:620.

38. Kluge MA, Williams JL, Wu CK, et al. Inadequate boston bowel preparation scale scores predict the risk of missed neoplasia on next colonoscopy. Gastrointest Endosc 2018;87:744.

39. Baxter NN, Sutradhar R, Forbes SS, et al. Analysis of administrative data finds endoscopist quality measures associated with postcolonoscopy colorectal cancer. Gastroenterology 2011;140:65–72.

40. Buchner AM, Shahid MW, Heckman MG, et al. High-definition colonoscopy detects colorectal polyps at a higher rate than standard white-light colonoscopy. Clin Gastroenterol Hepatol 2010;8:364–70.
41. Tziatzios G, Gkolfakis P, Lazaridis LD, et al. High-definition colonoscopy for improving adenoma detection: a systematic review and meta-analysis of randomized controlled studies. Gastrointest Endosc 2020;91:1027–36.e9.
42. Varughese S, Kumar AR, George A, et al. Morning-only one-gallon polyethylene glycol improves bowel cleansing for afternoon colonoscopies: a randomized endoscopist-blinded prospective study. Am J Gastroenterol 2010;105:2368–74.
43. Martel M, Barkun AN, Menard C, et al. Split-dose preparations are superior to day-before bowel cleansing regimens: a meta-analysis. Gastroenterology 2015;149:79–88.
44. Radaelli F, Paggi S, Hassan C, et al. Split-dose preparation for colonoscopy increases adenoma detection rate: a randomised controlled trial in an organised screening programme. Gut 2017;66:270–7.
45. Gupta S, Sussman DA, Doubeni CA, et al. Challenges and possible solutions to colorectal cancer screening for the underserved. J Natl Cancer Inst 2014;106: dju032.
46. Smith SG, von Wagner C, McGregor LM, et al. The influence of health literacy on comprehension of a colonoscopy preparation information leaflet. Dis Colon Rectum 2012;55:1074.
47. Calderwood A, Mahoney E, Jacobson B. A plan-do-study-act approach to improving bowel preparation quality. Am J Med Qual 2017;32:194–200.
48. Davis T, Hancock J, Morris J, et al. Impact of health literacy-directed colonoscopy bowel preparation instruction sheet. Am J Health Behav 2017;41:301–8.
49. Naylor K, Fritz C, Polite B, et al. Evaluating screening colonoscopy quality in an uninsured urban population following patient navigation. Prev Med Reports 2016;5:194–9.
50. Prakash SR, Verma S, McGowan J, et al. Improving the quality of colonoscopy bowel preparation using an educational video. Can J Gastroenterol 2013;27: 696–700.
51. El Bizri M, El Sheikh M, Lee G, et al. Mobile health technologies supporting colonoscopy preparation: a systematic review and meta-analysis of randomized controlled trials. PLoS One 2021;16:e0248679.
52. Bishay K, Causada-Calo N, Scaffidi MA, et al. Associations between endoscopist feedback and improvements in colonoscopy quality indicators: a systematic review and meta-analysis. Gastrointest Endosc 2020;92:1040.e9.
53. Kahi CJ, Ballard D, Shah AS, et al. Impact of a quarterly report card on colonoscopy quality measures. Gastrointest Endosc 2013;77:925–31.
54. Keswani RN, Yadlapati R, Gleason KM, et al. Physician report cards and implementing standards of practice are both significantly associated with improved screening colonoscopy quality. Am J Gastroenterol 2015;110:1134–9.
55. Fraser A, Rose T, Wong P, et al. Improved detection of adenomas and sessile serrated polyps is maintained with continuous audit of colonoscopy. BMJ Open Gastroenterol 2020;7:e000425.
56. Coe S, Crook J, Diehl N, et al. An endoscopic quality improvement program improves detection of colorectal adenomas. Am J Gastroenterol 2013;108:219–26.
57. Ussui V, Coe S, Rizk C, et al. Stability of increased adenoma detection at colonoscopy. Follow-up of an endoscopic quality improvement program-EQUIP-II. Am J Gastroenterol 2015;110:489–96.

58. Wallace MB, Crook JE, Thomas CS, et al. Effect of an endoscopic quality improvement program on adenoma detection rates: a multicenter cluster-randomized controlled trial in a clinical practice setting (EQUIP-3). Gastrointest Endosc 2017;85:538–45.e4.

59. Duloy A, Wood M, Benson M, et al. 126 Individualized feedback on colonoscopy skills improves group colonoscopy quality in providers with lower adenoma detection rates (ADR). Gastrointest Endosc 2019;89:AB53.

60. Kaminski M, Anderson J, Valori R, et al. Leadership training to improve adenoma detection rate in screening colonoscopy: a randomised trial. Gut 2016;65: 616–24.

61. Samadder NJ, Curtin K, Tuohy TMF, et al. Characteristics of missed or interval colorectal cancer and patient survival: a population-based study. Gastroenterology 2014;146:950–60.

62. Singh H, Nugent Z, Mahmud SM, et al. Predictors of colorectal cancer after negative colonoscopy: a population-based study. Am J Gastroenterol 2010; 105:663–73.

63. Singh H, Nugent Z, Demers AA, et al. Rate and predictors of early/missed colorectal cancers after colonoscopy in manitoba: a population-based study. Am J Gastroenterol 2010;105:2588–96.

64. Bressler B, Paszat LF, Chen Z, et al. Rates of new or missed colorectal cancers after colonoscopy and their risk factors: a population-based analysis. Gastroenterology 2007;132:96–102.

65. Hewett DG, Rex DK. Miss rate of right-sided colon examination during colonoscopy defined by retroflexion: an observational study. Gastrointest Endosc 2011; 74:246–52.

66. Chandran S, Parker F, Vaughan R, et al. Right-sided adenoma detection with retroflexion versus forward-view colonoscopy. Gastrointest Endosc 2015;81: 608–13.

67. Cohen J, Grunwald D, Grossberg LB, et al. The effect of right colon retroflexion on adenoma detection: a systematic review and meta-analysis. J Clin Gastroenterol 2017;51:818–24.

68. Keswani RN, Kahi CJ, Benson M, et al. Cecal retroflexion is infrequently performed in routine practice and the retroflexed view is of poor quality. BMC Gastroenterol 2021;21:307.

69. Kushnir VM, Oh YS, Hollander T, et al. Impact of retroflexion vs. second forward view examination of the right colon on adenoma detection: a comparison study. Am J Gastroenterol 2015;110:415.

70. Fuccio L, Frazzoni L, Hassan C, et al. Water exchange colonoscopy increases adenoma detection rate: a systematic review with network meta-analysis of randomized controlled studies. Gastrointest Endosc 2018;88:589–97.e11.

71. Barclay RL, Vicari JJ, Greenlaw RL. Effect of a time-dependent colonoscopic withdrawal protocol on adenoma detection during screening colonoscopy. Clin Gastroenterol Hepatol 2008;6:1091–8.

72. Desai M, Sanchez-Yague A, Choudhary A, et al. Impact of cap-assisted colonoscopy on detection of proximal colon adenomas: systematic review and meta-analysis. Gastrointest Endosc 2017;86:274–81.e3.

73. Rex D, Repici A, Gross S, et al. High-definition colonoscopy versus Endocuff versus EndoRings versus full-spectrum endoscopy for adenoma detection at colonoscopy: a multicenter randomized trial. Gastrointest Endosc 2018;88: 335–44.e2.

74. Rameshshanker R, Tsiamoulos Z, Wilson A, et al. Endoscopic cuff-assisted colonoscopy versus cap-assisted colonoscopy in adenoma detection: randomized tandem study-DEtection in Tandem Endocuff Cap Trial (DETECT). Gastrointest Endosc 2020;91:894–904.e1.

75. Rex DK, Slaven JE, Garcia J, et al. Endocuff vision reduces inspection time without decreasing lesion detection: a clinical randomized trial. Clin Gastroenterol Hepatol 2020;18:158–62.e1.

76. Patel HK, Chandrasekar VT, Srinivasan S, et al. Second-generation distal attachment cuff improves adenoma detection rate: meta-analysis of randomized controlled trials. Gastrointest Endosc 2021;93:544–53.e7.

77. Rex DK, Sagi SV, Kessler WR, et al. A comparison of 2 distal attachment mucosal exposure devices: a noninferiority randomized controlled trial. Gastrointest Endosc 2019;90:835–40.e1.

78. Shirin H, Shpak B, Epshtein J, et al. G-EYE colonoscopy is superior to standard colonoscopy for increasing adenoma detection rate: an international randomized controlled trial (with videos). Gastrointest Endosc 2019;89:545–53.

79. Hassan C, Spadaccini M, Iannone A, et al. Performance of artificial intelligence in colonoscopy for adenoma and polyp detection: a systematic review and meta-analysis. Gastrointest Endosc 2021;93:77–85.e6.

80. Leung FW, Hsieh YH. Artificial intelligence (computer-assisted detection) is the most recent novel approach to increase adenoma detection. Gastrointest Endosc 2021;93:86–8.

81. Repici A, Badalamenti M, Maselli R, et al. Efficacy of real-time computer-aided detection of colorectal neoplasia in a randomized trial. Gastroenterology 2020; 159:512–20.e7.

82. Shaukat A, Colucci D, Erisson L, et al. Improvement in adenoma detection using a novel artificial intelligence-aided polyp detection device. Endosc Int Open 2021;09:E263–70.

83. Pohl J, Schneider A, Vogell H, et al. Pancolonic chromoendoscopy with indigo carmine versus standard colonoscopy for detection of neoplastic lesions: a randomised two-centre trial. Gut 2011;60:485–90.

84. Kahi C, Anderson J, Waxman I, et al. High-definition chromocolonoscopy vs. high-definition white light colonoscopy for average-risk colorectal cancer screening. Am J Gastroenterol 2010;105:1301–7.

85. Bisschops R, East J, Hassan C, et al. Advanced imaging for detection and differentiation of colorectal neoplasia: European Society of Gastrointestinal Endoscopy (ESGE) Guideline - Update 2019. Endoscopy 2019;51:1155–79.

86. Repici A, Wallace MB, East JE, et al. Efficacy of per-oral methylene blue formulation for screening colonoscopy. Gastroenterology 2019;156:2198–207.e1.

87. Kidambi TD, Terdiman JP, El-Nachef N, et al. Effect of I-scan electronic chromoendoscopy on detection of adenomas during colonoscopy. Clin Gastroenterol Hepatol 2019;17:701–8.e1.

88. Aziz M, Desai M, Hassan S, et al. Improving serrated adenoma detection rate in the colon by electronic chromoendoscopy and distal attachment: systematic review and meta-analysis. Gastrointest Endosc 2019;90:721–31.e1.

89. Desai M, Viswanathan L, Gupta N, et al. Impact of electronic chromoendoscopy on adenoma miss rates during colonoscopy: a systematic review and meta-analysis. Dis Colon Rectum 2019;62:1124–34.

90. Dinesen L, Chua J, Kaffes AJ. Meta-analysis of narrow-band imaging versus conventional colonoscopy for adenoma detection. Gastrointest Endosc 2012; 75:604–11.

91. Atkins L, Hunkeler EM, Jensen CD, et al. Factors influencing variation in physician adenoma detection rates: a theory-based approach. Gastrointest Endosc 2016;83:617.

92. Xu L, Zhang Y, Song H, et al. Nurse participation in colonoscopy observation versus the colonoscopist alone for polyp and adenoma detection: a meta-analysis of randomized, controlled trials. Gastroenterol Res Pract 2016;2016: 7631981.

93. Aziz M, Weissman S, Khan Z, et al. Use of 2 observers increases adenoma detection rate during colonoscopy: systematic review and meta-analysis outcomes and statistical analysis. Clin Gastroenterol Hepatol 2020;18:1240–2.

94. Kaltenbach T, Anderson JC, Burke CA, et al. Endoscopic removal of colorectal lesions—recommendations by the us multi-society task force on colorectal cancer. Gastroenterology 2020;158:1095–129.

95. Choi J, Lee C, Park J, et al. Complete resection of colorectal adenomas: what are the important factors in fellow training? Dig Dis Sci 2015;60:1579–88.

96. Horiuchi A, Ikuse T, Tanaka N. Cold snare polypectomy: indications, devices, techniques, outcomes and future. Dig Endosc 2019;31:372–7.

97. Pohl H, Srivastava A, Bensen SP, et al. Incomplete polyp resection during colonoscopy—results of the complete adenoma resection (CARE) study. Gastroenterology 2013;144:74–80.e1.

98. Djinbachian R, Iratni R, Durand M, et al. Rates of incomplete resection of 1- to 20-mm colorectal polyps: a systematic review and meta-analysis. Gastroenterology 2020;159:904–14.e12.

99. Gupta S, Bassett P, Man R, et al. Validation of a novel method for assessing competency in polypectomy. Gastrointest Endosc 2012;75(3):568–75.

100. Gupta S, Anderson J, Bhandari P, et al. Development and validation of a novel method for assessing competency in polypectomy: direct observation of polypectomy skills. Gastrointest Endosc 2011;73:1232–9.e2.

101. Patel SG, Duloy A, Kaltenbach T, et al. Development and validation of a video-based cold snare polypectomy assessment tool (with videos). Gastrointest Endosc 2019;89:1222–30.e2.

102. Sedlack RE, Coyle WJ. Assessment of competency in endoscopy: establishing and validating generalizable competency benchmarks for colonoscopy. Gastrointest Endosc 2016;83:516–23.e1.

103. Ferlitsch M, Moss A, Hassan C, et al. Colorectal polypectomy and endoscopic mucosal resection (EMR): European Society of Gastrointestinal Endoscopy (ESGE) Clinical Guideline. Endoscopy 2017;49:270–97.

104. Kim JS, Lee B-I, Choi H, et al. Cold snare polypectomy versus cold forceps polypectomy for diminutive and small colorectal polyps: a randomized controlled trial. Gastrointest Endosc 2015;81:741–7.

105. Jung YS, Park CH, Nam E, et al. Comparative efficacy of cold polypectomy techniques for diminutive colorectal polyps: a systematic review and network meta-analysis. Surg Endosc 2018;32:1149–59.

106. Huh CW, Kim JS, Choi HH, et al. Jumbo biopsy forceps versus cold snares for removing diminutive colorectal polyps: a prospective randomized controlled trial. Gastrointest Endosc 2019;90:105–11.

107. Tutticci NJ, Kheir AO, Hewett DG. The cold revolution how far can it go? Gastrointest Endosc Clin N Am 2019;29:721–36.

108. Patel K, Rajendran A, Faiz O, et al. An international survey of polypectomy training and assessment. Endosc Int Open 2017;05:E190–7.

109. Rajendran A, Thomas-Gibson S, Bassett P, et al. Lower gastrointestinal polypectomy competencies in the United Kingdom: a retrospective analysis of Directly Observed Polypectomy Skills (DOPyS). Endoscopy 2021;53:629–35.

110. Duloy AM, Kaltenbach TR, Keswani RN. Assessing colon polypectomy competency and its association with established quality metrics. Gastrointest Endosc 2018;87:635–44.

111. Britto-Arias M, Waldmann E, Jeschek P, et al. Forceps versus snare polypectomies in colorectal cancer screening: are we adhering to the guidelines? Endoscopy 2015;47:898–902.

112. Pedersen I, Løberg M, Hoff G, et al. Polypectomy techniques among gastroenterologists in Norway – a nationwide survey. Endosc Int Open 2018;06:E812–20.

113. Kadle N, Westerveld DR, Banerjee D, et al. Discrepancy between self-reported and actual colonoscopy polypectomy practices for the removal of small polyps. Gastrointest Endosc 2020;91:655–62.e2.

114. van Doorn S, Bastiaansen B, Thomas-Gibson S, et al. Polypectomy skills of gastroenterology fellows: can we improve them? Endosc Int Open 2016;4:E182–9.

115. Kaltenbach TR, Patel S, Nguyen-Vu T, et al. ID: 3526237 Varied trainee competence in cold snare polypectomy (CSP): results of the complete randomized controlled trial - improving competency and metrics for polypectomy skills using evaluation tools and video feedback. Gastrointest Endosc 2021;93:AB65–6.

116. Patel K, Faiz O, Rutter M, et al. The impact of the introduction of formalised polypectomy assessment on training in the UK. Frontline Gastroenterol 2017;8:104–9.

117. Duloy AM, Kaltenbach TR, Wood M, et al. Colon polypectomy report card improves polypectomy competency: results of a prospective quality improvement study (with video). Gastrointest Endosc 2019;89:1212–21.

118. Ansell J, Hurley J, Horwood J, et al. The Welsh Institute for Minimal Access Therapy colonoscopy suitcase has construct and concurrent validity for colonoscopic polypectomy skills training: a prospective, cross-sectional study. Gastrointest Endosc 2014;79:490–7.

119. Ansell J, Arnaoutakis K, Goddard S, et al. The WIMAT colonoscopy suitcase model: a novel porcine polypectomy trainer. Color Dis 2013;15:217–23.

120. Jirapinyo P, Kumar N, Thompson CC. Validation of an endoscopic part-task training box as a skill assessment tool. Gastrointest Endosc 2015;81:967–73.

121. Haycock A, Youd P, Bassett P, et al. Simulator training improves practical skills in therapeutic GI endoscopy: results from a randomized, blinded, controlled study [Internet]. Gastrointest Endosc 2009;70:835–45.

122. Frimberger E, Klare P, Haller B, et al. Preliminary assessment of two novel mechanical colonoscopic polypectomy simulators: description, evaluation and validation. Endosc Int Open 2020;08:E1522–9.

123. Burgess NG, Bahin FF, Bourke MJ. Colonic polypectomy (with videos). Gastrointest Endosc 2015;81:813–35.

124. Keswani RN. Cold snare polypectomy: techniques and applications. Clin Gastroenterol Hepatol 2020;18:42–4.

125. Kucera W, Nealeigh M, Dunkin B, et al. The SAGES flexible endoscopy course for fellows: a worthwhile investment in furthering surgical endoscopy. Surg Endosc 2019;33:1189–95.

Patient Selection, Risks, and Long-Term Outcomes Associated with Colorectal Polyp Resection

Sanjeevani K. Tomar, MD[a],*, John A. Damianos, MD[b], Sultan Mahmood, MD[c]

KEYWORDS

- Colonoscopy • Complications • Risk factors • Polypectomy • Perforation
- Postpolypectomy bleeding • Postpolypectomy syndrome

KEY POINTS

- Adverse events from endoscopic mucosal resection and polypectomy, although rare, include immediate and delayed bleeding, perforation, and postpolypectomy syndrome, which can compromise the success of the procedure if not recognized and managed appropriately in a timely manner.
- Intraprocedural bleeding can be managed effectively with a variety of endoscopic modalities depending on the type of lesion, completeness of resection, device availability, and operator preference, whereas delayed postpolypectomy bleeding can be managed conservatively in most cases.
- For perforations, mucosal clip placement is the primary endoscopic therapy, although newer devices, such as the over-the-scope clip and endoscopic suturing, have expanded the options.
- Perforation closures should be monitored carefully with a multidisciplinary approach, with prompt surgical intervention in the case of clinical deterioration.
- Colonoscopy and polypectomy are associated with a significant reduction in risk of colon cancer. However, recurrent polyps and interval cancer remain a concern and can usually be attributed to incomplete resection and missed lesions.

 Video content accompanies this article at http://www.giendo.theclinics.com.

[a] Department of Internal Medicine, University at Buffalo, Erie County Medical Center, David K. Miller Building, 462 Grider Street, Buffalo, NY 14215, USA; [b] Department of Internal Medicine, Yale New Haven Health System, Yale School of Medicine, 333 Cedar Street-1080 LMP, New Haven, CT 06520-8019, USA; [c] Division of Gastroenterology, Hepatology & Nutrition, University at Buffalo, B6-13 Buffalo General Medical Center, 100 High Street, Buffalo, NY 14203, USA
* Corresponding author.
E-mail address: sktomar@buffalo.edu

Gastrointest Endoscopy Clin N Am 32 (2022) 351–370
https://doi.org/10.1016/j.giec.2021.12.011
1052-5157/22/© 2021 Elsevier Inc. All rights reserved.

giendo.theclinics.com

INTRODUCTION

Colonoscopies are routinely used to screen for colorectal cancer (CRC), enabling the detection and resection of colorectal polyps and thereby reducing the incidence of and mortality from CRC.[1] However, colonoscopy alone or in association with polyp removal can cause a spectrum of complications, including bleeding, perforation, and postpolypectomy syndrome (PPS).[2] Although no technique for colonoscopic polyp removal is entirely devoid of adverse events, they are relatively rare and their risk is generally outweighed by the benefits. Here, we review the patient selection criteria; complications; including their risk factors and management; and long-term outcomes associated with colorectal polyp resection to improve the risk-benefit analysis by physicians and facilitate a comprehensive informed consent process for patients.

RISK ASSESSMENT FOR PATIENT SELECTION

The vast majority (>85%) of serious colonoscopy complications result from polypectomy.[3] However, gastrointestinal (GI) endoscopists will almost certainly have patients who experience some type of iatrogenic adverse event, which are virtually unavoidable complications of endoscopy. Therefore, the goal should be to minimize the associated risks. Although serious adverse events can result in substantial morbidity and mortality, even minor events strain the patient-physician relationship. The objective of this article is to provide the endoscopist with approaches to reduce the risk of iatrogenic complications and to manage those that will inevitably occur.

The endoscopist should always question whether the procedure is truly indicated, not only from their own perspective but also from that of the patient. The endoscopist should then prepare for the procedure according to the following:

1. Know the patient's history in addition to any underlying comorbidities and medications
2. Know the polyp-related factors, including size, location, history, and morphology
3. Understand the complications that may arise due to the polyp removal technique and the equipment involved

When antithrombotic therapy is required for a short period of time (ie, after venous thromboembolism or bare metal stent insertion), polypectomy should be delayed until such therapy is no longer indicated. Once this period has elapsed, the decision to proceed with the procedure should be made after discussing the associated risks and benefits with the patient and relevant medical professionals.[4] In addition, the ability to withstand complications in older patients is much reduced, and so perforation or bleeding postpolypectomy is more likely to result in a poor outcome.[5] Thus, polypectomy should be avoided for polyps less than 1 cm in patients aged 80 years or older because of the very low likelihood of progression to cancer within their life expectancy. Removal of polyps greater than 1 cm should only be considered after careful assessment of the patient's underlying comorbidities and overall functional status and after deliberation with the patient.[6]

The level of training and expertise of the practitioner greatly influence the risk involved in any procedure. Even the best-prepared endoscopists, however, should know their capabilities and their limitations. According to the American Society for Gastrointestinal Endoscopy (ASGE) Quality Committee, an endoscopist experienced in advanced polypectomy should be enlisted for the removal of suspected benign colorectal lesions that are considered more complex, for example, polypectomy of stalked polyps greater than 2 cm (level 3) and colonic endoscopic submucosal resection (EMR) and endoscopic submucosal dissection (ESD) (level 4); level 2 competency, for example, removal of stalked polyps less than 2 cm, is recommended for independent basic practice.[7] The risk of adverse events increases with the complexity of the procedure. If the endoscopist does not feel confident in performing a procedure without incurring a serious adverse event, such as perforation or bleeding, an alternative clinically appropriate procedure should be considered or the patient should be referred to a more experienced endoscopist.[8]

The ASGE/American College of Gastroenterology Task Force on Quality in Endoscopy recommends that the postpolypectomy bleeding rate should be less than 1 of 100 procedures and the postcolonoscopy perforation rate for all examinations should be less than or equal to 1 of 500 colonoscopies; rates higher than these should initiate review by an endoscopy unit medical director or another expert to determine whether insertion or polypectomy practices are inappropriate.[9] Endoscopy units should strive for ongoing practice performance (quality) improvement. For example, endoscopists can present cases of adverse events at morbidity and mortality conferences and compare the rates in their unit with those reported across the country, such as with the GI Quality Improvement Consortium (GiQuIC), and/or enrolling in the ASGE Endoscopic Unit Recognition Program. By identifying trends associated with adverse events such as bleeding and perforation, the cause of a high adverse event rate can be more easily identified and addressed.

CONSENSUS-BASED DEFINITIONS

In 2010, the ASGE introduced standardized definitions for complications of endoscopy. An adverse event is defined as an event that prevents completion of the planned procedure and/or results in either admission to the hospital, a prolonged hospital stay, another procedure (needing sedation/anesthesia), or subsequent medical consultation. The complications can range from mild (requiring 3 or fewer nights' hospitalization) to severe (resulting in extended hospitalization, requiring surgical intervention, and resulting in permanent disability or even death).[10]

Bleeding is defined as a hemoglobin drop greater than 2 g/dL, although the requirement for blood transfusion has been proposed by others.[10,11] Perforation is determined by evidence of air or luminal contents outside the GI tract.[10]

ADVERSE EVENTS OF POLYPECTOMY

Although colonoscopy is generally considered safe, there are increased risks for several types of complications following polyp resection (**Box 1**), most of which are

---

Box 1
Complications of colonoscopy with polypectomy

- Hemorrhage
- Perforation
- Postpolypectomy syndrome
- Abdominal pain/discomfort
- Cardiopulmonary events/sedation related
- Rare: splenic hematoma or rupture, acute appendicitis, diverticulitis, incarcerated hernias, subcutaneous emphysema, intramural hematoma, ischemic colitis, chemical colitis, colonic explosion, infection, and death

largely self-limited or manageable with a conservative approach or endoscopy, although some can be life threatening and require surgery.[5] The complication rates reported by different studies are quite varied, likely as a result of different criteria, end points, and methods. In this section, we discuss some of the most common complications across all studies.

Hemorrhage

Hemorrhage is the most common adverse event of colonoscopy with polypectomy, with a reported average incidence rate of 9.8 of 1000 procedures for clinically significant bleeding compared with 2.4 of 1000 screening/surveillance colonoscopies.[12] Bleeding following endoscopic resection of polyps greater than or equal to 2 cm occurs in 6.5% of cases.[13] The rate of postcolonoscopy bleeding has declined from 6.4 of 1000 to 1.0 of 1000 colonoscopies from 2001 to 2015.[12] Most bleeding episodes are clinically trivial, whereas episodes requiring hospitalization, blood transfusion, repeat endoscopic intervention, or surgery are considered true complications.[10]

Risk factors
Several factors related to the polyp, the patient, and the resection technique can predict the risk of hemorrhage following polyp removal and are mentioned in **Box 2**.

Hemorrhage management
Bleeding can be immediate (intraprocedural bleeding or <24 hours) or delayed (postprocedural bleeding, generally occurring within 1–14 days, with presence of marked bloody stool after treatment or the requirement for hemostasis after treatment; caused by eschar slough, progressive tissue necrosis, and cautery-induced thermal spread).[11]

Immediate hemorrhage. Immediate polypectomy bleeding is generally not considered a true complication but can increase the complexity of the procedure by obscuring the visual field. Mild, transient oozing at the edge of an en bloc or piecemeal EMR generally does not require treatment, whereas ongoing active bleeding that interferes with completion of the procedure or oozing that persists by the end of the procedure requires immediate and aggressive endoscopic therapy, because intraprocedural bleeding is associated with clinically significant delayed bleeding after wide-field EMR.[27]

Delayed hemorrhage. Careful assessment of the patient and the severity of bleeding, based on clinical features such as hemodynamic instability, frequency of bloody bowel movements, comorbid conditions, patient age, resumption of antithrombotic agents, and so forth, is required for determining the best course of action in delayed postpolypectomy bleeding (**Fig. 1**).

More than half of all bleeding subsides spontaneously without any further intervention. Thus, in hemodynamically stable patients, expectant management is initially preferred and includes the following:

- Triage to the appropriate service (ward or intensive care unit) based on the severity of bleeding and patient comorbidities
- Fluid and blood transfusions as appropriate
- Withholding of anticoagulation and antiplatelet agents
- Correction of coagulopathy, if present
- If bleeding resolves spontaneously, the patients should be admitted to the hospital for observation and monitoring of hemoglobin, platelets, and coagulation profile for 24 hours before discharge.

Box 2
Risk factors for hemorrhage

Polyp-related factors

- Size greater than 1 cm[14–18]
- Location—right hemicolon,[18] cecum,[19] proximal to splenic flexure,[16] and rectum[20]
- Morphology—pedunculated with a thick stalk,[14] sessile,[21,22] and laterally spreading lesions[14]
- Histology—adenoma,[22] villous features,[23] and presence of adenocarcinoma[21,23]
- Multiple polyps (>4)[17]

Patient-related factor

- Age greater than 65 years[14]
- Male sex[17,20]
- Comorbidities—hypertension,[15] cardiac disease,[14,24] lung disease,[24] diabetes,[24] and renal disease[14]
- Medications—antiplatelet agents,[25] anticoagulants,[14,24,25] NSAIDs,[25] and steroids[25]

Technique-/device-related factors

- Hot-snare polypectomy in patients on warfarin[26]
- EMR,[27] ESD[19,25]—intraprocedural bleeding is associated with clinically significant delayed bleeding
- Pure cutting current—immediate bleeding[14]
- Electrosurgical current not controlled by a microprocessor[27]
- Blended current[a]—immediate bleeding[28]
- Suboptimal bowel preparation[14]
- Endoscopist less than 10 years since graduation,[17] less than 300 procedures performed[8,18]
- Procedure performed at ambulatory surgery centers[8]

NSAID, nonsteroidal anti-inflammatory drug

[a] A recent randomized controlled trial comparing blended and forced coagulation current for EMR found no significant difference in the occurrence of delayed bleeding.[28]

- If initial resuscitation measures fail, urgent intervention to achieve hemostasis should be attempted initially with colonoscopy, resorting to angiography for angioembolization or surgery if unsuccessful. Risk factors for ongoing bleeding or recurrence of bleeding requiring intervention include:
  - hematochezia hourly or every few minutes
  - hemodynamic instability
  - low hemoglobin on admission (<12 g/dL)
  - transfusion requirement
  - American Society of Anesthesiologists class II or higher

Endoscopic hemostasis techniques and devices It is important to visualize the field and identify the bleeding source. The transparent cap on the endoscope can be used to localize the bleeding vessel, and water pump irrigation can be used to identify the pinpoint source of bleeding (**Fig. 2**).

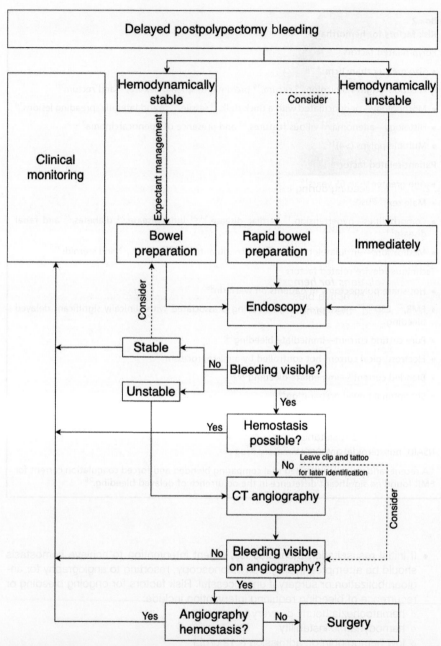

Fig. 1. Suggested management algorithm for delayed postpolypectomy bleeding. CT, computed tomography. (*Modified from* Werner DJ, Manner H, Nguyen-Tat M, et al. Endoscopic and angiographic management of lower gastrointestinal bleeding: review of the published literature. United European Gastroenterol J. 2018;6(3):337–42.)

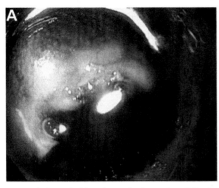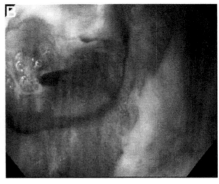

Fig. 2. (A) Brisk bleeding during ESD. (B) Pinpoint bleeding localized using the transparent cap and water flush.

After localizing the source, 1 of 4 hemostasis techniques, that is, injectable solutions, thermal devices, mechanical devices, or topical agents (**Box 3**), alone or in combination, can be used to control the bleeding, as discussed in the following sections.

Injectable solutions for hemostasis Injection of a 1:10,000 epinephrine-saline solution into the site of active bleeding will help achieve temporary hemostasis by vasoconstriction and the tamponade effect. However, epinephrine provides only temporary hemostasis and should be followed by more definitive therapy.

Thermal hemostatic devices Thermal devices can be contact (heater probe, gold probe, snare tip, and hemostatic forceps) or noncontact (argon plasma coagulation) and result in hemostasis by generating heat and causing edema, coagulation, and vessel constriction (Video 1). These, however, can extend the depth of tissue injury and should be used with caution. The electrocoagulation setting and argon plasma coagulation, where electrons flow through ionized argon gas, result in tissue desiccation, which creates resistance to further current flow, thus limiting injury.

An actively bleeding vessel within an EMR defect is best treated with grasping coagulation forceps (eg, Coagrasper, Olympus America (Center Valley, PA, USA) or with clip placement, with or without prior epinephrine injection. The Coagrasper device is a monopolar coagulation forceps designed for dual mechanical and thermal hemostasis. Although it is used primarily during ESD for coagulation of submucosal vessels, it can be used to grasp and seal bleeding vessels atop the resected stalk or polypectomy base, provided the grasped tissue can be tented.

Mechanical hemostatic devices Mechanical devices include endoscopic clips, which can be placed directly on the bleeding point or on the residual polypectomy stalk, and detachable loops, which are placed more easily over protuberant lesions such as a bleeding polypectomy stalk. The most popular method for endoscopic hemostasis is the application of through-the-scope clips (TTSCs). Mechanical hemostatic devices are preferred over thermal devices when technically feasible, because they do not extend the depth of tissue injury, which occurs with the use of thermal devices.

Topical hemostatic agents Three different topical hemostatic agents are commercially available, but only Hemospray (also known as TC-325; Cook Medical, Winston-Salem, NC, USA) is currently cleared by the US Food and Drug Administration for use in the United States. Hemospray is a hemostatic powder thought to cause hemostasis by sealing injured blood vessels and activating platelets and the intrinsic coagulation pathway.

> **Box 3**
> **Hemostatic therapies/devices**
>
> Injection
>
> - Dilute epinephrine (1:10,000 solution)
> - Pilodocanol
> - Fibrin glue
> - Histoacryl
> - EUS-guided angiotherapy
>
> Thermal (contact)
>
> - Heater probe
> - Bipolar electrocoagulation—gold probe, silver probe, BICAP
> - Monopolar electrocautery—snare tip cautery, hemostatic forceps
> - Coagulation grasper
> - Radiofrequency ablation
> - Cryotherapy
>
> Thermal (noncontact)
>
> - Argon plasma coagulation
> - Laser photocoagulation
>
> Mechanical
>
> - Grasp bleeding stalk with snare device and constrict
> - Band ligation
> - Detachable loop
> - TTSC or endoclip
> - OTSC, Padlock clip (STERIS Corp., Mentor, Ohio, USA)
> - Endoscopic suturing device (OverStitch, Apollo Endosurgery, Austin, TX, USA)
> - Flexible linear stapler
>
> Topical
>
> - Hemospray
> - Ankaferd Blood Stopper (ABS) (Ankaferd Health Products Ltd, Istanbul, Turkey)
> - EndoClot (EndoClot Plus, Inc, Santa Clara, CA, USA)
> - Pure-Stat (3D Matrix Europe SAS, Caluire-et-Cuire, France)
> - Oxidized cellulose
>
> BICAP, bipolar circumactive probe; EUS, endoscopic ultrasonography; OTSC, over-the-scope clip.
>
> *Modified from* Thirumurthi S, Raju GS. Management of polypectomy complications. Gastrointest Endosc Clin N Am 2015 Apr;25(2):335-57; with permission.

Box 4
Prevention of postpolypectomy bleeding

- Consider patient- and condition-related risk factors

- Ensure the lumen is adequately visible
  - Avoid blind dissection
  - Ensure that the correct layer is selected for dissection and verify the orientation in a tubular structure
  - Apply liberal water irrigation
  - Reschedule the procedure if bowel preparation was poor

- Patients on antithrombotics with a colorectal lesion greater than or equal to 2 cm should be individually assessed, with the risks of interrupting anticoagulation balanced against those of significant bleeding

- Use proper polypectomy technique
  - Avoid hot biopsy forceps
  - Treat intraprocedural bleeding during EMR/ESD, especially in the cecum, using endoscopic coagulation (eg, coagulation forceps or snare-tip soft coagulation) or mechanical therapy (eg, clip), with or without dilute epinephrine injection to prevent delayed bleeding
  - Use forced coagulation on thick vessels with the tip or shaft of the ESD knife to prevent bleeding
  - Consider prophylactic mechanical ligation of the stalk with a detachable loop or clips on pedunculated lesions with a head greater than or equal to 2 cm or with stalk thickness greater than or equal to 0.5 cm to reduce immediate and delayed bleeding.
  - Know when to refer to tertiary center for EMR (and do not attempt resection, biopsy the center of the polyp, or tattoo the polyp directly)

Prevention

The techniques for preventing postpolypectomy bleeding are summarized in **Box 4**.

Perforation

Immediate perforation occurs when the muscularis propria is grasped by a snare, whereas delayed perforation results from a deep cut or tissue necrosis from cautery.[29] According to a systematic review, the perforation rate is 0.8 of 1000 polypectomy procedures compared with 0.3 of 1000 colonoscopies for the screening/surveillance setting. However, the rate can be up to 5% following therapeutic procedures, such as ESD.[29,30] Perforations occurring during resection (eg, EMR and ESD) tend to be smaller (0.5 cm vs up to 2 cm for diagnostic colonoscopy)[31] and typically do not require laparotomy.[32,33]

Risk factors

Several factors related to the polyp, patient, and resection technique can predict the risk of perforation following polyp removal and are mentioned in **Box 5**.

Management of postpolypectomy perforation

When perforation is suspected, it can be helpful to devise a strategy (**Fig. 3**): preventing leakage of the intestinal contents by positioning the patient so that the defect is in a nondependent location and ensuring appropriate use of suction. Endoscopists should be comfortable with the various closure techniques.

Assessment of depth of resection for early recognition of perforation. Roughly one-third of perforations are detected during the colonoscopy,[34] apparent as a mucosal rent, shiny-appearing serosa, epiploic fat, or free intraperitoneal space. Submucosal

---

Box 5
Risk factors for perforation

Polyp-related factors

- Size greater than 2 cm[25]
- Location—cecum[34,35] and ascending colon[34]
- Morphology—nonpedunculated,[35] nonpolypoid,[36] and laterally spreading[36]
- Deeper layer involvement—Vienna classification 4 (noninvasive high-grade dysplasia) and 5 (invasive neoplasia)[37]
- Prior attempted polypectomy leading to submucosal fibrosis[38,39]

Patient-related factors

- Age greater than 75 years[40–42]
- Comorbidities—renal disease,[25] severe diverticulosis,[42] active severe colitis,[42] and adhesions from prior surgery[42]
- Male sex[25,40]
- Medications—warfarin, NSAIDS, and steroids[25,42]
- Prior radiation therapy[42]

Technique/device-related factors

- Mechanical injury
  - Tip of colonoscope—diverticula and tight/angulated turns (eg, in a redundant sigmoid or fixed by adhesions)[34]
  - Shaft of colonoscope—excessive looping or during retroflexion (eg, in a small rectum due to severe proctitis or pelvic radiation therapy)[34]
- Thermal injury—argon plasma coagulation and electrocautery[34]
- Barotrauma—air insufflation[34]
- Snare polypectomy—greater than 1 cm in right colon, greater than 2 cm in the left colon, or multiple polyps[34]
- ESR and ESD[25]
- Inadequate bowel preparation[42]
- No submucosal injection before snaring and electrocautery[34,36]
- Low-volume endoscopist, less than 300 procedures performed[8,30,40]
- Procedure performed at ambulatory surgery centers[8]
- Procedure performed by non-GI endoscopists (surgeons, family physicians, etc.)[43]

---

injection of a blue dye (eg, methylene blue or indigo carmine) can reveal the "target sign" of a probable perforation at the base of the resection site, that is, a white center (muscularis propria) surrounded by pinkish or bluish dye-stained submucosa. The underside of the resected specimen will appear as a reverse image. It is essential to detect these signs of perforation during the procedure rather than after clinical signs develop or radiography indicates the appearance of free air; this is particularly crucial during polypectomy, during which perforations can be treated endoscopically.

Endoscopic closure versus operative repair. The decision to manage the perforation conservatively with endoscopic closure or intervene operatively is influenced by many factors, summarized in **Box 6**.

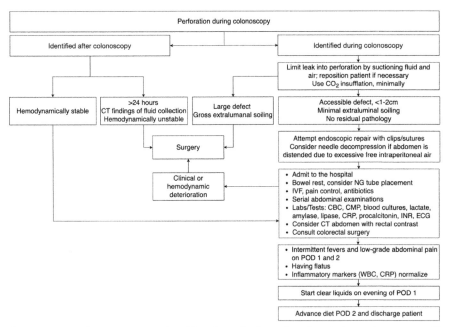

Fig. 3. Suggested management algorithm for colonic perforation during colonoscopy. *Abbreviations:* CT, computed tomography; CBC, complete blood cell count; CMP, comprehensive metabolic panel; CRP, C-reactive protein; ECG, electrocardiogram; INR, international normalized ratio; IVF, intravenous fluids; NG, nasogastric; POD, postoperative day; WBC, white blood cell count.

Endoscopic devices for perforation closure. When opting for endoscopic closure, the submucosa surrounding the perforation should be dissected to provide sufficient space for perforation closure. Endoscopic closure of perforation defects can be achieved with TTSCs (**Fig. 4**) (Video 2), over-the-scope clips (OTSCs), and endoscopic suturing devices (**Box 7**). The specific techniques of use are outside the scope of this review and are discussed more thoroughly by Raju.[44]

Postprocedural monitoring and management. Although the defect may appear to be sealed, the possibility of procedural failure due to incomplete clip closure, clip loss, or inaccurate/superficial stitch placement is not completely ruled out. Close monitoring in the period after endoluminal closure is crucial for early detection of failed clipping requiring surgical intervention. An evidence-based strategy for management of perforation after endoluminal closure is outlined in **Fig. 3** and summarized in **Box 8**.[47]

Prevention techniques
The techniques for preventing colonic perforation are discussed in depth by Rogart[42] and are summarized in **Box 9**.

Postpolypectomy Syndrome

PPS, also called postpolypectomy coagulation syndrome or transmural burn syndrome, occurs with localized serosal inflammation and peritonitis in up to 3% of patients undergoing hot snare polypectomy if there is full-thickness thermal injury of the bowel wall, without perforation.[48,49] PPS occurs most often after resection of large

---

Box 6
Indications for endoscopic and operative repair of perforation

Endoscopic repair

- Perforation defect less than 2 cm
- Adequate bowel preparation
- No extraluminal soiling
- No residual pathology
- Clinically stable patient
- Availability of devices
- Controlled access to the perforated site (the patient should be positioned so that the perforation is opposite the pooling of colonic contents, and CO_2 should be used for insufflation)
- Endoscopists' expertise

Operative repair

- Presence of a large perforation
- Inadequate bowel preparation
- Gross feculent peritoneal contamination
- Residual pathology (eg, incomplete EMR)
- Clinical deterioration on conservative management
- Failure to access and completely close the perforation
- Failed attempt at endoscopic closure

(>2 cm) sessile polyps, particularly in the thin-walled right colon, with prolonged application of electrosurgical current (coagulation mode). PPS has been associated with hypertension, large lesions, and nonpolypoid lesions.[48] Submucosal fluid cushions during EMR may reduce, but not eliminate, the risk of PPS.[50]

As a result of serosal irritation and localized peritonitis, patients can experience localized abdominal pain, fever, and leukocytosis, which mimic colonic perforation, within hours and up to 5 days postprocedure. Abdominal computed tomography is

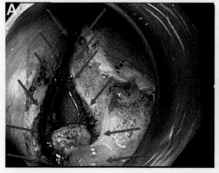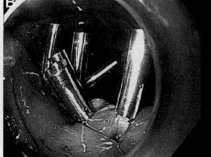

Fig. 4. (A) Perforation defect following EMR (red arrows). (B) TTSC closure of perforation in a zipper fashion.

Box 7
Closure devices

TTSC

- Readily available and easy to deploy for both the endoscopist and the assisting technician; most effective for perforation defects up to 2.5 cm in size, with noninflamed, nonfibrotic surrounding tissue, and treated within 24 hours

- Successfully approximate the mucosal and submucosal layers in a partial-thickness closure; restricted wingspan, low compression force, and potential for early detachment limits their usage with larger defects with gaping holes

- Avoid spillage of colon contents, because they can be deployed through the endoscope immediately after endoscopic recognition of perforation without leaving the operating field

- Successful in the closure of 90% of iatrogenic colon perforations[45]

OTSC

- Larger perforations (up to 3 cm), perforations with a fibrotic edge, and those not amenable to TTSC closure

- Grasp more tissue and apply a greater compressive force with the potential for single-layer, full-thickness closure

- Risks spillage of colon content, because the endoscope must be removed from the perforation site to load the device onto the end of the endoscope and then reinserted, followed by closure of the perforation; thus, the patient should be positioned so that the defect is in a nondependent location and the colon is fully decompressed before scope withdrawal to attach the OTSC

- Successful in the closure of 90% to 100% of iatrogenic colon perforations[45]

Over-the-scope suturing devices

- Prophylactic closure of very large (~4.25 cm to 5–8 cm) rectal EMR and ESD defects not amenable to standard clip closure for prevention of delayed perforation and bleeding; capable of deploying multiple interrupted or running stitches for accurate full-thickness closure[46]

---

optimal for distinguishing PPS from perforation, revealing localized colonic wall thickening and adjacent fat stranding without extraluminal air. PPS can be managed with bowel rest, intravenous fluids, antibiotics, and pain control or simply oral antibiotics and a day or two of a clear-liquid diet if symptoms are mild.

LONG-TERM OUTCOMES OF COLORECTAL POLYP RESECTION
Risk for Polyp Recurrence

Recurrence of adenomatous polyps following resection is common, occurring in 10.9%, 38.2%, and 52.6% of cases at 1, 3, and 5 years, respectively.[51] The primary cause of recurrence is incomplete polyp resection and, with an incomplete resection rate of 10.1% for all neoplastic polyps, is a risk factor for polyp progression to cancer.[52] Incomplete polyp resection may also lead to a buildup of scar tissue and fibrosis, making the subsequent resection more difficult. In addition, it increases incremental cost owing to the need for a follow-up resection. Factors related to incomplete polyp resection and recurrence are listed in **Box 10**. A submucosal lift can help delineate polyp margins and improve complete resection rates. The addition of a contrast dye agent to the submucosal injection solution can further help visualize the lesion and

---

Box 8
Postprocedural monitoring for perforations

- Perform serial abdominal examinations to monitor for tension pneumoperitoneum; if abdominal distension and respiratory distress are noted, perform percutaneous needle decompression with 18- or 20-gauge needle

- Maintain NPO status and consider nasogastric tube placement for decompression in the endoscopy room

- Start broad-spectrum intravenous antibiotics for aerobic and anaerobic coverage (eg, ciprofloxacin 400 mg every 12 hours + metronidazole 500 mg every 8 hours) and intravenous fluids

- Obtain blood work/tests, including complete blood cell count, comprehensive metabolic panel, lactate, amylase, lipase, C-reactive protein, and international normalized ratio, and an electrocardiogram

- Consult for colorectal surgery

- Coordinate admission to the hospital with medical and surgical team

- Consider ordering computed tomography of the abdomen and pelvis with rectal water-soluble contrast only; abdominal imaging may not be necessary if the patient is doing well clinically, because there is a tendency to treat the imaging findings and not the patient
  ○ No leak, continue conservative management
  ○ Leak present, surgery is required, especially if diagnosed after 24 hours

- Start oral intake with clear-liquid diet once pain and fever subside, appetite and bowel function return, and leukocytosis has resolved, which may be as early as postoperative day 1, followed by diet advancement and discharge on postoperative day 2

NPO, nil per os

Box 9
Prevention of postpolypectomy perforation

- Consider patient- and condition-related risk factors

- Ensure the lumen is adequately visible
  ○ Avoid pushing blindly
  ○ Use a smaller endoscope for severe diverticulosis or tight/sharp angulated colon
  ○ Apply liberal water irrigation
  ○ Reschedule the procedure if bowel preparation was poor

- Avoid excessive colonoscope looping, abdominal pressure, and position changes (keep lesion nondependent)

- Avoid retroflexion in small rectum

- Routinely decompress the colon; use CO_2 for insufflation

- Perform detailed inspection of the postresection mucosal defect to identify features for immediate or delayed perforation risk and perform endoscopic clip closure, accordingly

- Use proper polypectomy technique
  ○ Avoid hot biopsy forceps
  ○ Tent polyp away from wall when using snare cautery
  ○ Submucosal injection/lifting for larger sessile polyps
  ○ Consider piecemeal resection if polyp greater than 2 cm
  ○ Know when to refer to tertiary center for EMR (and do not attempt resection, biopsy the center of the polyp, or tattoo the polyp directly)

Modified from Rogart JN. Foregut and colonic perforations: practical measures to prevent and assess them. Gastrointest Endosc Clin N Am 2015;25(1):9–27; with permission.

Box 10
Risk factors for polyp recurrence

Polyp-related factors

- Size greater than or equal to 1 cm[54–56]
- Location—right hemicolon[55,56]
- Multiple polyps (>2)[55,56]
- Morphology—lesion occupying ≥75% of the luminal circumference[55]
- Histology—high-grade dysplasia, sessile serrated, villous, and tubulovillous features[54,55]

Patient-related factors

- Age greater than 60 years[55,56]
- Male sex[55]
- Obesity[55]
- Lifestyle—smoking,[56] alcohol use, low-fiber diet, red meat consumption[55]
- History of ulcerative colitis or inherited genetic predisposition for familial adenomatous polyposis[55]
- Low vitamin D and folate levels[55]
- Elevated serum homocysteine and ferritin levels[55]

Technique-/procedure-related factors.

- Cold biopsy forceps polypectomy[57]
- Piecemeal EMR and ESD resection[54,55]
- Suboptimal bowel preparation[55]
- Delayed postpolypectomy follow-up[55]
- Inexperienced endoscopist and/or endoscopy assistant[55]
- Missed diagnosis after the first colonoscopy[55]

---

distinguish normal tissue from polyp margins, especially in the case of sessile serrated adenomas/polyps. High-definition colonoscopes with imaging technologies such as chromoendoscopy, autofluorescence imaging, and confocal laser endomicroscopy have enabled endoscopists to make an in vivo optical diagnosis of colon polyp histology during colonoscopy. Additional tips and tricks to make the polypectomy process efficient and effective are discussed by Mahmood and colleagues.[53]

Risk for Colorectal Cancer

Despite the adverse events related to colonoscopy, the procedure can reduce the risk of CRC by ~70%.[1] Nevertheless, interval CRCs (ie, those that appear between serial colonoscopies) occur in 2.9% to 14% of cases and can arise from missed polyps (52%), incompletely resected polyps (19%), or de novo lesions (24%).[58,59] Risk factors for interval CRC are summarized in **Box 11**. The adenoma detection rate by endoscopists correlates inversely with interval CRC rates and death: each 1.0% increase in the adenoma detection rate is associated with a 3.0% decrease in the risk of cancer.[60] Although historically colonoscopy performance has been predicated on adenoma detection, it is detection combined with adequate resection that improves clinical

---

Box 11
Risk factors for interval colorectal cancer

Polyp-related factors

- Location—proximal colon[58,61]
- Prior polypectomy[61]
- Advanced adenomas[62]

Patient-related factors

- Age greater than 65 to 70 years[63]
- African American[64]
- Family history of CRC[58]
- Multiple comorbidities (≥3)[61,63]
- Previous diagnosis of diverticulosis[61,63]

Endoscopist-related factors

- Low adenoma detection rate[60]
- Performed few polypectomy procedures[61]
- High colonoscopy procedure volume[61]
- Specialty other than gastroenterology (eg, colorectal surgery, general surgery, internal medicine, or family practice)[61]

---

outcomes and consequences. Quality metrics should be implemented in all endoscopy centers and tracked over time to decrease the risk of interval cancer.[9]

SUMMARY

Endoscopic resection of polyps can result in complications, including those that are rare but devastating nonetheless. The risk for these can be minimized with appropriate recognition and consideration of the factors involved. Furthermore, adequate endoscopic training and cognizance of one's proficiency greatly influence the success of the procedure as well as the probability of complications. However, early recognition and assessment of complications that do occur provide the opportunity for prompt medical and/or surgical management, thereby promoting a successful outcome.

CLINICS CARE POINTS[65]

- Endoscopists should carefully assess all patient-, polyp-, and technique/device-related risk factors before attempting polypectomy to minimize complications.
- Endoscopic therapy is effective in managing most intraprocedural bleeding during EMR/ESD.
- Mechanical ligation of the stalk with a detachable loop or clips can be used for prophylaxis against immediate and delayed postpolypectomy bleeding on large pedunculated lesions.
- When removing nonpedunculated (≥2 cm) lesions, a contrast agent should be used, such as indigo carmine or methylene blue, in the submucosal injection solution to facilitate recognition of the submucosa from the mucosa and muscularis propria layers.
- Detailed inspection of the postresection mucosal defect should be performed to identify features for immediate or delayed perforation risk and perform endoscopic clip closure accordingly.

- Prophylactic closure of resection defects greater than or equal to 2 cm in size in the right colon should be used when feasible.
- CO_2 insufflation should be used instead of air during EMR to prevent barotrauma and perforation.
- Endoscopists should engage in a local (institution-, hospital-, or practice-based) quality assurance program, including measuring and reporting postpolypectomy adverse events.

DISCLOSURE

No conflicts of interest.

ACKNOWLEDGMENTS

We thank A. Aziz Aadam, MD, Director of Developmental Endoscopy, Director of Advanced Endoscopy Fellowship Program, and Associate Professor of Medicine, Northwestern University, Feinberg School of Medicine, Chicago for sharing the multimedia used in this article.

SUPPLEMENTARY DATA

Supplementary data related to this article can be found online at https://doi.org/10.1016/j.giec.2021.12.011.

REFERENCES

1. Brenner H, Stock C, Hoffmeister M. Effect of screening sigmoidoscopy and screening colonoscopy on colorectal cancer incidence and mortality: systematic review and meta-analysis of randomised controlled trials and observational studies. BMJ 2014;348:g2467.
2. Committee ASoP, Fisher DA, Maple JT, Ben-Menachem T, et al. Complications of colonoscopy. Gastrointest Endosc 2011;74:745–52.
3. Whitlock EP, Lin JS, Liles E, et al. Screening for colorectal cancer: a targeted, updated systematic review for the U.S. Preventive Services Task Force. Ann Intern Med 2008;149:638–58.
4. Committee ASoP, Acosta RD, Abraham NS, Chandrasekhara V, et al. The management of antithrombotic agents for patients undergoing GI endoscopy. Gastrointest Endosc 2016;83:3–16.
5. Ko CW, Dominitz JA. Complications of colonoscopy: magnitude and management. Gastrointest Endosc Clin N Am 2010;20:659–71.
6. Ahmed J, Landy J. PTH-006Shouldwe perform colonic polypectomy in patients over 80. Gut 2018;67:A14–5.
7. Cotton PB, Eisen G, Romagnuolo J, et al. Grading the complexity of endoscopic procedures: results of an ASGE working party. Gastrointest Endosc 2011;73:868–74.
8. Chukmaitov A, Bradley CJ, Dahman B, et al. Association of polypectomy techniques, endoscopist volume, and facility type with colonoscopy complications. Gastrointest Endosc 2013;77:436–46.
9. Rex DK, Schoenfeld PS, Cohen J, et al. Quality indicators for colonoscopy. Gastrointest Endosc 2015;81:31–53.
10. Cotton PB, Eisen GM, Aabakken L, et al. A lexicon for endoscopic adverse events: report of an ASGE workshop. Gastrointest Endosc 2010;71:446–54.

11. Tanaka S, Kashida H, Saito Y, et al. JGES guidelines for colorectal endoscopic submucosal dissection/endoscopic mucosal resection. Dig Endosc 2015;27: 417–34.

12. Reumkens A, Rondagh EJ, Bakker CM, et al. Post-colonoscopy complications: a systematic review, time trends, and meta-analysis of population-based studies. Am J Gastroenterol 2016;111:1092–101.

13. Hassan C, Repici A, Sharma P, et al. Efficacy and safety of endoscopic resection of large colorectal polyps: a systematic review and meta-analysis. Gut 2016;65: 806–20.

14. Kim HS, Kim TI, Kim WH, et al. Risk factors for immediate postpolypectomy bleeding of the colon: a multicenter study. Am J Gastroenterol 2006;101:1333–41.

15. Watabe H, Yamaji Y, Okamoto M, et al. Risk assessment for delayed hemorrhagic complication of colonic polypectomy: polyp-related factors and patient-related factors. Gastrointest Endosc 2006;64:73–8.

16. Liaquat H, Rohn E, Rex DK. Prophylactic clip closure reduced the risk of delayed postpolypectomy hemorrhage: experience in 277 clipped large sessile or flat colorectal lesions and 247 control lesions. Gastrointest Endosc 2013;77:401–7.

17. Blotiere PO, Weill A, Ricordeau P, et al. Perforations and haemorrhages after colonoscopy in 2010: a study based on comprehensive French health insurance data (SNIIRAM). Clin Res Hepatol Gastroenterol 2014;38:112–7.

18. Choung BS, Kim SH, Ahn DS, et al. Incidence and risk factors of delayed postpolypectomy bleeding: a retrospective cohort study. J Clin Gastroenterol 2014; 48:784–9.

19. Suzuki S, Chino A, Kishihara T, et al. Risk factors for bleeding after endoscopic submucosal dissection of colorectal neoplasms. World J Gastroenterol 2014; 20:1839–45.

20. Yan Z, Gao F, Xie J, et al. Incidence and risk factors of colorectal delayed postpolypectomy bleeding in patients taking antithrombotics. J Dig Dis 2021;22: 481–7.

21. Dobrowolski S, Dobosz M, Babicki A, et al. Blood supply of colorectal polyps correlates with risk of bleeding after colonoscopic polypectomy. Gastrointest Endosc 2006;63:1004–9.

22. Consolo P, Luigiano C, Strangio G, et al. Efficacy, risk factors and complications of endoscopic polypectomy: ten year experience at a single center. World J Gastroenterol 2008;14:2364–9.

23. Gimeno-Garcia AZ, de Ganzo ZA, Sosa AJ, et al. Incidence and predictors of postpolypectomy bleeding in colorectal polyps larger than 10 mm. Eur J Gastroenterol Hepatol 2012;24:520–6.

24. Sawhney MS, Salfiti N, Nelson DB, et al. Risk factors for severe delayed postpolypectomy bleeding. Endoscopy 2008;40:115–9.

25. Niikura R, Yasunaga H, Yamada A, et al. Factors predicting adverse events associated with therapeutic colonoscopy for colorectal neoplasia: a retrospective nationwide study in Japan. Gastrointest Endosc 2016;84:971–982 e6.

26. Horiuchi A, Nakayama Y, Kajiyama M, et al. Removal of small colorectal polyps in anticoagulated patients: a prospective randomized comparison of cold snare and conventional polypectomy. Gastrointest Endosc 2014;79:417–23.

27. Burgess NG, Metz AJ, Williams SJ, et al. Risk factors for intraprocedural and clinically significant delayed bleeding after wide-field endoscopic mucosal resection of large colonic lesions. Clin Gastroenterol Hepatol 2014;12:651–61.e1.

28. Pohl H, Grimm IS, Moyer MT, et al. Effects of blended (yellow) vs forced coagulation (blue) currents on adverse events, complete resection, or polyp recurrence

after polypectomy in a large randomized trial. Gastroenterology 2020;159: 119–28.e2.

29. Panteris V, Haringsma J, Kuipers EJ. Colonoscopy perforation rate, mechanisms and outcome: from diagnostic to therapeutic colonoscopy. Endoscopy 2009;41: 941–51.

30. Lohsiriwat V. Colonoscopic perforation: incidence, risk factors, management and outcome. World J Gastroenterol 2010;16:425–30.

31. Yang DH, Byeon JS, Lee KH, et al. Is endoscopic closure with clips effective for both diagnostic and therapeutic colonoscopy-associated bowel perforation? Surg Endosc 2010;24:1177–85.

32. Avgerinos DV, Llaguna OH, Lo AY, et al. Evolving management of colonoscopic perforations. J Gastrointest Surg 2008;12:1783–9.

33. Pissas D, Ypsilantis E, Papagrigoriadis S, et al. Endoscopic management of iatrogenic perforations during endoscopic mucosal resection (EMR) and endoscopic submucosal dissection (ESD) for colorectal polyps: a case series. Therap Adv Gastroenterol 2015;8:176–81.

34. Raju GS, Saito Y, Matsuda T, et al. Endoscopic management of colonoscopic perforations (with videos). Gastrointest Endosc 2011;74:1380–8.

35. Rutter MD, Nickerson C, Rees CJ, et al. Risk factors for adverse events related to polypectomy in the English Bowel Cancer Screening Programme. Endoscopy 2014;46:90–7.

36. Lee EJ, Lee JB, Choi YS, et al. Clinical risk factors for perforation during endoscopic submucosal dissection (ESD) for large-sized, nonpedunculated colorectal tumors. Surg Endosc 2012;26:1587–94.

37. Wada Y, Kudo SE, Tanaka S, et al. Predictive factors for complications in endoscopic resection of large colorectal lesions: a multicenter prospective study. Surg Endosc 2015;29:1216–22.

38. Kim ES, Cho KB, Park KS, et al. Factors predictive of perforation during endoscopic submucosal dissection for the treatment of colorectal tumors. Endoscopy 2011;43:573–8.

39. Takamaru H, Saito Y, Yamada M, et al. Clinical impact of endoscopic clip closure of perforations during endoscopic submucosal dissection for colorectal tumors. Gastrointest Endosc 2016;84:494–502.e1.

40. Rabeneck L, Paszat LF, Hilsden RJ, et al. Bleeding and perforation after outpatient colonoscopy and their risk factors in usual clinical practice. Gastroenterology 2008;135:1899–906, 1906.e1.

41. Lohsiriwat V, Sujarittanakarn S, Akaraviputh T, et al. What are the risk factors of colonoscopic perforation? BMC Gastroenterol 2009;9:71.

42. Rogart JN. Foregut and colonic perforations: practical measures to prevent and assess them. Gastrointest Endosc Clin N Am 2015;25:9–27.

43. Bielawska B, Day AG, Lieberman DA, et al. Risk factors for early colonoscopic perforation include non-gastroenterologist endoscopists: a multivariable analysis. Clin Gastroenterol Hepatol 2014;12:85–92.

44. Raju GS. Closure of defects and management of complications. Gastrointest Endosc Clin N Am 2019;29:705–19.

45. Verlaan T, Voermans RP, van Berge Henegouwen MI, et al. Endoscopic closure of acute perforations of the GI tract: a systematic review of the literature. Gastrointest Endosc 2015;82:618–628 e5.

46. Kantsevoy SV, Bitner M, Hajiyeva G, et al. Endoscopic management of colonic perforations: clips versus suturing closure (with videos). Gastrointest Endosc 2016;84:487–93.

47. Kowalczyk L, Forsmark CE, Ben-David K, et al. Algorithm for the management of endoscopic perforations: a quality improvement project. Am J Gastroenterol 2011;106:1022–7.

48. Cha JM, Lim KS, Lee SH, et al. Clinical outcomes and risk factors of post-polypectomy coagulation syndrome: a multicenter, retrospective, case-control study. Endoscopy 2013;45:202–7.

49. Hirasawa K, Sato C, Makazu M, et al. Coagulation syndrome: delayed perforation after colorectal endoscopic treatments. World J Gastrointest Endosc 2015;7: 1055–61.

50. Ferrara F, Luigiano C, Ghersi S, et al. Efficacy, safety and outcomes of 'inject and cut' endoscopic mucosal resection for large sessile and flat colorectal polyps. Digestion 2010;82:213–20.

51. Amonkar MM, Hunt TL, Zhou Z, et al. Surveillance patterns and polyp recurrence following diagnosis and excision of colorectal polyps in a medicare population. Cancer Epidemiol Biomarkers Prev 2005;14:417–21.

52. Pohl H, Srivastava A, Bensen SP, et al. Incomplete polyp resection during colonoscopy-results of the complete adenoma resection (CARE) study. Gastroenterology 2013;144:74–80 e1.

53. Mahmood Sultan MD, Anguila Enrik, MD MBA, ur Rahman Asad, et al. How to Approach Small Polyps in Colon. Tips and Tricks., Techniques and Innovations in Gastrointestinal Endoscopy 2021;328–35. https://doi.org/10.1016/j.tige.2021. 06.007.

54. Komeda Y, Watanabe T, Sakurai T, et al. Risk factors for local recurrence and appropriate surveillance interval after endoscopic resection. World J Gastroenterol 2019;25:1502–12.

55. Hao Y, Wang Y, Qi M, et al. Risk factors for recurrent colorectal polyps. Gut Liver 2020;14:399–411.

56. Harrington LX, Wei JW, Suriawinata AA, et al. Predicting colorectal polyp recurrence using time-to-event analysis of medical records. AMIA Jt Summits Transl Sci Proc 2020;2020:211–20.

57. Liu S, Ho SB, Krinsky ML. Quality of polyp resection during colonoscopy: are we achieving polyp clearance? Dig Dis Sci 2012;57:1786–91.

58. Samadder NJ, Curtin K, Tuohy TM, et al. Characteristics of missed or interval colorectal cancer and patient survival: a population-based study. Gastroenterology 2014;146:950–60.

59. Robertson DJ, Lieberman DA, Winawer SJ, et al. Colorectal cancers soon after colonoscopy: a pooled multicohort analysis. Gut 2014;63:949–56.

60. Corley DA, Jensen CD, Marks AR, et al. Adenoma detection rate and risk of colorectal cancer and death. N Engl J Med 2014;370:1298–306.

61. Cooper GS, Xu F, Barnholtz Sloan JS, et al. Prevalence and predictors of interval colorectal cancers in medicare beneficiaries. Cancer 2012;118:3044–52.

62. Click B, Pinsky PF, Hickey T, et al. Association of colonoscopy adenoma findings with long-term colorectal cancer incidence. JAMA 2018;319:2021–31.

63. Singh S, Singh PP, Murad MH, et al. Prevalence, risk factors, and outcomes of interval colorectal cancers: a systematic review and meta-analysis. Am J Gastroenterol 2014;109:1375–89.

64. Fedewa SA, Flanders WD, Jemal A, et al. Racial and ethnic disparities in interval colorectal cancer incidence. Ann Intern Med 2018;168:80.

65. Kaltenbach T, Anderson JC, Burke CA, et al. Endoscopic removal of colorectal lesions: recommendations by the US Multi-Society Task Force on Colorectal Cancer. Am J Gastroenterol 2020;115:435–64.

Surveillance Recommendation for Colonoscopy after Polypectomy

Charles Muller, MD[a], Vijaya L. Rao, MD[b],*

KEYWORDS

• Colonoscopy • Surveillance • Polyp • Polypectomy

KEY POINTS

• . Patients with advanced adenomas on index colonoscopy benefit most from surveillance exams with regard to reduction in CRC risk.
• Resection of low-risk lesions on index colonoscopy is associated with reduced CRC compared to those not screened, with less certain incremental benefit from subsequent surveillance.
• In practice, surveillance colonoscopy is often overutilized by individuals at lowest risk of advanced neoplasia or CRC and underutilized by those at highest risk.

INTRODUCTION

Colorectal cancer (CRC) is the third leading cause of cancer and cancer-related mortality in the United States, with an estimated 148,000 new cases annually in 2020.[1] CRC incidence and mortality, however, have declined over the past several decades,[2] largely due to improvement and uptake in screening, particularly with colonoscopy.[3–8] Colonoscopy allows for the modification of CRC outcomes not only by the identification of CRC at an earlier, more treatable stage but also by allowing for the identification of colorectal polyps, premalignant lesions from which the most CRCs arise.[9] Although the benefits of endoscopic polyp detection are in part due to the identification of individuals at increased risk of CRC who would benefit from heightened surveillance, endoscopic removal of premalignant colorectal polyps also has the potential to reduce the incidence of[10] and mortality from CRC.[4,11]

The most common type of colorectal polyps is adenomas, which are premalignant lesions that can progress through a well-described adenoma–carcinoma sequence

a Division of Gastroenterology & Hepatology, Northwestern Memorial Hospital, 259 East Erie, Suite 1600, Chicago, IL 60611, USA; b Section of Gastroenterology, Hepatology & Nutrition, University of Chicago Medicine, 5841 South Maryland Avenue, Rm S-401, Chicago, IL 60637, USA
* Corresponding author.
E-mail address: vijayarao@medicine.bsd.uchicago.edu
Twitter: @cmmuller7 (C.M.); @VijayaRaoMD (V.L.R.)

Gastrointest Endoscopy Clin N Am 32 (2022) 371–384
https://doi.org/10.1016/j.giec.2021.12.012
1052-5157/22/© 2021 Elsevier Inc. All rights reserved.

that takes several years.[9] Carcinogenesis in adenomatous polyps follows a stepwise series of molecular changes, characterized by progressive *APC* then *KRAS* and *p53* mutations. Adenomas are often stratified by endoscopic and histologic features that impact the risk of CRC. High-risk adenomas (HRAs) or advanced adenomas include those greater than 10 mm in size or those with villous histology or high-grade dysplasia, whereas low-risk (LRA) or nonadvanced adenomas include those less than 10 mm in size and lacking advanced histologic features. Increasing recognition is also being given to the malignant potential of serrated polyps, comprising hyperplastic polyps, sessile serrated polyps (SSPs), and traditional serrated adenomas (TSAs),[12] which are characterized by *BRAF* mutations, disruptions to the Wnt signaling pathway, and widespread methylation of CpG islands.[13,14] Serrated polyps are thought to be precursor lesions in up to 30% of CRC cases.[15-18]

Despite the efforts to tailor colonoscopy and surveillance strategies based on environmental or genetic risk factors,[19,20] current practice in the United States relies nearly entirely on personal polyp history along with the family history of CRC or polyps as the only factor to inform surveillance intervals for individuals without a known hereditary CRC syndrome or inflammatory bowel disease.[21-23] Given that colonoscopies are invasive and expensive procedures and that polyp-related factors can result in recommended surveillance intervals ranging from 1 to 10 years,[23] the public health and economic impact of recommendations for colonoscopy surveillance after polypectomy are significant. Current estimates suggest that approximately 25% of colonoscopies in the United States are performed for surveillance purposes.[24] Moreover, evidence has shown that in practice, surveillance colonoscopy is often overutilized by individuals at lowest risk of advanced neoplasia (AN) or CRC and underutilized by those at highest risk,[25-27] highlighting the importance of defining individual risk of metachronous neoplasia after colonoscopy to inform the equitable allocation of health care resources and maximize their yield. The US Multi-Society Task Force (MSTF) on CRC published guidelines for surveillance after polypectomy in 2012,[28] which were updated in 2020 with some important changes (**Table 1**).[23] This review will provide an updated overview of evidence and outcomes of surveillance after polypectomy.

SURVEILLANCE AFTER POLYPECTOMY OF ADENOMAS
Metachronous Colorectal Cancer Risk

Adenomatous polyps, which are found in 25% to 50% of screening colonoscopies,[29-31] are the most common polyps with malignant potential found during colon cancer screening. Individuals with adenomas tend to develop additional adenomas throughout life, with approximately 40% to 50% of individuals undergoing polypectomy developing recurrence of polyps within 5 years and up to 60% to 70% after 10 years.[32-35] Despite undergoing polypectomy, individuals with adenomas appear to be at increased risk of CRC than the general population.[36,37] When stratified by adenoma subtype, it appears that observed CRC risk is driven primarily by those with advanced adenomas.[37] A population-based study from the United Kingdom found that individuals with an adenoma found on colonoscopy (of any size) had a standardized incidence ratio (SIR) of 1.26 for subsequent CRC than the general population.[37] However, the SIR for CRC for individuals with an advanced adenoma was 2.23, whereas 0.68 for those without an advanced adenoma, providing further evidence that polypectomy for nonadvanced adenoma is in fact protective against CRC while polypectomy for advanced adenoma helps to identify individuals at elevated risk of metachronous CRC.[37] A Norwegian cohort study with a median of 7 years of follow-up found similarly divergent influences of removal of LRAs and HRAs on risk of

Table 1
Summary of changes in US MSTF polyp surveillance guidelines from 2012 to 2020

US MSTF Post-polypectomy Surveillance Recommendations	2012[28]	2020[23]
Adenoma		
1–2 adenomas <10 mm	5–10 y	7–10 y
3–4 adenomas <10 mm	3 y	3–5 y
5–10 adenomas <10 mm	3 y	3 y
Adenoma >10 mm; villous histology; high-grade dysplasia	3 y	3 y
10 or more adenomas	<3 y	1 y
Piecemeal EMR adenoma >20 mm	<1 y[a]	6 mo
Serrated lesions		
HP <10 mm	10 y[b]	10 y
1–2 SSP <10 mm	5 y	5–10 y
3–4 SSP <10 mm	3 y[b]	3–5 y
5–10 SSP <10 mm	3 y[b]	3 y
SSP >10 mm; dysplasia	3 y	3 y
HP >10 mm	3–5 y[c]	3–5 y
TSA	3 y	3 y
Piecemeal EMR SSP >20 mm	<1 y[a]	6 mo

Abbreviations: EMR, endoscopic mucosal resection; HP, hyperplastic polyp; SSP, sessile serrated polyp; TSA, traditional serrated adenoma; US MSTF, United States Multi-Society Task Force on Colorectal Cancer.
[a] 2012 Guidelines recommend early follow-up colonoscopy for piecemeal resection of adenoma or SSP greater than 15 mm if concern for incomplete removal.
[b] Recommendations for surveillance of certain serrated lesions derived from Rex and colleagues, 2012.[64]
[c] 2012 expert consensus by Rex and colleagues[64] recommends 5 y surveillance for HP >.5 mm proximal to sigmoid. Some advocate that all HP >10 mm proximal to sigmoid be treated as SSP.

CRC-related mortality.[38] Findings from the large Prostate Lung Colorectal and Ovarian Cancer (PLCO) cohort demonstrated that index HRA was associated with a nearly threefold increased risk of CRC and CRC-related mortality, whereas no such risks were seen in individuals with baseline LRA.[39]

In spite of the increased risk of CRC associated with adenomas, evidence suggests that polypectomy with the resection of adenomatous tissue can reduce this risk. Two large case-control studies of CRC in the United States and Germany found that compared to individuals without prior colonoscopy, individuals with colonoscopy and polypectomy within the previous 5 years had significantly reduced risk of CRC.[5,40] No significant durable protection from CRC incidence for individuals with polypectomy in the preceding 6 to 10 years was found in either study.[5,40] In the same studies, among those with the removal of advanced adenomas, an attenuated protective effect of polypectomy on CRC incidence was seen for up to 5 years as well.[5,40] Findings from the National Polyp Study cohort, with a median of approximately 16 years of follow-up, found that in addition to reducing the incidence of CRC, polypectomy of individuals with adenomatous polyps resulted in 48% reduction in CRC-related mortality than the general population, to a level similar to that of individuals in the study without adenomatous polyps.[11]

Although evidence has supported the notion that baseline endoscopic findings and removal of adenomas appear to influence subsequent CRC risk, the influence of surveillance colonoscopy on CRC incidence has been less clearly understood. A large cohort study from the United Kingdom sought to determine the influence of surveillance endoscopy among individuals following baseline polypectomy of intermediate-risk adenomas (1–2 adenomas larger than 10 mm or 3–4 small adenomas).[41] With a median of 8 years of follow-up, individuals with 1 to 2 surveillance procedures were nearly half as likely to be diagnosed with CRC than those without any surveillance.[41] Subgroup analysis of individuals without surveillance after baseline polypectomy revealed that individuals with large (20 mm) or high-grade adenomas or proximal polyps had a higher incidence of CRC than the general population, whereas CRC incidence was lower than the general population among those without those index features not undergoing surveillance.[41] An additional cohort study found that among individuals with advanced adenomas at baseline, exposure to one surveillance colonoscopy resulted in a CRC risk approaching the general population, whereas those without surveillance had a fourfold increased risk of CRC.[37] Among the group with LRAs at baseline, those with and without surveillance had reduced CRC risk than the general population.[37] Together, these studies demonstrate that the benefits for surveillance colonoscopy, at least with respect to CRC risk, appear to be limited to those with advanced adenomas at baseline. Those with LRAs at baseline are at reduced risk of CRC than the general population, with less certain incremental benefit from subsequent surveillance.

Metachronous Advanced Neoplasia Risk

Given the paucity of surveillance studies using CRC as an end point, a great deal of the evidence supporting surveillance intervals following polypectomy is derived from the studies of AN risk after polypectomy as a surrogate for CRC risk.[23,28,42–45] AN typically refers to a composite end point including advanced adenoma and/or CRC. Several studies have demonstrated that individuals with advanced adenomas at baseline are at greater risk of metachronous AN development than individuals with LRAs at baseline,[35,42,46–48] with about 20% of individuals developing high-risk neoplastic lesions on surveillance examinations, compared to 5% to 10% of those with low-risk findings at baseline.[46–48]

Although those with prior LRAs (1–2 adenomas <10 mm) are at the risk of development of recurrent polyps,[32,33] risk of AN in this population does not appear to be markedly elevated compared to those with no polyps at baseline, paralleling the trend seen for CRC risk with low-risk polyps. In a Korean cohort, 45% of those with LRAs developed recurrent polyps within 5 years of surveillance than 28% of those without baseline polyps, but rates of advanced adenoma at 5 years were similar between the 2 groups (2.4% and 2%, respectively).[35] Two large meta-analyses found a small absolute risk of metachronous AN development among individuals with LRAs at index colonoscopy than those with a normal index colonoscopy with up to 5 years of follow-up.[30,48] These findings informed the decision to expand surveillance intervals from 5 to 10 to 7 to 10 years following polypectomy for LRAs in the updated MSTF polyp surveillance guidelines.[23] Despite the strong evidence suggesting that those with LRAs are at similar, if not reduced risk, for CRC or AN than those without polyps, the observation that exposure to surveillance has the potential to reduce CRC risk further for those with LRAs[38] prevented a recommendation for 10-year surveillance in this group as is currently recommended for those without polyps.[23]

In comparison to the modest AN risk among those with baseline LRAs, the previously mentioned meta-analysis demonstrated a 17% AN risk within 5 years among those with advanced adenoma at baseline.[48] Cohort studies have demonstrated a 2 to 4-fold increased risk of metachronous AN in follow-up.[49,50] In addition to higher risk of recurrent AN compared to lower risk groups, those with baseline advanced adenoma appear to develop high-risk lesions within shorter time intervals as well. Although Chung and colleagues found an advanced adenoma recurrence rate of 12.2% within 5 years for those with baseline advanced adenoma, they importantly found that the majority (9.6%) of recurrences were found within 3 years.[35] Furthermore, a model of cost-effectiveness of low-intensity surveillance (10 years for LRA and 5 years for HRA) versus high-intensity surveillance (5 years for LRA and 3 years for HRA) found that high-intensity surveillance resulted in modest clinical improvements in CRC incidence (in addition to other clinical parameters) at an acceptable cost.[51] These findings support the continued recommendation for short-interval initial surveillance following polypectomy for high-risk lesions.[23,28]

Intermediate-Risk (3–4<10 mm) Adenomas

Individuals with 3 or more small adenomas at baseline have been shown to be at increased risk of AN or CRC than those with fewer or no adenomas.[49,50,52–54] Whereas the 2012 guidelines placed individuals with 3 or more small (<10 mm) adenomas in the same risk category as individuals with HRA, recent work has demonstrated that individuals with these intermediate features at baseline have approximately half the risk of metachronous HRA on surveillance as those with HRA at baseline.[46] Furthermore, a large retrospective study found that individuals with 3 to 4 LRAs at baseline had a similar metachronous HRA risk as those with 1 to 2 LRAs at baseline, whereas the presence of any number of HRA at baseline resulted in increased metachronous HRA risk compared to those with 4 or less LRAs at baseline.[55] The large PLCO cohort further demonstrated that individuals with 3 to 4 nonadvanced adenomas had similar CRC risk and CRC-related mortality as those with 1 to 2 adenomas with more than 10 years of follow-up.[39] These data contributed to the recommendation that individuals with 3 to 4 small adenomas could undergo surveillance at a longer interval (3–5 years) than those with HRA at baseline (3 years).[23] Contributing to the rationale for prolonged interval surveillance for those with 3 to 4 adenomas is the hypothesis that attention to adenoma detection rate and wide adoption of high-definition colonoscopy has contributed to enhanced identification of small adenomas that may have previously been missed. Thus, those with 3 to 4 small adenomas in the current era may more closely resemble those with 1 to 2 small adenomas in a previous era.

Impact of Serial Surveillance For Adenomas

For individuals undergoing more than one surveillance colonoscopy, it is important to determine whether subsequent AN risk is perpetually influenced by baseline examination findings or whether the most recent surveillance examination findings are more informative of downstream AN risk, thus allowing recommendations for surveillance interval to "reset" with each colonoscopy. In a study of individuals with 2 surveillance colonoscopies after baseline polypectomy, individuals with baseline high-risk features but low-risk features on first surveillance had subsequent AN risk (11%) similar to an individual with baseline low risk features (12%).[47] Furthermore, in the 12% of low-risk baseline patients who had high risk features at first surveillance, subsequent AN risk was 18%, similar to AN risk at first surveillance for those with baseline high risk features.[47] Although these findings suggest that low-risk findings on surveillance colonoscopy are predictive of lower future neoplasia risk, a Korean study of individuals with at least 2 surveillance colonoscopies found that individuals with low-risk or high-risk polyps at baseline were 3 and 8 times more likely to harbor AN during their second surveillance colonoscopy as those with normal baseline examination, even when no polyps were found at first surveillance.[32] Together, these findings support continued intensive surveillance of individuals with any prior history of high risk neoplasms despite lower risk findings at surveillance, whereas for those without history of high-risk lesions, findings at the most recent colonoscopy can likely safely inform future surveillance intervals. The updated MSTF polyps surveillance guidelines reflect these principles, with a recommendation for a minimum 5-year surveillance intervals for any individuals with a history of high-risk neoplasia.[23]

SURVEILLANCE AFTER POLYPECTOMY OF SSPs

In contrast to adenomatous polyps, about which a great deal is known about natural history, surveillance, and risk of CRC or advanced colorectal neoplasia, much less is known about the CRC or AN risk for serrated polyps, a heterogeneous group of lesions with related histology. Although it is well described that individuals with serrated polyposis syndrome are at increased risk of CRC (20%–30% lifetime),[56–59] literature describing CRC risk for serrated polyps is less robust, likely in part due to the historical under-recognition of their precancerous potential, subtle endoscopic findings, and heterogeneity among pathologists and endoscopists in reporting such lesions.[60–62] The malignant potential of SSPs in particular, which can be found in 5% to 10% of screening colonoscopies,[57] is increasingly recognized, while by comparison, hyperplastic polyps are felt not to confer an increased risk of CRC when diminutive and located in the rectosigmoid colon.[16,63–66] Surveillance after polypectomy for SSPs is thus generally recommended.[23]

Evidence is mounting that individuals with SSPs have a CRC risk that is similar to those with adenomatous polyps. A Danish case-control study found that compared to those without polyps, individuals with SSPs had a slightly higher CRC risk (OR 3.07) than those with adenomatous polyps (OR 2.50).[16] Although CRC risk was particularly elevated for SSPs with dysplasia (OR 4.76) or proximally located SSPs (OR 12.42), modest CRC case numbers resulted in wide estimates of risk.[16] A Norwegian cohort study demonstrated similar findings of comparable CRC risk between large serrated polyps and advanced adenomas.[67] Strikingly, 23 large serrated polyps (only 5 of which were hyperplastic polyps) were only biopsied and left in situ in the cohort, none of which developed into malignancy with median 11 years of follow-up.[67] This observed prolonged "dwell time" to carcinogenesis of SSPs compared to adenomas has been replicated by additional studies,[68,69] whereas others have suggested more rapid progression to invasive cancer, occasionally within months.[70,71] Accumulation of mutations and molecular changes may explain prolonged stability of SSPs over years followed by rapid progression to malignancy.[69] Thus, while serrated polyps appear to potentially be associated with elevated CRC risk, the exact mechanism of this association and its relation to the natural history of serrated polyps remains uncertain. For example, while specific serrated polyps may not progress to cancer, it is possible that the presence of serrated polyps may serve as a marker of field effect for at-risk colon for future carcinogenesis.

Studies of SSP surveillance using AN as an end point have demonstrated conflicting results. Some studies have demonstrated the increased risk of AN, particularly with large SSPs or lesions proximal to the splenic flexure.[66,70,72–74] A study of a large Chinese screening cohort found that the presence of SSPs conferred a similar risk of synchronous AN as the presence of LRAs, while the presence of large SSPs, but not the multiplicity of SSPs, was associated with even greater AN risk.[72] A smaller US study also demonstrated that SSPs (regardless of size) conferred significantly greater risk on metachronous AN than LRA alone with similar AN risk to HRA at baseline.[74]

The combination of serrated polyps and adenomas at baseline may increase the risk of neoplasia at surveillance than either lesion alone. In a large cohort, the presence of

SSPs alone at baseline was predictive of future large serrated polyps during surveillance but not of future HRAs. Synchronous SSP and HRA at baseline, however, resulted in nearly a fourfold increased risk of HRA in surveillance than those with just an HRA at baseline.[29] Additional studies have demonstrated the synergistic influence of SSPs and synchronous advanced adenomatous polyps on metachronous AN.[73–75] However, other studies with CRC as an end point have failed to provide evidence of this synergy.[16] Thus, SSPs appear to be a risk factor for future SSPs, but data demonstrating the risk of metachronous HRA or CRC with only SSP at baseline are weak and conflicting.

TSAs are the least common serrated polyp, comprising between 0.5% and 1.9% of all colorectal polyps.[76] Histologically, ectopic crypt foci distinguish TSA from SSP, and these lesions are more likely to occur in the distal colon.[76] Given their rarity, estimates of the malignant potential of TSA are lacking although previous reports have demonstrated high rates of dysplasia, and it is generally believed that they are premalignant lesions.[16,77] Evidence that up to half of TSAs appear to develop from microvesicular hyperplastic polyps or SSP as precursor lesions has led to a theory that TSA may represent a more advanced premalignant lesion on the serrated carcinoma pathway.[76] A Danish case-control study found that the presence of TSA was associated with a fourfold increased risk of future CRC than those without polyps, which was comparable to the risk of those with SSP with dysplasia and nearly double that of those with conventional adenomas.[16] An additional study found increased risk of AN among individuals with TSA than those with conventional adenomas.[78] These limited findings support the recommendation to pursue surveillance after the removal of TSA within 3 years, regardless of size. The data supporting this recommendation, however, are weak.[23]

INFLUENCE OF ENDOSCOPIC QUALITY PARAMETERS ON SURVEILLANCE

Increasing evidence has suggested failure to perform high-quality colonoscopy is a risk factor for interval CRC, which has prompted the description and adoption of quality benchmarks for colonoscopy including cecal intubation, adenoma detection, bowel prep, and polyp resection technique.[79,80] In a large pooled analysis of interval CRC cases, approximately 50% were thought to be caused by probable missed lesions,[81] for which endoscopist ADR, bowel prep quality, and withdrawal time are important factors. An additional 20% were likely related to incomplete resection or prior lesions,[81] highlighting the importance of preresection endoscopic inspection, resection technique, and postresection inspection. Additional studies have similarly shown that a small minority (5%) of metachronous CRCs are felt to arise from de novo lesions.[82] A large cohort study of more than 300,000 patients found that individuals with an endoscopist in the highest quintile of ADR were half as likely to develop or die from interval CRC as those with endoscopists in the lowest ADR quintile.[83] Moreover, each 1% increase in ADR was associated with 3% decreased risk of interval CRC.[83] An additional study found that the increase in ADR over time resulted in reduced interval CRC incidence and CRC-related mortality.[84]

Polypectomy technique is an important factor for subsequent neoplasia risk and thus for surveillance recommendations. A provocative study found that when adjacent tissue was biopsied after polypectomy, residual neoplastic tissue was found in 10% of polypectomies.[85] Incomplete resection was even higher for large (10–20 mm) polyps (17%) and SSPs (33%), with significant variability incomplete resection rates between endoscopists.[85] In an additional cohort, Brenner and colleagues found that incomplete polyp resection was among the most significant risk factors for incidence

CRC.[40] Further highlighting the importance of resection technique, a study of individuals undergoing surveillance after the resection of large (10–20 mm) polyps found that metachronous neoplasia arose from incomplete resection of 18% of nonpedunculated polyps.[86] Moreover, incomplete resection occurred in 29% of polyps removed piecemeal, compared to 9% of those removed en-bloc.[86]

Additional colonoscopy-related factors significantly influence neoplasia risk after polypectomy. In their large UK cohort, Atkin and colleagues demonstrated that among individuals with baseline polypectomy not undergoing surveillance, incidence of CRC was higher among those without high-quality baseline examination (complete colonoscopy with adequate bowel prep) than that of the general population, while for those with high-quality baseline examination, CRC incidence was lower than the general population.[41] A study from the Netherlands of surveillance colonoscopy after baseline polypectomy found that incomplete colonoscopy and inadequate bowel prep were associated with higher metachronous AN risk (threefold) than polyp size, multiplicity or high risk histologic features.[49] A Korean study similarly found poor bowel prep to be an independent risk factor for AN after polypectomy.[87] These findings support the notion that high-quality baseline examination influences subsequent neoplasia risk and that the ability to safely recommend an increased interval for surveillance is dependent on the quality of the index examination.

SURVEILLANCE FOR OLDER ADULTS

Decisions surrounding cancer screening in older individuals are complicated and must take into consideration cancer incidence, cost-effectiveness, and mortality benefit of screening in individuals with limited life expectancy. Cancer screening is even more complicated in this population when screening involves an invasive procedure as with CRC screening and colonoscopy. Although guidelines recommend the consideration of stopping screening for individuals at average risk of CRC at age 75,[21,88,89] guidance for continuing surveillance of older individuals with a history of polyps is notably lacking.[23] A retrospective study including individuals over the age of 75 undergoing surveillance colonoscopy found that age greater than 75 was associated with significantly lower risk of CRC in surveillance and was independently associated with increased risk of postprocedural complications resulting in hospitalization.[90] Moreover, older individuals are more likely to have incomplete colonoscopies because of inadequate bowel prep.[91] Given that most estimates suggest the progression from small adenoma to CRC takes at least 10 years,[92,93] it is generally not recommended to continue surveillance if a patient's life expectancy is not at least 10 years.[31] Multiple calculator tools exist to help quantify a patient's life expectancy based on comorbidities and to help weigh benefits and risks of given screening tests within that context, including for colonoscopy.[91] Understanding the limitations to surveillance colonoscopy in older individuals, in addition to considering prior polyp history and presence of significant comorbidities, is important when making a recommendation. Furthermore, it is critical to elicit patient understanding and values and to communicate recommendations to both patients and other stakeholder health care providers when coming to a shared decision to either continue or stop surveillance.[91]

SUMMARY

Greatly expanded literature over the past 2 decades have deepened our understanding of the risk of future polyps or CRC after polypectomy in addition to the influence of surveillance on these risks to allow for greater precision in surveillance colonoscopy recommendations. Resection of low-risk lesions is associated with reduced CRC and AN risk than those not screened, whereas the resection of high-risk polyps identifies a group at elevated risk who benefit from intensive surveillance. A growing body of evidence suggests that serrated polyps, particularly SSPs, are premalignant lesions that should be treated similarly to adenomatous polyps. Increasing attention to colonoscopy quality has the potential to improve outcomes and strengthen recommendations for surveillance. Future directions for polypectomy surveillance include the incorporation of demographic, polyp-related, or genetic factors into models that could provide further precision for interval recommendations while more data are needed to inform surveillance in older adults (age >75) and in particular younger adults (age <50), a group undergoing colonoscopy with greater frequency and at increasing risk of CRC.

CLINICS CARE POINTS

- Individuals with 1 to 2 small adenomas can undergo surveillance colonoscopy in 7 to 10 years as opposed to the prior recommendation of 5 years.
- Individuals with 3 to 4 small adenomas should undergo surveillance colonoscopy in 3 to 5 years, rather than 3 years.
- Individuals with an HRA (greater than 1 cm in size, villous histology, or high-grade dysplasia) should undergo surveillance colonoscopy in 3 years.
- The decision to screen for CRC after the age of 75 should be individualized to each patient based on functional status, co-morbidities, and prior history of CRC or adenomatous polyps.

DISCLOSURE

The authors have no disclosures

REFERENCES

1. Siegel RL, Miller KD, Jemal A. Cancer statistics, 2020. CA Cancer J Clin 2020; 70:7–30.
2. Siegel RL, Fedewa SA, Anderson WF, et al. Colorectal cancer incidence patterns in the United States, 1974-2013. J Natl Cancer Inst 2017;109:djw322.
3. Edwards BK, Ward E, Kohler BA, et al. Annual report to the nation on the status of cancer, 1975-2006, featuring colorectal cancer trends and impact of interventions (risk factors, screening, and treatment) to reduce future rates. Cancer 2010;116: 544–73.
4. Levin TR, Corley DA, Jensen CD, et al. Effects of organized colorectal cancer screening on cancer incidence and mortality in a large community-based population. Gastroenterology 2018;155:1383–91.e5.
5. Nishihara R, Wu K, Lochhead P, et al. Long-term colorectal-cancer incidence and mortality after lower endoscopy. N Engl J Med 2013;369:1095–105.
6. Doubeni CA, Corley DA, Quinn VP, et al. Effectiveness of screening colonoscopy in reducing the risk of death from right and left colon cancer: a large community-based study. Gut 2018;67:291–8.
7. Shaukat A, Mongin SJ, Geisser MS, et al. Long-term mortality after screening for colorectal cancer. N Engl J Med 2013;369:1106–14.
8. Doubeni CA, Weinmann S, Adams K, et al. Screening colonoscopy and risk for incident late-stage colorectal cancer diagnosis in average-risk adults: a nested case-control study. Ann Intern Med 2013;158:312–20.

9. Fearon ER, Vogelstein B. A genetic model for colorectal tumorigenesis. Cell 1990; 61:759–67.

10. Winawer SJ, Zauber AG, Ho MN, et al. Prevention of colorectal cancer by colonoscopic polypectomy. The National Polyp Study Workgroup. N Engl J Med 1993; 329:1977–81.

11. Zauber AG, Winawer SJ, O'Brien MJ, et al. Colonoscopic polypectomy and long-term prevention of colorectal-cancer deaths. N Engl J Med 2012;366:687–96.

12. Snover D, Ahnen D, Burt R. Serrated polyps of the colon and Rectum and serrated polyposis syndrome. Lyon, France: International Agency for Research on Cancer; 2010.

13. Crockett SD, Nagtegaal ID. Terminology, molecular features, epidemiology, and management of serrated colorectal neoplasia. Gastroenterology 2019;157: 949–66.e4.

14. Gervaz P, Bucher P, Morel P. Two colons-two cancers: paradigm shift and clinical implications. J Surg Oncol 2004;88:261–6.

15. Huang CS, Farraye FA, Yang S, et al. The clinical significance of serrated polyps. Am J Gastroenterol 2011;106:229–40 [quiz 241].

16. Erichsen R, Baron JA, Hamilton-Dutoit SJ, et al. Increased risk of colorectal cancer development among patients with serrated polyps. Gastroenterology 2016; 150:895–902.e5.

17. Snover DC. Update on the serrated pathway to colorectal carcinoma. Hum Pathol 2011;42:1–10.

18. Samowitz WS, Albertsen H, Herrick J, et al. Evaluation of a large, population-based sample supports a CpG island methylator phenotype in colon cancer. Gastroenterology 2005;129:837–45.

19. Peng L, Weigl K, Boakye D, et al. Risk scores for predicting advanced colorectal neoplasia in the average-risk population: a systematic review and meta-analysis. Am J Gastroenterol 2018;113:1788–800.

20. Jeon J, Du M, Schoen RE, et al. Determining risk of colorectal cancer and starting age of screening based on lifestyle, environmental, and genetic factors. Gastroenterology 2018;154:2152–64.e19.

21. Rex DK, Boland CR, Dominitz JA, et al. Colorectal cancer screening: recommendations for physicians and patients from the U.S. multi-society task force on colorectal cancer. Gastroenterology 2017;153:307–23.

22. Syngal S, Brand RE, Church JM, et al. ACG clinical guideline: genetic testing and management of hereditary gastrointestinal cancer syndromes. Am J Gastroenterol 2015;110:223–62 [quiz 263].

23. Gupta S, Lieberman D, Anderson JC, et al. Recommendations for follow-up after colonoscopy and polypectomy: a consensus update by the US multi-society task force on colorectal cancer. Am J Gastroenterol 2020;115:415–34.

24. Lieberman DA, Williams JL, Holub JL, et al. Colonoscopy utilization and outcomes 2000 to 2011. Gastrointest Endosc 2014;80:133–43.

25. Laiyemo AO, Pinsky PF, Marcus PM, et al. Utilization and yield of surveillance colonoscopy in the continued follow-up study of the polyp prevention trial. Clin Gastroenterol Hepatol 2009;7:562–7 [quiz 497].

26. Personal communications.

27. Djinbachian R, Dubé AJ, Durand M, et al. Adherence to post-polypectomy surveillance guidelines: a systematic review and meta-analysis. Endoscopy 2019; 51:673–83.

28. Lieberman DA, Rex DK, Winawer SJ, et al. Guidelines for colonoscopy surveillance after screening and polypectomy: a consensus update by the US multisociety task force on colorectal cancer. Gastroenterology 2012;143:844–57.
29. Anderson JC, Butterly LF, Robinson CM, et al. Risk of metachronous high-risk adenomas and large serrated polyps in individuals with serrated polyps on index colonoscopy: data from the New Hampshire colonoscopy registry. Gastroenterology 2018;154:117–27.e2.
30. Hassan C, Gimeno-García A, Kalager M, et al. Systematic review with meta-analysis: the incidence of advanced neoplasia after polypectomy in patients with and without low-risk adenomas. Aliment Pharmacol Ther 2014;39:905–12.
31. Rutter MD, East J, Rees CJ, et al. British Society of Gastroenterology/Association of Coloproctology of Great Britain and Ireland/Public Health England post-polypectomy and post-colorectal cancer resection surveillance guidelines. Gut 2020;69:201–23.
32. Park HW, Han S, Lee JY, et al. Probability of high-risk colorectal neoplasm recurrence based on the results of two previous colonoscopies. Dig Dis Sci 2015;60:226–33.
33. Laiyemo AO, Doubeni C, Brim H, et al. Short- and long-term risk of colorectal adenoma recurrence among whites and blacks. Gastrointest Endosc 2013;77:447–54.
34. Avidan B, Sonnenberg A, Schnell TG, et al. New occurrence and recurrence of neoplasms within 5 years of a screening colonoscopy. Am J Gastroenterol 2002;97:1524–9.
35. Chung SJ, Kim YS, Yang SY, et al. Five-year risk for advanced colorectal neoplasia after initial colonoscopy according to the baseline risk stratification: a prospective study in 2452 asymptomatic Koreans. Gut 2011;60:1537–43.
36. Coleman HG, Loughrey MB, Murray LJ, et al. Colorectal cancer risk following adenoma removal: a large prospective population-based cohort study. Cancer Epidemiol Biomarkers Prev 2015;24:1373–80.
37. Cottet V, Jooste V, Fournel I, et al. Long-term risk of colorectal cancer after adenoma removal: a population-based cohort study. Gut 2012;61:1180–6.
38. Løberg M, Kalager M, Holme Ø, et al. Long-term colorectal-cancer mortality after adenoma removal. N Engl J Med 2014;371:799–807.
39. Click B, Pinsky PF, Hickey T, et al. Association of colonoscopy adenoma findings with long-term colorectal cancer incidence. JAMA 2018;319:2021–31.
40. Brenner H, Chang-Claude J, Rickert A, et al. Risk of colorectal cancer after detection and removal of adenomas at colonoscopy: population-based case-control study. J Clin Oncol 2012;30:2969–76.
41. Atkin W, Wooldrage K, Brenner A, et al. Adenoma surveillance and colorectal cancer incidence: a retrospective, multicentre, cohort study. Lancet Oncol 2017;18:823–34.
42. Martínez ME, Baron JA, Lieberman DA, et al. A pooled analysis of advanced colorectal neoplasia diagnoses after colonoscopic polypectomy. Gastroenterology 2009;136:832–41.
43. Lieberman DA, Weiss DG, Harford WV, et al. Five-year colon surveillance after screening colonoscopy. Gastroenterology 2007;133:1077–85.
44. Laiyemo AO, Murphy G, Albert PS, et al. Postpolypectomy colonoscopy surveillance guidelines: predictive accuracy for advanced adenoma at 4 years. Ann Intern Med 2008;148:419–26.
45. Miller HL, Mukherjee R, Tian J, et al. Colonoscopy surveillance after polypectomy may be extended beyond five years. J Clin Gastroenterol 2010;44:e162–6.

46. Kim JY, Kim TJ, Baek SY, et al. Risk of metachronous advanced neoplasia in patients with multiple diminutive adenomas. Am J Gastroenterol 2018;113:1855–61.

47. Morelli MS, Glowinski EA, Juluri R, et al. Yield of the second surveillance colonoscopy based on the results of the index and first surveillance colonoscopies. Endoscopy 2013;45:821–6.

48. Dubé C, Yakubu M, McCurdy BR, et al. Risk of advanced adenoma, colorectal cancer, and colorectal cancer mortality in people with low-risk adenomas at baseline colonoscopy: a systematic review and meta-analysis. Am J Gastroenterol 2017;112:1790–801.

49. van Heijningen EM, Lansdorp-Vogelaar I, Kuipers EJ, et al. Features of adenoma and colonoscopy associated with recurrent colorectal neoplasia based on a large community-based study. Gastroenterology 2013;144:1410–8.

50. Fairley KJ, Li J, Komar M, et al. Predicting the risk of recurrent adenoma and incident colorectal cancer based on findings of the baseline colonoscopy. Clin Transl Gastroenterol 2014;5:e64.

51. Meester RGS, Lansdorp-Vogelaar I, Winawer SJ, et al. High-intensity versus low-intensity surveillance for patients with colorectal adenomas: a cost-effectiveness analysis. Ann Intern Med 2019;171:612–22.

52. Park SK, Song YS, Jung YS, et al. Do surveillance intervals in patients with more than five adenomas at index colonoscopy be shorter than those in patients with three to four adenomas? A Korean Association for the Study of Intestinal Disease study. J Gastroenterol Hepatol 2017;32:1026–31.

53. Bjerrum A, Milter MC, Andersen O, et al. Risk stratification and detection of new colorectal neoplasms after colorectal cancer screening with faecal occult blood test: experiences from a Danish screening cohort. Eur J Gastroenterol Hepatol 2015;27:1433–7.

54. Brenner H, Chang-Claude J, Jansen L, et al. Role of colonoscopy and polyp characteristics in colorectal cancer after colonoscopic polyp detection: a population-based case-control study. Ann Intern Med 2012;157:225–32.

55. Vemulapalli KC, Rex DK. Risk of advanced lesions at first follow-up colonoscopy in high-risk groups as defined by the United Kingdom post-polypectomy surveillance guideline: data from a single U.S. center. Gastrointest Endosc 2014;80:299–306.

56. Muller C, Yamada A, Ikegami S, et al. Risk of colorectal cancer in serrated polyposis syndrome: a systematic review and meta-analysis. Clin Gastroenterol Hepatol 2021.

57. IJspeert JEG, Bevan R, Senore C, et al. Detection rate of serrated polyps and serrated polyposis syndrome in colorectal cancer screening cohorts: a European overview. Gut 2017;66:1225–32.

58. Carballal S, Rodríguez-Alcalde D, Moreira L, et al. Colorectal cancer risk factors in patients with serrated polyposis syndrome: a large multicentre study. Gut 2016;65:1829–37.

59. Bleijenberg AG, IJspeert JE, van Herwaarden YJ, et al. Personalised surveillance for serrated polyposis syndrome: results from a prospective 5-year international cohort study. Gut 2020;69:112–21.

60. Tinmouth J, Henry P, Hsieh E, et al. Sessile serrated polyps at screening colonoscopy: have they been under diagnosed? Am J Gastroenterol 2014;109:1698–704.

61. Kahi CJ, Hewett DG, Norton DL, et al. Prevalence and variable detection of proximal colon serrated polyps during screening colonoscopy. Clin Gastroenterol Hepatol 2011;9:42–6.

62. Schachschal G, Sehner S, Choschzick M, et al. Impact of reassessment of colonic hyperplastic polyps by expert GI pathologists. Int J Colorectal Dis 2016;31:675–83.
63. IJspeert JE, Rana SA, Atkinson NS, et al. Clinical risk factors of colorectal cancer in patients with serrated polyposis syndrome: a multicentre cohort analysis. Gut 2017;66:278–84.
64. Rex DK, Ahnen DJ, Baron JA, et al. Serrated lesions of the colorectum: review and recommendations from an expert panel. Am J Gastroenterol 2012;107: 1315–29 [quiz 1314, 1330].
65. IJspeert JE, Vermeulen L, Meijer GA, et al. Serrated neoplasia-role in colorectal carcinogenesis and clinical implications. Nat Rev Gastroenterol Hepatol 2015; 12:401–9.
66. Hazewinkel Y, de Wijkerslooth TR, Stoop EM, et al. Prevalence of serrated polyps and association with synchronous advanced neoplasia in screening colonoscopy. Endoscopy 2014;46:219–24.
67. Holme Ø, Bretthauer M, Eide TJ, et al. Long-term risk of colorectal cancer in individuals with serrated polyps. Gut 2015;64:929–36.
68. Lash RH, Genta RM, Schuler CM. Sessile serrated adenomas: prevalence of dysplasia and carcinoma in 2139 patients. J Clin Pathol 2010;63:681–6.
69. Bettington M, Walker N, Rosty C, et al. Clinicopathological and molecular features of sessile serrated adenomas with dysplasia or carcinoma. Gut 2017;66:97–106.
70. Li D, Jin C, McCulloch C, et al. Association of large serrated polyps with synchronous advanced colorectal neoplasia. Am J Gastroenterol 2009;104:695–702.
71. Nakamura H, Fu K, Parra-Blanco A, et al. A sessile colonic polyp showing striking morphological changes within a 2-month period. Endoscopy 2007;39(Suppl 1): E279–80.
72. Ng SC, Ching JY, Chan VC, et al. Association between serrated polyps and the risk of synchronous advanced colorectal neoplasia in average-risk individuals. Aliment Pharmacol Ther 2015;41:108–15.
73. Schreiner MA, Weiss DG, Lieberman DA. Proximal and large hyperplastic and nondysplastic serrated polyps detected by colonoscopy are associated with neoplasia. Gastroenterology 2010;139:1497–502.
74. Melson J, Ma K, Arshad S, et al. Presence of small sessile serrated polyps increases rate of advanced neoplasia upon surveillance compared with isolated low-risk tubular adenomas. Gastrointest Endosc 2016;84:307–14.
75. Pereyra L, Zamora R, Gómez EJ, et al. Risk of metachronous advanced neoplastic lesions in patients with sporadic sessile serrated adenomas undergoing colonoscopic surveillance. Am J Gastroenterol 2016;111:871–8.
76. Bettington ML, Chetty R. Traditional serrated adenoma: an update. Hum Pathol 2015;46:933–8.
77. Kim KM, Lee EJ, Kim YH, et al. KRAS mutations in traditional serrated adenomas from Korea herald an aggressive phenotype. Am J Surg Pathol 2010;34:667–75.
78. Yoon JY, Kim HT, Hong SP, et al. High-risk metachronous polyps are more frequent in patients with traditional serrated adenomas than in patients with conventional adenomas: a multicenter prospective study. Gastrointest Endosc 2015; 82:1087–93.e3.
79. Rex DK, Schoenfeld PS, Cohen J, et al. Quality indicators for colonoscopy. Gastrointest Endosc 2015;81:31–53.
80. Keswani RN, Crockett SD, Calderwood AH. AGA clinical practice update on strategies to improve quality of screening and surveillance colonoscopy: expert review. Gastroenterology 2021;161:701–11.

81. Robertson DJ, Lieberman DA, Winawer SJ, et al. Colorectal cancers soon after colonoscopy: a pooled multicohort analysis. Gut 2014;63:949–56.
82. le Clercq CM, Winkens B, Bakker CM, et al. Metachronous colorectal cancers result from missed lesions and non-compliance with surveillance. Gastrointest Endosc 2015;82:325–33.e2.
83. Corley DA, Jensen CD, Marks AR, et al. Adenoma detection rate and risk of colorectal cancer and death. N Engl J Med 2014;370:1298–306.
84. Kaminski MF, Wieszczy P, Rupinski M, et al. Increased rate of adenoma detection associates with reduced risk of colorectal cancer and death. Gastroenterology 2017;153:98–105.
85. Pohl H, Srivastava A, Bensen SP, et al. Incomplete polyp resection during colonoscopy-results of the complete adenoma resection (CARE) study. Gastroenterology 2013;144:74–80.e1.
86. Adler J, Toy D, Anderson JC, et al. Metachronous neoplasias arise in a higher proportion of colon segments from which large polyps were previously removed, and can be used to estimate incomplete resection of 10-20 mm colorectal polyps. Clin Gastroenterol Hepatol 2019;17:2277–84.
87. Jang HW, Park SJ, Hong SP, et al. Risk factors for recurrent high-risk polyps after the removal of high-risk polyps at initial colonoscopy. Yonsei Med J 2015;56:1559–65.
88. Bibbins-Domingo K, Grossman DC, Curry SJ, et al. Screening for colorectal cancer: us preventive services task force recommendation statement. JAMA 2016;315:2564–75.
89. The Lancet Gastroenterology Hepatology. USPSTF recommends expansion of colorectal cancer screening. Lancet Gastroenterol Hepatol 2021;6:1.
90. Tran AH, Man Ngor EW, Wu BU. Surveillance colonoscopy in elderly patients: a retrospective cohort study. JAMA Intern Med 2014;174:1675–82.
91. Maratt JK, Calderwood AH, Saini SD. When and how to stop surveillance colonoscopy in older adults: five rules of thumb for practitioners. Am J Gastroenterol 2018;113:5–7.
92. Stryker SJ, Wolff BG, Culp CE, et al. Natural history of untreated colonic polyps. Gastroenterology 1987;93:1009–13.
93. Sekiguchi M, Otake Y, Kakugawa Y, et al. Incidence of advanced colorectal neoplasia in individuals with untreated diminutive colorectal adenomas diagnosed by magnifying image-enhanced endoscopy. Am J Gastroenterol 2019;114:964–73.

Printed and bound by CPI Group (UK) Ltd, Croydon, CR0 4YY

08/05/2025

01864723-0002